PHARMACEUTICAL DRUG PRODUCT DEVELOPMENT AND PROCESS OPTIMIZATION

Effective Use of Quality by Design

PHARMACEUTICAL DRUG PRODUCT DEVELOPMENT AND PROCESS OPTIMIZATION

Effective Use of Quality by Design

Edited by

Sarwar Beg, PhD
Mahfoozur Rahman, PhD
Syed Sarim Imam, PhD
Nabil K. Alruwaili, PhD
Majed Al Robaian, PhD
Sunil Kumar Panda, PhD

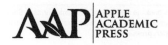

APPLE
ACADEMIC
PRESS

Apple Academic Press Inc.
4164 Lakeshore Road
Burlington ON L7L 1A4
Canada

Apple Academic Press Inc.
1265 Goldenrod Circle NE
Palm Bay, Florida 32905
USA

© 2020 by Apple Academic Press, Inc.

First issued in paperback 2021

Exclusive worldwide distribution by CRC Press, a member of Taylor & Francis Group
No claim to original U.S. Government works

ISBN 13: 978-1-77463-496-7 (pbk)
ISBN 13: 978-1-77188-872-1 (hbk)

Library and Archives Canada Cataloguing in Publication

Title: Pharmaceutical drug product development and process optimization : effective use of quality by design / edited by Sarwar Beg, PhD, Mahfoozur Rahman, PhD, Syed Sarim Imam, PhD, Nabil K. Alruwaili, PhD, Majed Al Robaian, PhD, Sunil Kumar Panda, PhD.

Names: Beg, Sarwar, 1987- editor. | Rahman, Mahfoozur, 1984- editor. | Imam, Syed Sarim, editor. | Alruwaili, Nabil K., editor. | Majed Al Robaian, editor. | Panda, Sunil Kumar, editor.

Description: Includes bibliographical references and index.

Identifiers: Canadiana (print) 20200180398 | Canadiana (ebook) 20200180452 | ISBN 9781771888721 (hardcover) | ISBN 9780367821678 (ebook)

Subjects: LCSH: Drug development.

Classification: LCC RM301.25 .P53 2020 | DDC 615.1/9—dc23

Library of Congress Cataloging-in-Publication Data

Names: Beg, Sarwar, 1987- editor.

Title: Pharmaceutical drug product development and process optimization : effective use of quality by design / edited by Sarwar Beg [and five others].

Description: Palm Bay, Florida : Apple Academic Press, [2020] | Includes bibliographical references and index. | Summary: "Pharmaceutical manufacturers are constantly facing quality crises of drug products, leading to an escalating number of product recalls and rejects. Due to the involvement of multiple factors, the goal of achieving consistent product quality is always a great challenge for pharmaceutical scientists. This volume, Pharmaceutical Drug Product Development and Process Optimization: Effective Use of Quality by Design, addresses this challenge by using the Quality by Design (QbD) concept, which was instituted to focus on the systematic development of drug products with predefined objectives to provide enhanced product and process understanding. This volume presents and discusses the vital precepts underlying the efficient, effective, and cost-effective development of pharmaceutical drug products. It focuses on the adoption of systematic quality principles of pharmaceutical development, which is imperative in achieving continuous improvement in end-product quality and also leads to reducing cost, time, and effort, while meeting regulatory requirements. The volume covers the important new advances in the development of solid oral dosage forms, modified release oral dosage forms, parenteral dosage forms, semisolid dosage forms, transdermal drug, delivery systems, inhalational dosage forms, ocular drug delivery systems, nanopharmaceutical products, and nanoparticles for oral delivery. Providing an abundance of knowledge, this volume will be valuable for those who are engaged in pharmaceutical product development, including new drugs and generic drug products. Key features Reviews a vast collection of literature on applicability of systematic product development tools Discusses various dosage forms where challenges are very high Provides regulatory guidance related to specific dosage form development Covers the major types of drug products, including enteral, parenteral, and other (including transdermal, inhalation, etc.)"-- Provided by publisher.

Identifiers: LCCN 2020005168 (print) | LCCN 2020005169 (ebook) | ISBN 9781771888721 (hardcover) | ISBN 9780367821678 (ebook)

Subjects: MESH: Drug Development | Quality Control

Classification: LCC RM301.25 (print) | LCC RM301.25 (ebook) | NLM QV 745 | DDC 615.1/9--dc23

LC record available at https://lccn.loc.gov/2020005168

LC ebook record available at https://lccn.loc.gov/2020005169

Apple Academic Press also publishes its books in a variety of electronic formats. Some content that appears in print may not be available in electronic format. For information about Apple Academic Press products, visit our website at **www.appleacademicpress. com** and the CRC Press website at **www.crcpress.com**

About the Editors

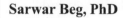

Sarwar Beg, PhD

Department of Pharmaceutics,
School of Pharmaceutical Education and Research,
Jamia Hamdard, New Delhi, India

Sarwar Beg, PhD, is currently serving as Assistant Professor of Pharmaceutics & Biopharmaceutics at the School of Pharmaceutical Education and Research, Jamia Hamdard University, New Delhi, India (rank #1 in pharmacy as per the Govt. of India). Prior to joining Jamia Hamdard, Dr. Beg worked with Jubilant Generics Limited, Noida, India, as Research Scientist, where he was solely responsible for implementation of Quality by Design (QbD) in formulation development and analytical development of generic products. He has nearly a decade of experience in systematic development and characterization of novel and nanostructured drug delivery systems using QbD paradigms, including Design of Experiments (DoE), Quality Risk Management (QRM), Multivariate Chemometric Approaches, Advanced Biopharmaceutics, and Pharmacokinetic. In addition, Dr Sarwar has acquired know-how of applying advanced release kinetic modeling, pharmacokinetic modeling, and *in vitro/in vivo* correlation (IVIVC) for efficient development of drug products.

To date, he has authored over 150 publications, including research and review papers in high-impact peer-reviewed journals, ten journal special issues, twelve books, and over 45 book chapters, and he holds three Indian patent applications. He has very good citation record with Google Scholar (*H-Index* 26, i-10 index 70) and has been cited over 2,800 times. He is serving as the Regional Editor (Asia) of the *journal Current Nanomedicine* (Bentham Science) and is an editorial board member of several other journals. Dr. Beg has also participated and presented his research work and delivered lectures at several conferences held at India, China, Bangladesh, Canada, and USA, earning several best paper awards. He has also been awarded with an "Innovative Pharma Researcher Award—2016" by SIPRA Lab (Hyderabad), "Eudragit® Award 2014" in

South-Asia by M/s Evonik (Germany), "Budding QbD Scientist Award 2014" and "Budding ADME Scientist Award 2013" by M/s Select Biosciences (UK), and "Novartis Biocamp Award 2012" (Hyderabad). In 2017, Dr. Beg was distinguished by the Honorable Union Health Minister of India and Managing Director, Sun Pharmaceutical Industries, with prestigious the "Sun Pharma Science Foundation" Award.

Mahfoozur Rahman, PhD

Department of Pharmaceutical Sciences,
Faculty of Health Science,
Sam Higginbottom University of Agriculture,
Technology & Sciences (SHUATS), Allahabad, India

Mahfoozur Rahman, PhD, is an Assistant Professor in the Department of Pharmaceutical Sciences, Faculty of Health Science, Sam Higginbottom University of Agriculture, Technology & Sciences (SHUATS), Allahabad, India. His major areas of research interest include development and characterization of nanosized drug delivery systems for inflammatory disorders including psoriasis, arthritis, neurodegenerative disorders, and cancer, etc. In addition, he is also working on amalgamation of herbal medicinal plants with modern therapeutics in order to deliver a scientifically acceptable therapy for various diseases management. To date he has published over 90 publications in peer-reviewed journals, including *Seminars in Cancer Biology, Drug Discovery Today, Nanomedicine, Expert Opinion on Drug Delivery.* He has also published book chapters, several international books, and three articles in international magazine with various reputed publishers. Overall, he has earned a highly impressive publishing and cited record in Google Scholar (H-index of 18, total citations: 1,050). Dr. Rahman has received travel grants for various international congresses, such as the International Association of Parkinsonism and Related Disorders, Movement Disorder Association, Nano Today Conferences, and KSN 2019. He is also serving as a Guest Editor for *Seminar Cancer Biology, Recent Patents on Anti-Infective Drug Discovery, and Current Nanomedicine,* and he is an editorial member of many prestigious journals.

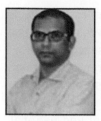

Syed Sarim Imam, PhD

Department of Pharmaceutics, College of Pharmacy, King Saud University, Saudi Arabia

Syed Sarim Imam, PhD, is working as Associate Professor at the College of Pharmacy, King Saud University, Saudi Arabia. Dr. Imam earned his PhD from the Faculty of Pharmacy, Jamia Hamdard, New Delhi, India. He received his research fellowship from the Indian Council of Medical Research, New Delhi, during his doctorate tenure. He has more than 10 years of teaching and research experience. His research interests include drug delivery, brain targeting, formulation optimization, and lipid-based delivery systems. Dr. Imam has a list of more than 60 research/review manuscripts published in journals of international repute. He has very good citation record with Google Scholar (H-index of 15, and i10-index of 26) to his credit. Dr. Imam has also participated and presented his research work at several conferences held in India and abroad. He has contributed over 20 book chapters in books published by in several publishers, including Elsevier, CRC. and Springer. Dr. Imam is a reviewer to a large number of international and national journals of repute and a member or life member of many Indian scientific organizations.

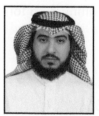

Nabil K. Alruwaili, PhD

Pharmaceutics Department, School of Pharmacy, Jouf University, Sakaka, Saudi Arabia

Nabil K. Alruwaili, PhD, is an Assistant Professor of Pharmaceutics Department, School of Pharmacy, Jouf University, Sakaka, Saudi Arabi, where he is the chairman of the Pharmaceutics Department. He obtained both his BSc (Pharmaceutical Sciences, 2008) and MSc (Quality Control of Pharmaceutics, 2011) degrees from the College of Pharmacy at King Saud University (KSU), Riyadh, Saudi Arabia. He was awarded his PhD (Pharmaceutics, 2017) from Massachusetts College of Pharmacy and Health Sciences University, Boston, USA. Previously, Dr. Alruwaili worked at the Saudi Food and Drug Authority (SFDA) in product evaluation and standards-setting administration, in Riyadh for three years. He has significant experience in assessment and registration dossiers submitted by companies for a variety of pharmaceutical products. There are many aspects to be assessed in such files, including the Drug Master File (DMF), which involves drug design and manufacturing. Dr. Alruwaili is effective in building successful projects through open channels of communication and synergistic relationships across research disciplines in order to motivate others on all levels in the achievement of individual and organizational goals. He has several published articles and has presented papers at international and national scientific conferences.

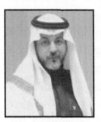

Majed Al Robaian, PhD

Faculty of Pharmacy, Taif University, Saudi Arabia

Majed Al Robaian, PhD, is the Dean of the Faculty of Pharmacy at Taif University, Saudi Arabia. He obtained his BSc from King Saud University in Riyadh, Saudi Arabia, and his MSc in Pharmaceutical Sciences from Strathclyde University, United Kingdom, in 2010 and his PhD from the same university in 2014. His research interests focus on drug delivery and, in particular, the delivery of therapeutic genes for the treatment of cancer. Before obtaining his PhD, he worked as Director of Pharmacy at King Abdulaziz Hospital, Saudi Arabia. Currently, he is appointed as the Science Faculty Ambassador for Strathclyde University, UK. He is also a member of a number of committees in the Saudi Commission for Health Specialties.

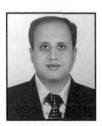

Sunil Kumar Panda, PhD

Director of Research & Development,
Menovo Pharmaceuticals, People's Republic of China

Sunil Kumar Panda, PhD, serves as a Director of Research & Development at Menovo Pharmaceuticals (a Shanghai stock exchange listed company) in the People Republic of China. He is a native of Berhampur, Odisha India. Dr. Sunil has degree in Pharmaceutical Science and earned his PhD at Berhampur University, Odisha India. He completed his postgraduation in business management from the premier Indian Institute of Management, Trichy. His dissertation work is on novel formulation design for few cardiovascular disorders. He has rich research work experience with top Indian pharmaceutical companies, such as Zydus Cadila, Dr. Reddy's Laboratories, Jubilant, and Unichem. His professional research work has focused on complex generics and, in particular, has looked at multi-unit particle systems (MUPS), extended release dosage forms, and nanosuspension. He has an intellectual WIPO patent on delayed release suspension as well as several international publications in peer-reviewed journal. His current research work involves 505 b (2) and Para IV invalidation for products in the USA market. His primary interest includes work on extended release pellets and delayed release capsules. He is academic consultant to the Government College of Engineering and Technology, Bhubaneswar, India. He has a research experience of over 14 years in India and abroad. He has received many international grants for pursuing his research. He is listed as a foreign research expert in People's Republic of China. He has interest in both academia as well as industry.

Contents

Contributors

Farhan Jalees Ahmad
Department of Pharmaceutics, School of Pharmaceutical Education and Research, Jamia Hamdard, Hamdard Nagar, New Delhi – 110062, India

Sadat Ali
Department of Pharmacy, Kanpur Institute of Technology, Kanpur, India

Saima Amin
Formulation Research Lab, Department of Pharmaceutics,
School of Pharmaceutical Education and Research, Jamia Hamdard, New Delhi, India

Chettupalli Anand
Department of Pharmaceutics, Anurag Group of Institutions, School of Pharmacy, Venkatapur, Ghatkesar, Telangana- 500088, India

Mohammed Tahir Ansari
Pharmaceutics Division, Universiti Kuala Lumpur Royal College of Medicine Perak, Ipoh, Malaysia |
School of Pharmacy, University of Nottingham Malaysia, Semenyih, Selangor, Malaysia

Sarwar Beg
Department of Pharmaceutics, School of Pharmaceutical Education and Research, Jamia Hamdard, New Delhi – 110062, India

Sanjay Chuhan
Glocal School of Pharmacy, Glocal University, Saharanpur, Mirzapur Pole, 247121, U.P., India

Syed Azizullah Ghori
Department of Pharmacy Practice, College of Clinical Pharmacy,
Imam Abdulrahman Bin Faisal University, P.O. Box 1982, Dammam – 31441, Saudi Arabia

Sadaf Jamal Gilani
College of Pharmacy, Aljouf University, Aljouf, Sakaka, Kingdom of Saudi Arabia

Mayank Handa
Department of Pharmaceutics, National Institute of Pharmaceutical Education and Research, Raebareli, Lucknow, Uttar Pradesh – 226002, India

Mohammad Saquib Hasnain
Department of Pharmaceutics, College of Pharmacy, Shri Venkateshwara University, Gajraula, Uttar Pradesh-244236, India

Syed Sarim Imam
Department of Pharmaceutics, College of Pharmacy, King Saud University, Riyadh–11451, Saudi Arabia

Mohammed Jafar
Department of Pharmaceutics, College of Clinical Pharmacy,
Imam Abdulrahman Bin Faisal University, P.O. Box 1982, Dammam – 31441, Saudi Arabia

Mohammed Asadullah Jahangir
Department of Pharmaceutics, Nibha Institute of Pharmaceutical Sciences, Rajgir–803116, Nalanda,
Bihar, India

Gaurav Kumar Jain
Department of Pharmaceutics, School of Pharmaceutical Education & Research, Jamia Hamdard,
Hamdard Nagar, New Delhi – 110062, India

Goutam Kumar Jena
Department of Pharmaceutics, Roland Institute of Pharmaceutical Sciences, Berhampur,
Odisha – 760010, India

Dheeraj Kumar
Department of Pharmaceutics, National Institute of Pharmaceutical Education and Research,
Raebareli, Lucknow, Uttar Pradesh–226002, India

Shahnaz Majeed
Pharmaceutics Division, Universiti Kuala Lumpur Royal College of Medicine Perak, Ipoh, Malaysia

Abdul Muheem
School of Pharmaceutical Education and Research, Jamia Hamdard, New Delhi–110062, India

Sunil Kumar Panda
Research & Development, Menovo Pharmaceuticals, People's Republic of China

Vishwas P. Pardhi
Department of Pharmaceutics, National Institute of Pharmaceutical Education and Research,
Raebareli, Lucknow, Uttar Pradesh – 226002, India

Rabinarayan Parhi
Department of Pharmaceutical Sciences, Susruta School of Medical and Paramedical Sciences,
Assam University (A Central University), Silchar, Assam

Ch Niranjan Patra
Department of Pharmaceutics, Roland Institute of Pharmaceutical Sciences, Berhampur,
Odisha – 760010, India

Mahfoozur Rahman
Department of Pharmaceutical Sciences, Faculty of Health Science, Sam Higginbottom University
of Agriculture, Technology & Sciences (SHUATS), Allahabad, India

Mohd. Moshahid Alam Rizvi
Genome Biology Lab, Department of Biosciences, Faculty of Natural Sciences,
Jamia Millia Islamia, New Delhi, India

Md. Rizwanullah
Formulation Research Lab, Department of Pharmaceutics,
School of Pharmaceutical Education and Research, Jamia Hamdard, New Delhi, India

A. A. Sallam
Al-Taqaddom Pharmaceutical Industries, Amman, Jordan

Farheen Mohd Sami
Pharmaceutics Division, Universiti Kuala Lumpur Royal College of Medicine Perak,
Ipoh, Malaysia

Rahul Shukla
Department of Pharmaceutics, National Institute of Pharmaceutical Education and Research, Raebareli, Lucknow, Uttar Pradesh–226002, India

Ajit Singh
Department of Pharmaceutics, National Institute of Pharmaceutical Education and Research, Raebareli, Lucknow, Uttar Pradesh–226002, India

Nidhi Singh
Department of Pharmaceutics, National Institute of Pharmaceutical Education and Research, Raebareli, Lucknow, Uttar Pradesh–226002, India

Mohamad Taleuzzaman
Glocal School of Pharmacy, Glocal University, Saharanpur, Mirzapur Pole, 247121, U.P., India

Musarrat Husain Warsi
College of Pharmacy, Taif University, Taif–21431, Saudi Arabia

Sobiya Zafar
Nano Research Laboratory, School of Pharmaceutical Education & Research, Jamia Hamdard, Hamdard Nagar, New Delhi – 110062, India

Abbreviations

3D	three-dimensional
3DP	3D printing
4-ASA	4-aminosalicylic acid
4-MSK	4-methoxysalicylate
ADHD	attention-deficit hyperactivity disorder
AEA	aminoacetate
AFM	atomic force microscopy
AI	artificial intelligence
ALS	alendronate sodium
AMD	associated macular degeneration
ANDA	abbreviated new drug application
ANNs	artificial neural networks
ANOVA	analysis of variance
APAT	application of process analytical technology
APEs	average percent errors
API	active pharmaceutical ingredients
APSD	aerodynamic particle size distribution
ATR	attenuated total reflectance
AUC	area under the curve
BBB	blood-brain barrier
BBD	Box-Behnken design
BSA	bovine serum albumin
BSE	bovine spongiform encephalopathy
BZ	benznidazole
CAD	computer aided design
CAE	computer-aided engineering
CAF	caffeine
CAPA	corrective and preventive action
CAPE	computer-aided production engineering
CAQ	computer-aided quality
CBB	coomassie brilliant blue R-250
CBZ	carbamazepine
CC	candesartan cilexetil

CCD	central composite design
CDER	Center for Drug Evaluation and Research
CFCs	chlorofluorocarbon
CGG	carboxymethyl guar gum
Chol	cholesterol
CL	cutaneous leishmaniasis
CMAs	critical material attributes
CMC	chemistry, manufacturing and chemistry
CMS	carboxymethyl starch
CNS	central nervous system
COPD	chronic obstructive pulmonary disease
CoPECs	compact polyelectrolyte complexes
CoQ10	coenzyme Q10
CPF	ciprofloxacin
CPMP	Committee for Proprietary Medicinal Products
CPPs	critical process parameters
CQAs	critical quality attributes
CRM	customer relationship management
CS	chitosan
D-NE	darunavir encapsulated nanoemulsion
DCN	diacerein
DDU	delivered dose uniformity
DESE	double emulsion solvent evaporation
DL	drug loading
DMS	derma membrane structure
DMSO	dimethyl sulfoxide
DoE	design of experiments
DOX	doxorubicin hydrochloride
DPI	dry powder inhalers
DPPC	dipalmitoylphophatidylcholine
DPPS	dipalmitoylphosphatidylserine
DSC	differential scanning calorimetry
DTX	docetaxel
DZ	dacarbazine
EA	3-O-ethyl-ascorbic acid
EC	ethylcellulose
EE	entrapment efficiency
EHM	ethylhexyl methoxycinnamate

EM	enalapril maleate
EMEA	The European Agency for the Evaluation of Medicinal Products
ER	extended-release
ERP	enterprise resource planning
Et	ethanol
FBRM	focused beam reflectance measurements
FCCD	face centered cubic design
FDA	Food and Drug Administration
FDM	fused deposition modeling
FPD	fine particle dose
FPF	fine particle fraction
FR&D	formulation research & development
FTIR	Fourier transform infrared spectroscopy
G	glycerol
GALT	gut-associated lymphoid tissue
GAs	genetic algorithm
GBP	gabapentin
GI	gastrointestinal
GSK	GlaxoSmithKline
HAP	hydroxyapatite
HC	hydrocortisone
HCT	hydrochlorothiazide
HFA	hydrofluoroalkane
HME	hot-melt extrusion
HPC	hydroxypropyl cellulose
HPH	high-pressure homogenization
HPMC	hydroxypropyl methylcellulose
HT	hydroxytyrosol
HTS	high throughput screening
i.m.	intramuscularly
ICD	irritant contact dermatitis
IDDS	implantable drug delivery systems
IM	intramuscular
iNAM	isonicotinamide
IND	investigational new drug
INH	isoniazid
IPEC	interpolyelectrolyte complexes

IPM	isopropyl myristate
IR	immediate-release
ISA	isostearyl alcohol
IV	intravenous
IVIVC	in vitro-in vivo correlation
IVIVR	in vitro-in vivo relationship
KBE	knowledge-based engineering
LCTT	lower critical transition temperature
LDH	layered double hydroxides
LLCs	lyotropic liquid crystals
LMGA	low mass gelling agents
LUV	large unilamellar vesicles
MA	madecassoside
MAD	monoolein aqueous dispersion
MC	methyl cellulose
MDDS	multiparticulate drug delivery systems
ME	membrane emulsification
MLV	multilamellar lipid vesicles
MOX	moxifloxacin hydrochloride
MR	modified-release
MRO	maintenance, repair, and operations management
MTG	mitiglinide calcium
MTM	manometric temperature measurement
MTX	methotrexate
MWCNT	multiwalled carbon nanotubes
NAM	nicotinamide
NCE	new chemical entity
NDA	new drug application
NDLs	nano-deformable liposomes
NDT	nondestructive testing
NE	nanoemulsion
NIR	near infrared spectroscopy
NLC	nanolipid carriers
NLPs	nanoliposomes
NMP	N-methyl pyrrolidone
NMR	nuclear magnetic resonance
NPX	naproxen
NSAIDs	non-steroidal anti-inflammatory agents

NSVs	nonionic surfactant vesicles
NTD	nitrendipine
ODT	orally disintegrating tablets
OM	olmesartanmedoxomil
OSDrC®	one step dry coating
P-gp	P-glycoprotein
PAA	poly (acrylic acid)
PAAm	polyacrylamide
PAT	process analytical technology
PBD	Plackett-Burman design
PC	phosphatidylcholine
PCL	poly (caprolactone)
PDES	process development execution systems
PDI	polydispersity index
PDR	product design report
PEC	polyelectrolyte complexes
PEG	polyethylene glycol
PEGDA	polyethylene glycol diacrylate
PEHVs	preparing hybridized vesicles
PEO	polyethylene oxide
PG	polyethylene glycol
Pg	propylene glycol
PHBV	poly (3-hydroxybutyrate-co-3-hydroxyvalerateacid)
PL	phospholipid
PLA	poly (dl-lactic acid)
PLCM	pharmaceutical lifecycle management
PLGA	poly (lactic-co-glycolic acid)
PLM	product lifecycle management
PLO	pluronic lecithin organogels
pMDI	pressurized metered-dose inhaler
PMMA	poly (methyl methacrylate)
PNIPAAM	poly (N-isopropyl acrylamide
PNPs	polymeric nanoparticles
POL	poloxamer
PPLM	product and process lifecycle management
PPO	polypropylene oxide
PQLI	product quality lifecycle implementation
PR	pulsatile release

PS	phosphatidylserine
PVA	poly (vinyl alcohol)
PYR	pyrazinamide
PZNLCs	pioglitazone loaded nanostructured lipid carriers
QbD	quality by design
QC	quality control
QRM	quality risk management
QTPP	quality target product profile
R&D	research and development
RAs	risk assessments
RLD	reference listed drug
RO	rosemary oil
RSM	response surface methodology
SC	subcutaneous
SCM	supply chain management
SD	sildenafil
SE	self-emulsifying
SEDDS	self-emulsifying drug delivery systems
SEM	scanning electron microscopy
SLA	stereolithography
SLD	sildenafil citrate
SLM	solid lipid microparticles
SLN	solid lipid nanoparticles
SMGA	small molecule gelling agents
SNEDDS	self-nanoemulsifying drug delivery systems
SNLCs	supramolecular nano-engineered lipidic carriers
SSG	stibogluconate
SUA	serum uric acid
SUPAC	scale-up and post-approval changes
SUV	small unilamellar vesicles
TBA	tert-butanol
TD	Taguchi design
TDD	transdermal drug delivery
TDDS	transdermal drug delivery system
TDLAS	tunable diode laser absorption spectroscopy
TEM	transmission electron microscopy
TPH	theophylline
TPP	target product profile

TPQP	target product quality profile
TQ	thymoquinone
TSC	tri sodium citrate
TSE	transmissible spongiform encephalopathy
UCTT	upper critical transition temperature
ULV	unilamellar lipid vesicles
USFDA	United States Food and Drug Administration
USP	United States Pharmacopoeia
XRD	X-ray diffractometer
XRPD	X-ray powder diffraction

Preface

For decades the pharmaceutical sector has been considered as one of the most regulated markets across the globe, which continuously strives to deliver quality products for the patient's benefit. Usually, pharmaceutical product development involves diverse varieties of functional and nonfunctional substances, including active ingredients, excipients, polymers, etc., along with the entire manufacturing process that constitutes of multistep operations and is associated with multiple factors that need to be controlled for producing drug products with desired quality. Due to the involvement of multiple factors, the goal of achieving consistent product quality is always a great challenge for pharmaceutical scientists. Several regulatory initiatives have been undertaken so far to maintain the quality of drug products manufactured with utmost batch-to-batch consistency. One of the most vital initiatives was made by federal regulatory agencies, the United States Food and Drug Administration (USFDA) and International Conference on Harmonization (ICH) the implemented quality practices into manufacturing. In this regard, the concept of Quality by Design (QbD) was instituted as a relatively newer pharma paradigm, which particularly focuses on the systematic development of drug products with predefined objectives to provide enhanced product and process understanding. QbD has ultimate utility in the systematic development of drug products with consistent quality and minimal defects in the end.

Being inspired by the concept of QbD, several drug formulations manufactured by pharmaceutical industries across the globe have been optimized. These include solid, semisolid, ocular, inhalational, topical, injectable dosage forms, and many more. The key objective behind the adoption of systematic quality principles has now turned to be highly useful for improving quality, reducing cost, time and efforts, leading to enormous regulatory satisfactions.

Looking into the current scenario of pharmaceutical development from the past few decades, it is very clear that the manufacturers are continuously facing a quality crisis, leading eventually to the escalating number of product recalls and rejects. Thus, optimizations of the product and process performance are the two key objectives of pharmaceutical development, which can certainly be helpful in achieving continuous improvement in the end product quality. This book, in this context, is an endeavor towards the compilation of vital precepts underlying efficient, effective, and cost-effective, development of pharmaceutical products with ultimate benefits to three major stakeholders: patients, industry, and regulatory agencies.

The present book comprises of a total of 11 chapters contributed by international experts on diverse types of pharmaceutical dosage forms. A brief account on the contents of each chapter and their importance has been provided below.

Chapter 1, entitled *Introduction to Pharmaceutical Product Development,* provides an overview account of the holistic aspects of product development, various steps involved in the manufacturing process with a journey from lab scale to commercial-scale development, and regulatory challenges associated with approval of the drug products.

Chapter 2, entitled *Systematic Product and Process Development Tools in Life Cycle Management,* provide details on current progress in the technologies used for the development of drug products with the ultimate saving of time, efforts and resources. Also, the chapter highlights the application of systematic tools like experimental designs and multivariate testing in efficient product development.

Chapter 3, entitled *Recent Advances in the Development of Solid Oral Dosage Forms,* provides an insight into current progress and opportunities for efficient development of solid dosage forms with the ultimate goal of consistent end-product quality in mind.

Chapter 4, entitled *Recent Advances in the Development of Modified Release Oral Dosage Forms,* provides an insight into current progress and opportunities for efficient development of aforesaid dosage forms with the ultimate goal of consistent end-product quality in mind.

Chapter 5, entitled *Recent Advances in the Development of Parenteral Dosage Forms,* provides an insight into current progress and opportunities for efficient development of injectable preparations with the ultimate goal of consistent end-product quality in mind.

Chapter 6, entitled *Recent Advances in the Development of Semi-Solid Dosage Forms,* provides an insight into current progress and opportunities for efficient development of such preparations with the ultimate goal of consistent end-product quality in mind.

Chapter 7, entitled *Recent Advancements in the Transdermal Drug Delivery,* provides an insight into current progress and opportunities for efficient development of transdermal products with the ultimate goal of consistent end-product quality in mind.

Chapter 8, entitled *Recent Advances in the Formulation Development of Inhalational Dosage Forms,* provides an insight into current progress and opportunities for efficient development of inhalation preparations with the ultimate goal of consistent end-product quality in mind.

Chapter 9, entitled *Recent Advances in the Development of Novel Ocular Drug Delivery Systems,* provides an insight into current progress and opportunities for efficient development of ocular preparation with the ultimate goal of consistent end-product quality in mind.

Chapter 10, entitled *Recent Advances in the Development of Nanopharmaceutical Products,* provides an insight into current progress and opportunities for efficient development of nanotechnology-based products with the ultimate goal of consistent end-product quality in mind.

Chapter 11, entitled *Recent Advances in the Development of Nanoparticles for Oral Drug Delivery,* provides an insight into current progress and opportunities for efficient development of nanotechnology-based products with the ultimate goal of consistent end-product quality in mind.

CHAPTER 1

Introduction to Pharmaceutical Product Development

RAHUL SHUKLA*, MAYANK HANDA, and VISHWAS P. PARDHI

Department of Pharmaceutics, National Institute of Pharmaceutical Education and Research, Raebareli, Lucknow, Uttar Pradesh – 226002, India

Corresponding author. E-mail: rahulshuklapharm@gmail.com

1.1 INTRODUCTION

The development of a new pharmaceutical product is the need of time to address the rising pressure on pharmaceutical industries for introducing new clinical candidates in the drug discovery pipeline. The number of pharmaceutical products in the market is increasing at a tremendous rate and the pharmaceutical industry is playing an immense role in it. After the discovery of a new chemical entity (NCE), it is handed over to the product development team of the industry for further development of the dosage form (Bauer and Brönstrup, 2014). The newly discovered NCEs can be developed as an immediate release product, sustained-release product, injectable, topical or transdermal and so many other forms by considering the factors such as nature of the disease (acute or chronic), site of action, the onset of action, patient condition and critical physicochemical properties of the NCE. Table 1.1 provides information on the annual revenue of top-ranked pharmaceutical companies globally. The giant pharmaceutical companies are mainly indulging in drug discovery programs most of the time encounter a problem of product failure while producing the commercial batch if sufficient biopharmaceutical factors are not considered during the developmental phase. These factors lead to economy loss, manpower and time to identify the root cause and rectification of product failure. Thus, the development of new drug products necessitates thorough knowledge of pharmaceutical sciences to avoid such losses (U.S. Department of Health and Human Services Food and Drug Administration, 2009). Figure 1.1 provides an illustrative presentation of drug discovery.

TABLE 1.1   Annual Revenue of Globally Top Ranked Pharmaceutical Companies

Global Ranking	Company	Revenue in year 2017 (in US billion $)*
1	Pfizer	52.54
2	Roche	44.36
3	Sanofi	36.66
4	Johnson & Johnson	36.30
5	Merck	35.40
6	Novartis	33.00
7	AbbVie	28.22
8	Gilead Sciences	25.65
9	GlaxoSmithKline (GSK)	24.00
10	Amgen	22.85

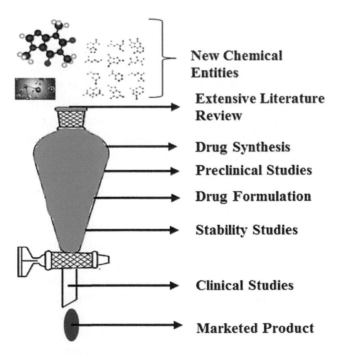

FIGURE 1.1   Illustrative presentation of drug product development.

Product development is a broad term that covers a wide spectrum of the products varies from different pharmaceuticals, medical devices, diagnostic kits, and surgical products. There are many products available in the market with different prices from different manufacturers according to the need of the customers (Politis et al., 2017). In the case of pharmaceutical products, a single NCE can be available in the different dosage forms depending upon the target population based on gender, age, patient conditions, and clinical needs. Pharmaceutical product development is a multistep process that initiates from the triggering of an idea followed by the conception which finally leads to the formation of the product. It usually takes approximately 20 years of time and the expenditure of a huge amount of money for a drug product to reach in the market through the vast process of drug discovery, clinical phase, and product development. In simple words, we can say that pharmaceutical product development is the process of development of converting the NCE into the drug product which can be comfortably consumed by the patient with a dose to elicit the desired therapeutic effect (Program et al., 2008). Table 1.2 provides information on top-selling brands and its revenue globally.

1.2 DRUG DISCOVERY

The sojourn journey of the NCEs which are therapeutically applicable in mitigation and cure of diseases from discovery laboratories to the shelf of retail shops and in the hands of the patient is the successful drug discoveries. Efforts of drug discovery start very first from the initial stage of identifying the biological target and identification of lead molecules which paves the foundation stone for the synthesis of molecules and finally leads to product development. Drug discovery is a multistep process starting from target identification to the lead optimization followed by pre-clinical and clinical trials. First of all, an effective biological target is selected which plays an important role in the disease (Bauer and Brönstrup, 2014). The next step in the process of drug discovery is the synthesis of the compounds, characterization of compounds, *in vitro* screening followed by pre-clinical and clinical trials. The average time for drug development is 10–15 years and the average cost of drug development varies from US\$ 1.5 billion to US\$ 1.9 billion. Due to the high cost of R&D and human clinical trials, the process of drug discovery and development is very costly (Zhao et al., 2006a). A graph depicting various stages in the product life cycle is mentioned in Figure 1.2. Table 1.3 is the information

TABLE 1.2   Annual Revenue of Top Most Selling Brands Globally

Global Ranking	Brand	NCEs	Company	Revenue in year 2017 (in US billion $)*
1	Humira	Adalimumab	AbbVie Inc. (USA)	18.43
2	Eylea	Aflibercept	Bayer (Germany) & Regeneron Pharmaceuticals (USA)	8.23
3	Revlimid	Lenalidomide	Celgene (USA)	8.19
4	Rituxan	Rituximab	Biogen & Roche	8.11
5	Enbrel	Etanercept	Amgen Inc. (USA) & Pfizer (Europe)	7.98
6	Herceptin	Trastuzumab	Roche	7.55
7	Eliquis	Apixaban	Bristol-Myers Squibb (USA) & Pfizer (USA)	7.40
8	Avastin	Bevacizumab	Roche	7.21
9	Remicade	Infliximab	Johnson & Johnson (USA) & Merck (USA)	7.16
10	Xarelto	Rivaroxaban	Bayer (Germany) & Johnson & Johnson (USA)	6.54
11	Januvia/ Janumet	Sitagliptin	Merck	5.90
12	Lantus	Insulin glargine	Sanofi	5.65
13	Prevnar 13/ Preventer	Pneumococcal 13-valent conjugate Vaccine	Pfizer	5.60
14	Opdivo	Nivolumab	Bristol-Myers Squibb	4.95
15	Neulasta/ Peglasta and Neupogen/ Gran	Pegfilgrastim and Filgrastim	Amgen (USA) & Kyowa Hakko Kirin (Japan)	4.56
16	Lyrica	Pregabalin	Pfizer	4.51
17	Harvoni	Ledipasvir/ Sofosbuvir	Gilead Sciences	4.37
18	Advair/ Seretide	Fluticasone and Salmeterol	GlaxoSmithKline	4.36
19	Tecfidera	Dimethyl fumarate	Biogen	4.21
20	Stelara	Ustekinumab	Johnson & Johnson	4.01

of patented molecules going to expire in the year 2018. In the current era, the developing countries are suffering from many infectious diseases and the number of treatments available for these diseases is very less. It was noted in the past that most of the drugs are discovered either by traditional methods of drug discovery from natural resources or by serendipity. At present, novel approaches of drug discovery are followed which starts with target identification based on the disease by employing various tools such as combinatorial chemistry, cell-based assays, high throughput screening and computer-based (*in-silico*) studies (Zhao et al., 2006a; Katsila et al., 2016). Various phases of product development are given in Figure 1.3.

TABLE 1.3 Brands Whose Patent Tenure is Over or Going to Expire in the Year 2018

Brand	Company
Finacea	Bayer
Fortesta	Endo Pharmaceuticals Inc.
Cialis	Eli Lilly
Levitra	Bayer
Lotronex	Abbott
Makena	AMAG Pharmaceuticals Inc.
Promacta	Novartis
Rapaflo	Allergan
Tikosyn	Pfizer
Vesicare	Astellas Pharma Inc.

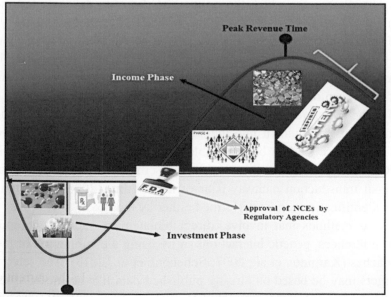

FIGURE 1.2 Graph showing various phases of drug development.

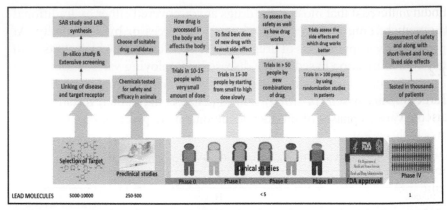

FIGURE 1.3   Diagrammatic representation of various phases involved in drug product development.

The steps involved in modern drug discovery are discussed in the following sections.

1.2.1   TARGET IDENTIFICATION

The first step in the process of modern drug discovery is target identification. The disease for which the drug to be discovered is selected thoroughly and a suitable target having a significant effect in the pathology of the disease is chosen. Target selection should be such that the drug should bind to it effectively with proper confirmation to elicit the desired response (Charoo and Ali, 2013). The drug target is generally a biomolecule, which may be a receptor, ion channel, protein or nucleic acid (Schenone et al., 2013). The structure of the biological target should be such that the new chemical entity should fit into the structure to show therapeutic action, such targets are said to be druggable targets and provide druggability to NCE. Generally, the target plays a very crucial role in the pathology or signal transduction pathway (Carson and Wilms, 2006). The step of target identification can be performed either by employing any one of the following methods that involve, direct biochemical method, computational inferences, genetic interactions or by using a combination of these approaches (Karginov et al., 2007; Schenone et al., 2013). The selection of targets may be based on already published data like scientific articles or patents and from the omic studies such as transcriptional profiling and proteomics. These methods for selection of biological target helps in finding altered expression patterns of gene or protein in disease condition (Lomenick et al., 2009).

1.2.2 TARGET VALIDATION

Target validation is the process by which the utility of the target in the drug discovery is justified. Target validation is an early step of drug discovery in which various techniques are used to justify the utility of the target (Charoo and Ali, 2013). Target validation tells us whether the target has the ability to act as a target in the drug discovery process. The process of target validation includes determination of the structure-activity relationship of developed NCE, determination of NCE resistant mutant of the predetermined target, i.e., overexpression or knockdown of the speculated target and tracking the downstream signaling system of the target (Titov and Liu, 2012). There are some techniques for validating the target which involve model interaction, sense reversal, proteomics and *in vivo* target validation (Smith, 2003; Karginov et al., 2007).

1.2.3 LEAD DISCOVERY

Once the target has been optimized, the next step in the ladder of the drug discovery process is lead discovery which includes identification of ligand with high affinity for the validated biological target. In the process of lead discovery various compounds are synthesized and checked for activity and potency using various animal models. Generally, knock-out and knock-in models are used in the process for activity testing in animal models (Tung, 2013). Libraries of the compounds are obtained using combinational synthesis. High throughput screening and *in silico* screening are also used for screening of a large number of synthesized compounds towards the target (Titov and Liu, 2012). Screening by using NMR (Nuclear magnetic resonance) techniques is a new screening strategy that greatly improves the lead finding the step of drug discovery (Hajduk and Burns, 2002). Eventually, the compounds which bind to the target with high affinity and show activity are further processed as lead molecules (Prašnikar and Škerlj, 2006).

1.2.4 LEAD OPTIMIZATION

Lead optimization is the next step in drug discovery after the lead molecule has been identified. After the completion of this phase of drug discovery, the best analog will be obtained to process further for drug development. The lead compounds are chemically and structurally modified in order to make it more suitable to act as a drug (Bauer and Bronstrup, 2014). The process of lead optimization includes replicative rounds of synthesis and characterization of the potential lead molecule to manifest how chemical structure and the activities are interconnected in terms of its targets and its biotransformation (Lomenick et al., 2009). The lead molecules are extensively characterized for various pharmacodynamic properties such as potency and efficacy, pharmacokinetic properties and toxicological aspects (Cheng et al., 2007).

1.2.5   PRE-CLINICAL AND CLINICAL DEVELOPMENT

1.2.5.1   PRE-CLINICAL DEVELOPMENT

Preclinical studies also known as non-clinical studies. These studies are performed on the animals to check the safety and efficacy of the drug. Pre-clinical studies on animals include animal safety studies, repeat dose toxicity studies, carcinogenicity studies, metabolism studies, and dose escalation studies till the toxic dose is achieved (Edwards et al., 2015). The drug compound is also tested on the various cell lines or animal models (rodents and non-rodents) in order to obtain preliminary data on the safety, efficacy and pharmacokinetic information of the drug (Bauer and Bronstrup, 2014).

1.2.5.2   CLINICAL DEVELOPMENT

After the successful completion of pre-clinical trials, the drug molecule enters into the clinical phase in which the drug is tested on humans (Weng et al., 2014). The very first step before going for clinical studies is the deter-mination of dose which is being administered to humans by extrapolating the animal dose to the human dose more appropriately by considering the body surface area (Shin et al., 2010). In the clinical developmental phase, the drug is tested both on the healthy volunteers as well as patients to determine the safety and efficacy (Mani et al., 2011).

Clinical developmental phase can be divided into different sub-phases as described below:

Phase 0—Phase 0 of the clinical trials also known as micro-dosing and these are ExpIND studies (Exploratory Investigational New Drug) which are performed before the standard phase 1 dose-escalation drug safety and tolerability testing (Gupta et al., 2011). This phase of the clinical trial tells us whether the drug molecule with therapeutic activity in the pre-clinical trials is showing anticipated activity in humans or not (Haines, 1978; Kinders et al., 2007).

Phase 1—Phase 1 clinical trials are usually small trials where only a few subjects are recruited. Generally, 20-100 healthy volunteers are selected to assess the safety, tolerability, pharmacokinetics, and pharmacodynamics of the drug (Toumazi et al., 2018). The criterion of healthy volunteers is an exception for anticancer drugs where the drug is evaluated in patients. In this phase, the variability of the dose is followed to decide the therapeutic dose for further processing. Initially, the first few patients are given with very low dose and after confirmation of tolerability, the next group will have a slightly higher dose with further gradual increment to each next group till the best tolerable dose is found (Bauer and Brönstrup, 2014). Pharmacokinetic parameters of the drug such as absorption, metabolism, and excretion of the drug are also tested in this phase. Approximately, 70 % of the drug candidate passes this phase (Ursino et al., 2017).

Phase 2—Phase 2 trials are larger than phase 1 trials which often performed on 100-300 patients. In this phase, mainly the efficacy of the drug is evaluated and along with that, some more information regarding side effects as well as the best therapeutic dose to be selected is obtained. The second phase of the clinical trials lasts from several months to two years (Bauer and Brönstrup, 2014). The clinical studies in this phase are performed in a randomized manner where the patients are randomly allocated for treatment and/or control groups. After the completion of phase 2 clinical trials, the pharmaceutical company and regulatory authorities have enough information about the safety and efficacy of the drug. Approximately one-third of the drug candidate passes phases 1 and 2 of the clinical trial (Floyd, 1999).

Phase 3—This phase of the clinical trial involves many more patients as compared to phase 1 and phase 2. The number of patients selected for this phase ranges from 300–1000 and compares the new treatment with contemporary standard treatment. The reason for selecting a large group of patients population is because the differences in success rate might be small and thus, trials in a larger number of patients are able to show the difference (Weng et al., 2014). Most of phase 3 clinical trials are randomized and are usually conducted with the main purpose of definitive estimation of the efficacy. In this phase, the specific side effects of the drug are also monitored. Generally, two successful phases 3 clinical trials are required by the USFDA to get the marketing approval. After the successful completion of phase 3 of a clinical trial, USFDA gives its final node to the marketing of drug products to the innovator company (Berridge, 2004).

Phase 4—Phase 4 of the clinical trials is also known as *Post Marketing Surveillance*. The principle objective for running a phase 4 trial is to get more about side effects and safety of the drug, long term risk, and benefits and to know the drug performance in the variable gene pool (Speck-Planche et al., 2017). Once the company got marketing approval for the drug, the drug reaches the market but the post-launch safety monitoring being a mandatory criterion as per the USFDA guidelines. The drug can be withdrawn from the market on the basis of the results of Phase 4 (Proteins and Technology, 2015).

1.3   NEED OF PRODUCT DEVELOPMENT

It is the tendency of human nature that leads to innovations from time to time. A product that is highly useful at a point of time may prove insignificant at another time point. Pharmaceutical companies have to introduce new features into the product to fulfill patient demand. Continuous introduction of high efficacy antibiotics with time is an example of a change of needs of patients. Pharmaceutical companies keep on developing new antibiotics with higher efficacy and low MIC (Minimum Inhibitory Concentration) (Dara and Tiwari, 2014). The need for the development of a novel drug delivery system is a demand of time. For example, pills were the most common delivery system in the past but with the advancement of technology and changing needs of patient more effective dosage forms are developed. For example, enteric-coated tablets, buccal tablets and orally dispersible tablets (ODTs). In order to avoid the frequent administration of the drug (dosing frequency), sustained-release formulations of the drug were also developed (Kauss et al., 2013).

The extensive growth rate of pharmaceutical industries and an increase in competition among them is also one of the attributing factors for the development of the new product. In order to survive in the market, pharmaceutical companies are trying to develop new products with more patient convenience to attract more and more customers and to increase their income source. Also with the advancement of technology, the process of development of new drug products became easier (Bauer and Brönstrup, 2013). The development of new drug products is also associated with an image of the company. Companies always try to pump new drugs into the market to maintain their image and reputation (Yousefi et al., 2017).

1.4   OBSTACLES IN PRODUCT DEVELOPMENT

Pharmaceutical product development is a tedious process and needs a huge investment of time and money (Khatri et al., 2014). Figure 1.4 highlights some of the obstacles in pharmaceutical product development are:

- Unknown pathophysiology of diseases, which makes the process of target identification challenging.
- Difference in the genotype of the different patients may lead to chances of the unexpected response of the drug in different patients, which eventually leads to the product failure.
- Current stringent regulatory processes for new drug approval such as Investigational New Drug (IND), New Drug Application (NDA), and Abbreviated New Drug Application (ANDA).
- Inability to rely on the published data is also one of the obstacles in the development of new products. In such cases, reproducibility remains a criterion for isolation. There are great chances of failure in the replication of the published data from one lab to another, as sometimes false or fake data is reported in the literature (International Conference on Harmonization of Technical Requirements for Registration of Pharmaceuticals for Human Use, 2009).

1.5   TYPES OF PHARMACEUTICAL PRODUCTS

1.5.1   BREAKTHROUGH PRODUCTS

Breakthrough products are those which are new to the world and create new market value and huge money. For example, vaccines for cancer or AIDS which are in various phases of clinical trials can be a breakthrough product in the near future. Other breakthrough products in the near future can be products for malaria and psoriasis treatment (Halbert, 2002).

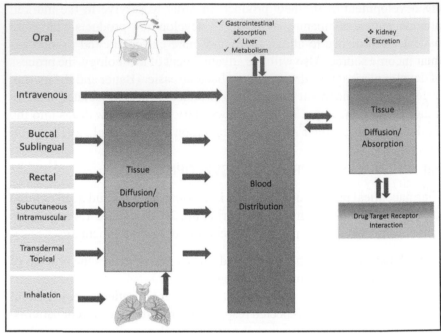

FIGURE 1.4   Flow diagram of various dosage forms going through various processes in the body.

1.5.2   INCREMENTAL PRODUCTS

Extension products of the existing products are known as incremental products. The new dosage form of the already available product called incremental products. For example, if a product is available in the form of gel and its spray or some other dosage form is prepared, then it is said to be the incremental product of that gel (Mire-Sluis et al., 2012).

1.5.3   NICHE PRODUCTS

Niche products are the products with features that are urgently needed to a particular market subgroup. Model niche products are easily distinguished from other products and are produced and sold for specialized uses inside its corresponding niche market. In pharma industries, niche products are the generic drug products with minimum competition in the market

(Dolgin, 2010). An example of such a product is Shelcal and Shelcal-CT, a calcium supplement product targeted at women's which was launched by Elder Pharmaceuticals, an Indian based pharmaceutical company head-quartered in Mumbai, Maharashtra (Shah and Difalco, 2016).

1.6 QUALITY BY DESIGN (QBD) APPROACH IN PRODUCT DEVELOPMENT

The concept of applying statistical analysis at the initial research stages rather than at the end was introduced by Sir Ronald Fisher in the early 20th century. The application of statistical analysis at the design phase helps to build quality into the finished product. The QbD approach had been adopted by the pharmaceutical industry in the later phases as compared to other sectors (N. Politis et al., 2017). Over a recent decade, pharmaceutical product development by using QbD approach in the area of thrust for the pharmaceutical industry and regulatory authorities. USFDA and ICH are giving special emphasis on the use of QbD for the new product development in the industry (Charoo and Ali, 2013; Beg et al., 2019). Implementation of QbD principles in product development leads to a rise in the success rate of product and prevent product failure, reduced validation burden, prompt regulatory pathway, and reduced post-marketing changes. Target product quality profile, critical quality attributes, risk assessments, design space, control strategy, product lifecycle management are the key elements of the QbD. Design of Experiments (DoE) is the commonly used statistical method in the pharmaceutical industry amongst all other mathematical models in QbD (Khatri et al., 2014; Singh et al., 2013).

QbD is the newer approach of pharmaceutical product development which requires a thorough understanding of product quality attributes and processes. Traditionally, pharmaceutical products are manufactured to meet the quality tests which are given in the specifications of the product. If any manufactured batch failed to comply with these tests, it is rejected or sent for reprocessing (Weissman and Anderson, 2015; Beg et al., 2017). The process of QbD in the industry involves multivariate experiments that utilize process analytical technology (PAT) and the identification of critical quality attributes (CQAs) by performing various tests. Before applying the QbD approach in the manufacturing process, the effect of all process variables on the final product is studied (Zhao et al., 2006a). The application of QbD in pharmaceutical product development is given in Figure 1.5.

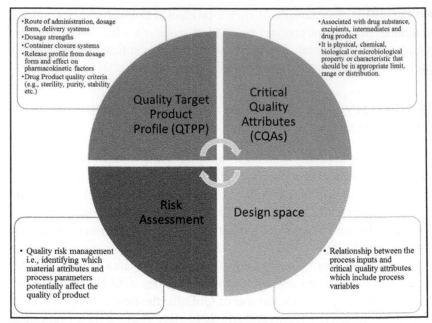

Route of administration, dosage
form, delivery systems
Dosage strengths
Container closure systems
Release profile from dosage
form and effect on
pharmacokinetic factors
Drug Product quality criteria
(e.g., sterility, purity, stability
etc.)

Quality Target Product Profile (QTPP)

Associated with drug substance,
excipients, intermediates and
drug product
It is physical, chemical,
biological or microbiological
property or characteristic that
should be in appropriate limit,
range or distribution.

Critical Quality Attributes (CQAs)

Risk Assessment

Quality risk management
i.e., identifying which
material attributes and
process parameters
potentially affect the
quality of product

Design space

Relationship between the
process inputs and
critical quality attributes
which include process
variables

FIGURE 1.5   Flow chart showing the application of QbD in product development.

Target product profile (TPP), target product quality profile (TPQP), design and development of product, developing the manufacturing process, identifying the CQAs, assessment and management of the risks involved in the process, establishment of design space and control strategy for product quality are the important components of product development by employing QbD. The regulatory guidelines such as ICH Q8, ICH Q9, and ICH Q10 deals with the quality of the product by delineating the principles of QbD (Politis et al., 2017).

Design of Experiments is a software-based approach used for establishing the relationship between the factors affecting the process and the output of the experiment. Numbers of designs are used to plan the experiments of which some of the commonly used experimental designs are as below:

1.6.1   COMMONLY USED EXPERIMENTAL DESIGNS

1.6.1.1   FULL FACTORIAL DESIGNS

In full factorial design, every level of every factor with every level of every other factor is considered. High, medium, or low levels are assigned for each factor. The number of experiments depends on the number of factors and the number of levels for each factor. For example, in Table 1.4 if the number of independent factors is "n" and each factor having two levels, then the number of experiments can be calculated as 2^n (Politis et al., 2017).

TABLE 1.4 Number of Runs for 2^n Full Factorial Design

Sr. No.	Number of factors	Total number of Run/Experiment
1.	2	4
2.	3	8
3.	4	16
4.	5	32
5.	6	64

1.6.1.2 FRACTIONAL FACTORIAL DESIGNS

In the case of full factorial design, large numbers of the run are generated, if the numbers of factors considered are more than three. So to cut-short the number of the run, the fractional factorial design is selected. On the basis of applicability only a few experiments are performed (Allen, 2008).

So the numbers of runs in case of fractional factorial design are determined by equation:

$$N = 2^{k-p}$$

where, N is the number of runs generated; k is the treatment factor; and p is the number of blocks.

1.6.1.3 PLACKETT–BURMAN DESIGNS

A Plackett-Burman design is a type of screening design that is useful to find out which factors of the experiment are significantly affecting the response variables. Plackett-Burman design helps us to eliminate the noise (unimportant factors). In this type of design, a large number of factors are evaluated with the minimum number of runs. This type of design is very useful in a situation where only some of the factors are important and avoid the data obtained from the non-relevant experiments (Allen, 2010).

1.6.1.4 RESPONSE SURFACE DESIGNS

Response surface design is a type of DoE that is used to refine our experiment by determining the important factors in our experiment especially if there is the possibility of curvature in the experiment (Charoo and Ali, 2013).

The only small difference between the equation of response surface design and the equation of factorial design is the addition of squared (or quadratic) in the equation of response surface design. The response surface design is helpful in:

- finding the level of variables to optimize the process; and
- selecting the best conditions for the experiment.

One limitation with the response surface design is that it can be used only if there are up to eight factors.

1.7 INDUSTRIAL PRODUCT DEVELOPMENT

Development of pharmaceutical product in the industry is a tedious and long term process which requires a huge investment of time and money. The pharmaceutical industry is further divided into sub-departments and all of these department works in coordination with each other in the development of the pharmaceutical product (Malay K. Das and Chakraborty, 2015). Pharmaceutical product development starts with market research where the medical and marketing teams of the company do the research to know the need of consumers. On the basis of data obtained from the market research, the Research and Development (R&D) team of the company works for the development of the Active Pharmaceutical Ingredient (API). Once the R&D team is able to synthesize the desired API with the desired activity, its safety and efficacy studies are also conducted (Singh et al., 2018). After the establishment of the safety and efficacy of the API, it is handed over to the Formulation Research & Development (FR&D) team for the development of dosage form. After the various trials by the FR&D team, the most suitable dosage form is selected for further processing. After the finalization of the dosage form technology transfer (Tech Transfer) team comes in the picture which works on the requirement and transfer of the technology for manufacturing of the same dosage form at the commercial scale. After the successful technology transfer, the manufacturing team manufactures the product on a large scale (Das and

Chakraborty, 2015). Manufactured products are then sent to the quality control (QC) department for testing the quality of the product. After the successful establishment of the quality of the product, it is handed over to the packaging and labeling department. Then after the establishment of the stability of the product, the market launch of the stabilized batch is handed over to the marketing department and sent to the market (Henry, 2005). Teams and various department indulge in pharmaceutical product development is given diagrammatically in Figure 1.6.

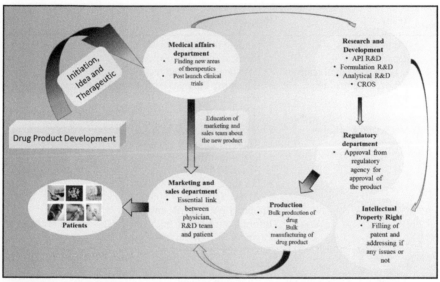

FIGURE 1.6 Diagrammatic flow representing the various departments and teams of pharmaceutical organizations involved in the process of product development.

The common steps involved in the development of pharmaceutical products are discussed in the following subsections.

1.7.1 MARKET RESEARCH

Market research is the first and most important step in product development. The medical and marketing team of the company tries to collect data from various sources to know the needs of the consumers (Zhao et al., 2005). The medical research team of the company conducts surveys and meets medical prescriptioners to know about the current market trends and requirements (Narayan, 2011). The medical affairs department of the company conducts research at both the local market and the global market. After getting the data from various sources and surveys, it is compiled and given to the R&D team for further processing (Zhao et al., 2006b). Table 1.5 enlists various team of pharmaceutical organization involved in product development.

TABLE 1.5   Various teAm of Pharmaceutical Organization Involved Directly or Indirectly in Product Development

S. No.	Team	Responsibilities
1.	Medical affairs department • Global medical team • Local medical team	• Finding the new areas of therapeutics • Medical Information services • Post-launch clinical trials • Educating the marketing team about new therapeutics and products • Health economics and outcomes of research
2.	Marketing and sales department	Five principles for which market team works: • Right products • Right quantity • At the right place • For the right price • At the right time Product flow towards customer Information flow on both sides Payment flow towards the provider Assists physicians in matching drug therapy to patients
3.	Research & Development • API R&D • F-R&D • A-R&D • CROs	• Literature review • Identification of lead molecules • Synthesis of new molecules and its stability • Pre-clinical studies to know the efficacy of molecules • Pre-formulation studies • Route of administration as well as the development of suitable dosage form • Stability of developed dosage form • Analytical method development • Toxicity and Pharmacokinetic studies of new molecules
4.	Regulatory department	Approval from the various regulatory agency for clinical trials and after clinical trial approval various market approval from different unions and nations
5.	Intellectual Property Department	Filing of patents and rectification of IPR related issues

1.7.2   SYNTHESIS OF API

Once the medical research team gives the compiled data to the R&D team of the company, the API–R&D team of the company works for the development of the desired molecule (Proteins and Technology, 2015). Large numbers of the molecules are synthesized by utilizing the principles of combinational chemistry. These molecules are then screened using high throughput screening (HTS) to get the lead molecule. This lead molecule is further checked for its safety and efficacy. Once the safety and efficacy of the molecule are established, it is finalized and synthesized at a large scale to use in the final product (Devalapally et al., 2007).

1.7.3   DEVELOPMENT OF DOSAGE FORM

Once the API is synthesized by the API-R&D team, it is handed over to the FR&D team for the development of a suitable dosage form. Different trials are conducted with the drug for the formulation of different dosage forms. Different excipients are tried at a different concentration for the different dosage forms (Ahmed and Kasraian, 2002). Dosage form development starts firstly with the preformulation studies which areas described below.

1.7.3.1   PREFORMULATION STUDIES

Preformulation studies play a vital role in drug discovery and development. Preformulation studies mainly determine the physicochemical properties of a drug such as pKa, log P, log D, and other properties. These studies provide significant information about the ability of a drug or compound to be used on commercial or research scale by considering technical and financial aspects during lead identification and lead optimization (Singh et al., 2017). The preformulation studies initially identified and optimize the lead molecule, and then these lead molecules are moved towards the formulation developmental phase. The formulation developmental phase is carried out by considering different guidelines about manufacturing, formulation development, and evaluation. The obtained preformulation data contributes to different groups and departments of the pharmaceutical industry (Allen, 2010). For the pharmaceutical industry and formulator, reformulation studies give significant and sufficient data for optimization of the chemical structure with relevant solubility, log P and stability of the compound. It also provides a notion about the futuristic pharmacokinetic and toxicological profile of the drug (Huang et al., 2009). The same data obtained from preformulation studies further provided to the analytical department for the development of stability-indicating assays as well as analytical methods. In the manufacturing of the drug, preformulation study data on salt selection, purity of compound, polymorphism, particle size, and shape provides idea about suitable manufacturing method of a compound which subsequently helps in the design of appropriate dosage form (Durig and Fassihi, 1991). For clinical evaluation of compound, preformulation data is needed along with data from preclinical testing in animal studies for evaluation of absorption, distribution, metabolism, and excretion of the drug in humans through the therapeutic absorbed dose (Pharmaceutical, 2006). Therefore, preformulation studies are critical in drug discovery and development of a drug as it enables the reduction of time and cost for the development of new drugs. Preformulation studies also involve salt selection, polymorphism study, crystal habits modifications, the study of bulk properties of the drug, hygroscopicity, drug stability, and drug solubility, etc. These preformulation parameters are further elaborated to have a clear idea of the concept.

1.7.3.2   SALT SELECTION

For the successful development of dosage form, various physicochemical and biological properties have to be considered. Some of these properties are beneficial while some are unwanted like poor solubility, dissolution rate and stability (Ich, 2009). These unwanted properties can be overcome by converting them to salt form. The suitable salt form of drugs helps to enhance the bioavailability and stability of drugs. The salt forms are more prominently employed for the enhancement of aqueous solubility, however, selected salt forms alters other properties of API such as melting point, mechanical properties, chemical stability, hygroscopicity, and crystal form. The salt form which exists in hydrates is problematic particularly during the wet granulation process (Allen Jr., 2008).

1.7.3.3   POLYMORPHISM STUDY

Polymorphism is the existence of API or drug in more than one crystal forms and these different forms are known as polymorphs. Polymorph identification is a crucial step in dosage form development. The polymorphs with higher melting points are suitable for pharmaceutical product development. The process of conversion of one unstable polymorph into another polymorph is called polymorphic phase transitions. These phase transitions mostly occur in solid dosage forms that affect the drug release. The polymorphic phase transitions are always problematic when determined in the late phase of development. The polymorphism phase transitions affect the bioavailability of drugs by increasing or decreasing the solubility and also affects the stability by converting the original stable form into an unstable form (Bauer and Brönstrup, 2014).

1.7.3.4   CRYSTAL HABIT MODIFICATION

In pharmaceutical industries, it is very important to develop a stable and robust dosage form. For this purpose crystal engineering is a very helpful tool that modifies the physicochemical properties of the drug by changing the crystal habit of the drug. The change in solid-state properties of the drug ultimately affects the physicochemical properties which have impacts on solubility, dissolution rate, flow properties and compressibility of drugs (Zhao et al., 2006a).

1.7.3.5   STUDY OF BULK PROPERTIES

Bulk properties of the drug include flow properties, particle size, and size distribution. The particle size and shape have an impact on the dissolution rate of drugs. The smaller size of a drug provides greater surface area to volume ratio which subsequently improves the saturation solubility and dissolution properties of the drug. The solubility and dissolution are key aspects during the formulation development process because they affect the bioavailability of drugs. The critical quality attributes of the product such as disintegration testing, *in vitro* dissolution studies, friability test and content uniformity are influenced by the bulk properties of drugs (Karande et al., 2006).

1.7.3.6   HYGROSCOPICITY

The hygroscopicity and deliquescence of drug substances are parameters which are taken into consideration in the development of drug product.

The study of the hygroscopic nature of a drug plays a crucial role as solids with residual moisture shows changes in various physicochemical properties in relation to their dry state. The moisture absorb by drug from the environment are responsible for different chemical reaction and it also affects the stability of the drug substances by undergoing polymorphic transformations (Durig and Fassihi, 1991).

1.7.3.7   DRUG STABILITY

The storage conditions of pharmaceutical dosage form affect the stability of drug substances. Thus, compound handling and storage conditions requirements decided in accordance with the stability of the drug. The stability screening studies data provide information for the enhancement of stabilization strategies. The standard stability testing procedure for developed formulation should be in compliance with the ICH stability guidelines for new drug substances and products, i.e., Q1A (R2).

1.7.3.8   DRUG SOLUBILITY

The absorption of the drug depends on the solubility and permeability of drugs. The solubility and permeability are two opposite term but for effective absorption, they should be balanced. The poor solubility of the drug is having a great impact on the bioavailability of drug which intern affects the efficacy. The solubility of poorly soluble drug can be improved by different strategies which include physicochemical modification of drug and various other methods such as crystal engineering, size reduction (micronization), salt formation, amorphization, micellar solubilization, solid dispersion, complexation and many more (Savjani et al., 2012).

After all these preformulation studies actually formulation optimization process starts and the process of formulation development ends with a satisfactory *in vivo* performance. Drug-excipient and excipient-excipient compatibility studies are also considered during formulation development in order to avoid any interaction among drug and excipients in the final dosage form. The best formulation from the different trials is selected for scale-up (Dave et al., 2015). Table 1.6 highlights various parameters and methods in pharmaceutical product development.

TABLE 1.6 Parameters and Methods in Pharmaceutical Product Development

S. No.	Procedures	Dosage Form	
1.	**Bulk Active Characterization**	**Tablet**	**Parenterals**
	a) **Physical characterization from bulk batch**	• Polymorphism • Bacterial Endotoxin Test • Particle size distribution • Bulk density • Microscopic observation	• Polymorphism • Bacterial Endotoxin Test • Particle size distribution • Bulk density • Solubility
	b) **Chemical characterization**	• Assay • Stressed Analysis • Impurity Profile • Optical rotation • Enantiomeric purity	• Assay • Stressed Analysis • Impurity Profile • Optical rotation • Enantiomeric purity
2.	**Excipients**	Excipient compatibility using Differential Scanning calorimetry methods and stability assessment	Excipient compatibility using Differential Scanning calorimetry methods and stability assessment
3.	**Container closure system**	• Material composition • Type of thermoplastic resin and resin pigments	• Compatibility with a rubber stopper and glass containers
4.	**Manufacturing process**	**Loss on drying limits** **Wet granulation:** • Aqueous/ Non-aqueous • High shear/ low shear mixing • Drying time in Fluidized bed dryer **Dry granulation:** • Slugging/Deslugging • Torque/endpoint **Direct Compression:** • Mixing time	**Pyrogen free** **Aqueous preparation:** • Viscosity • pH • Stabilizers/ Buffers • Heating required/ not • Sterilization method • Osmolarity • Antioxidant & Preservatives **Non-aqueous preparation:** • Osmolarity • Viscosity • Sterilization method • Preservatives & Antioxidant **Lyophilized preparation:** • Use of cryoprotectant • Drying time • Type of solvents used • Residual solvent • Solubility of lyophilized powder

TABLE 1.6   *(Continued)*

S. No. Procedures	Dosage Form	

	Lubrication:	**Filtration:**
	• Pre lubrication time & post lubrication time	• Aseptic filtration • Type of filter paper • Compatibility with filter paper
	Granulation:	**Storage:**
	• Flow properties • Density • Particle size distribution • Compressibility	• Specify the storage condition • Type of glass used amber colored or clear
	Compression:	
	• Weight • Thickness • Hardness • Friability • Disintegration • Dissolution	

1.7.4   REGULATORY APPROVAL AND PATENT FILING

Once the best dosage form is decided for further development, regulatory approval has to be taken from the regulatory authorities. For conducting the clinical trials, the IND application is filed to the regulatory authority. The IND application includes essential information which includes preclinical animal study data (safety, efficacy and toxicity data), drug profile and pharmacokinetics data (Jones, 2008). After the evaluation of the submitted data by the regulatory authority, based on the fulfillment of the criterion of the regulatory agency, the application is either rejected or approved for a clinical trial is given to the respective company. After the successful completion of clinical trials, NDA is filed to get approval for the marketing of drug products (Gregory and Ho, 1981). In the case of generic products, ANDA is filed to get the marketing approval. At the same time, the Intellectual Property Department of the company may file a patent in one or more countries to get marketing exclusivity (Andrews, 2007).

1.7.5   TECHNOLOGY TRANSFER

After getting approval for the optimized batches of products from the regulatory authority, the industry has to go for the large scale manufacturing of the product. In simple words, it can be said that the technology transfer is, when the industry switches from pilot plant scale to full manufacturing scale or from one manufacturing site to another manufacturing site (Acharya et al., 2018). The main role of the tech transfer team in the pharmaceutical industry is to provide sufficient information to the large scale manufacturer on the basis of information received from the R&D team. Technology transfer is an integral product of new product development.

Technology transfer is the link between the R&D team and the production plant of the pharmaceutical company (Sinha and Vohora, 2018).

1.7.6 LARGE-SCALE MANUFACTURING

After the successful technology transfer by tech transfer, the company is ready for the production of the final product on a large scale. In the pharmaceutical company, all the manufacturing process is done according to the guidelines of GMP and GLP. The manufacturing process of product development varies depending on the type of product we are manufacturing (Niazi, 2009). Manufacturing of pharmaceutical company is generally a multistep process and require the attention of the production officer and operator. The manufacturing of sterile dosage forms is carried out in an aseptic area (class 10) while the production of non-sterile products is carried out in class 100 area. The quality of the product is checked at the various checkpoints by the IPQA (In Process Quality Assurance) department of the quality control (US Department of Health and Human Services et al., 1997). After the production of the final product, it is handed over to the packaging department for the packaging which is an essential part of pharmaceutical product manufacturing (Allen, 2008).

1.7.7 QUALITY TESTING

The quality of the manufactured product is tested by the quality control team of the company. Few samples are taken randomly after the manufacturing of the product and sent to the quality control lab for testing of products (US Department of Health and Human Services et al., 1997). The manufactured product should complies with the limits of the test given in the respective pharmacopeia (Andrews, 2007). Different quality tests are carried out to check the quality of the product which varies from product to product which includes hardness test, friability test, disintegration test and dissolution test in case of oral solid dosage forms (FDA/CDER, 1997). Similarly, other quality control tests like sterility test, pyrogen test, pH determination, and osmolarity test are the common tests performed for the sterile preparations (Arambulo, 1979; Chorghade, 1995).

1.7.8   PACKAGING AND LABELING

Packaging and labeling is the final step in the development of a pharmaceutical product. Pharmaceutical products are generally packed in glass, plastic, stainless steel or aluminum containers (Allen Jr., 2008). Tablets and capsules are generally packed in the form of aluminum strips pack, blister pack or alu-alu packs. Injectable products are generally packed in the glass vials or ampoules which are usually made of type 1 glass (Borosilicate glass). Topical preparations like gels are packed in aluminum or plastic collapsible tubes (Andrews, 2007). Pharmaceutical packaging is of two types, namely primary packaging and secondary packaging. Primary packing materials are those which are in immediate contact with the product. For example, glass vials, plastic tubes, aluminum strips, etc. On the other hand, secondary packing materials are those in which the primary packing materials packed; for example, cartons (Organization, 2002). Figure 1.7 provides a diagrammatic representation of various phases of dosage form in process of product development.

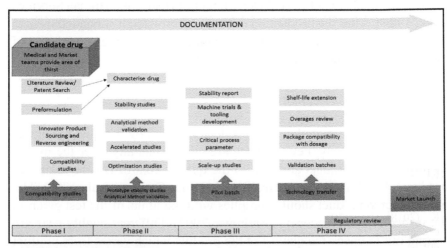

FIGURE 1.7   Diagrammatic representation showing various phases of the dosage form in the process of product development.

1.8 CONCLUDING REMARKS

Successful product development requires criticality and thorough knowledge of each subject of pharmacy from the very development step. The use of modern techniques like studying the SAR and using a computer-based model provides very early prediction to consider selective molecule for the future or not. With the advent of modern development techniques like QbD enables product development with accuracy and leaving nil chances of product failure in future or later development stages. QbD also helpful in preventing economy loss bypassing the exhaustive validation techniques and provide risk assessment. So, nowadays pharmaceutical companies use modern techniques to get targeted results. Regulatory agencies that act as a watchdog in product approval are emphasized on minimal side effects of new drug products in clinical Phase-IV trials and keep a tap on the data submitted by innovator companies. Regulatory long approval processes shorten the market phase of innovator products and increase the competition from other pharmaceutical companies. At last product development is a complete pack of knowledge, risk in terms of life as well as the economy as the cost of product development is increasing as days passes.

KEYWORDS

- **lead molecule**
- **drug discovery**
- **phase-IV**
- **product development**
- **parameters**
- **approval**
- **regulatory**

REFERENCES

Acharya, P. C., Shetty, S., Fernandes, C., Suares, D., Maheshwari, R., & Tekade, R. K., (2018). Chapter 1—Preformulation in drug research and pharmaceutical product development. In: *Dosage Form Design Considerations* (pp. 1–55). doi: https://doi. org/10.1016/B978-0-12-814423-7.00001-0 (Accessed on 19 November 2019).

Ahmed, I., & Kasraian, K., (2002). Pharmaceutical challenges in veterinary product development. *Advanced Drug Delivery Reviews*. doi: 10.1016/S0169-409X (02)00074-1.

Allen, Jr. L. V., (2008). Dosage form design and development. *Clinical Therapeutics, 30*, 2102–2111. doi: 10.1016/j.clinthera.2008.11.015. http://dx.doi.org/10.1016/j.clinthera.2008.11.015 (Accessed on 19 November 2019).

Allen, L. V., (2010). *Dosage Form Design: Pharmaceutical and Formulation Considerations*. Ansel's Pharmaceutical Dosage Forms and Drug Delivery Systems.

Andrews, G. P., (2007). Advances in solid dosage form manufacturing technology. *Philosophical Transactions: Mathematical, Physical and Engineering Sciences, 365*, 2935–2949. doi: 10.1098/rsta.2007.0014.

Arambulo, A. S., (1979). In process quality control in the manufacture of essential drugs. *Drug Development and Industrial Pharmacy*. doi: 10.3109/03639047909055678.

Bauer, A., & Brönstrup, M., (2013). Industrial natural product chemistry for drug discovery and development. *Natural Product Reports, 31*, 35–60. doi: 10.1039/c3np70058e.

Bauer, A., & Bronstrup, M., (2014). Industrial natural product chemistry for drug discovery and development. *Natural Product Reports, 31*, 35–60. doi: 10.1039/c3np70058e.

Berridge, J. C., (2004). ICH Q8: Pharmaceutical development. *Pharmaceutical Quality Forum*, 1–22.

Beg, S., Rahman, M., Kohli, K., (2019). Quality-by-design approach as a systematic tool for the development of nanopharmaceutical products. *Drug Discovery Today*. 24(3), 717–725.

Beg, S., Rahman, M., Panda, S.S., (2017). Pharmaceutical QbD: Omnipresence in the product development lifecycle. *European Pharmaceutical Review*. 22(1), 2–8.

Carson, J. W., & Wilms, H., (2006). Development of an international standard for shear testing. *Powder Technology, 167*. doi: 10.1016/j.powtec.2006.04.005.

Charoo, N. A., & Ali, A. A., (2013). Quality risk management in pharmaceutical development. *Drug Development and Industrial Pharmacy, 39*, 947–960. doi: http://dx.doi.org/10.3109/03639045.2012.699065 (Accessed on 19 November 2019).

Cheng, K.-C., Korfmacher, W. A., White, R. E., & Njoroge, F. G., (2007). Lead optimization in discovery drug metabolism and pharmacokinetics/case study: The hepatitis C virus (HCV) protease inhibitor SCH, 503034. *Perspectives in Medicinal Chemistry, 1*, 1177391X0700100001.

Chorghade, S. M., (1995). Drug discovery and development. *Pharmaceutical Biology, 33*, 1. doi: 10.3109/13880209509067080.

Dara, S. K. A., & Tiwari, R. N., (2014). Pharmaceutical process validation: An industrial perspective. *Research Journal of Pharmacy and Technology*.

Das, M. K., & Chakraborty, T., (2015). ANN in pharmaceutical product and process development. In: *Artificial Neural Network for Drug Design, Delivery and Disposition*, pp. 277–293. doi: 10.1016/B978–0–12–801559–9.00014–4.

Dave, V., Haware, R. A., Sangave, N., Sayles, M., & Popielarczyk, M., (2015). *Drug-Excipient Compatibility Studies in Formulation Development: Current Trends and Techniques*.

Devalapally, H., Chakilam, A., & Amiji, M. M., (2007). Role of nanotechnology in pharmaceutical product development. *Journal of Pharmaceutical Sciences*. doi: 10.1002/jps.20875.

Dolgin, E., (2010). *Big Pharma Moves from 'Blockbusters' to 'Niche Busters'*. Nature Publishing Group.

Drakeman, D. L., (2014). Benchmarking biotech and pharmaceutical product development. *Nature Biotechnology*. doi:10.1038/nbt.2947.

Durig, T., & Fassihi, A. R., (1991). Preformulation study of moisture effect on the physical stability of pyridoxal hydrochloride. *International Journal of Pharmaceutics, 77*, 315–319. doi: 10.1016/0378–5173 (91)90333-J.

Edwards, A. M., Arrowsmith, C. H., Bountra, C., Bunnage, M. E., Feldmann, M., Knight, J. C., Patel, D. D., et al., (2015). Preclinical target validation using patient-derived cells. *Nature Reviews Drug Discovery*. doi: 10.1038/nrd4565.

FDA/CDER, (1997). *Guidance for Industry*. Dissolution testing of immediate release solid oral dosage forms, Food and Drug Administration, Center for Drug Evaluation and Research.

Floyd, A. G., (1999). Top ten considerations in the development of parenteral emulsions. *Pharmaceutical Science and Technology Today*. doi: 10.1016/S1461–5347 (99)00141–8.

Gregory, G. K. E., & Ho, D. S. S., (1981). *Pharmaceutical Dosage Form Packages* (pp. 2–7). United States Patent 4,305,502.

Gupta, U., Bhatia, S., Garg, A., Sharma, A., & Choudhary, V., (2011). Phase 0 clinical trials in oncology new drug development. *Perspectives in Clinical Research*. doi: 10.4103/2229–3485.76285.

Haines, B. A., (1978). Worldwide regulations and legislation, their effects on pharmaceutical product development. *Drug Development and Industrial Pharmacy, 4*, 1–30. doi: 10.3109/03639047809055637.

Hajduk, P. J., & Burns, D. J., (2002). Integration of NMR and high-throughput screening. *Combinatorial Chemistry & High Throughput Screening, 5*, 613–621.

Halbert, G., (2002). 2: Pharmaceutical development. In: *The Textbook of Pharmaceutical Medicine (*pp. 96–127).

Henry, J. A., (2005). Development of a new pharmaceutical product. *Clinical Toxicology, 43*, 434.

Huang, J., Kaul, G., Cai, C., Chatlapalli, R., Hernandez-Abad, P., Ghosh, K., & Nagi, A., (2009). Quality by design case study: an integrated multivariate approach to drug product and process development. *Int. J. Pharm*. doi: S0378–5173 (09)00507–9 [pii]\n10.1016/j.ijpharm.2009.07.031.

Ich, (2009). Pharmaceutical development Q8. *ICH Harmonized Tripartite Guideline, 8*, 1–28.

International Conference on Harmonization of Technical Requirements for Registration of Pharmaceuticals for Human Use, (2009). *Q8 (R2)—Pharmaceutical Development*. ICH Harmonized Tripartite Guideline.

Jones, D., (2008). Pharmaceutical solutions for oral administration. *Pharmaceutics: Dosage Form and Design,* 1–24.

Karande, P., Jain, A., & Mitragotri, S., (2006). Insights into synergistic interactions in binary mixtures of chemical permeation enhancers for transdermal drug delivery. *Journal of Controlled Release, 115*, 85–93. doi: 10.1016/j.jconrel.2006.07.001.

Karginov, F. V., Conaco, C., Xuan, Z., Schmidt, B. H., Parker, J. S., Mandel, G., & Hannon, G. J., (2007). A biochemical approach to identifying microRNA targets. *Proceedings of the National Academy of Sciences, 104*, 19291–19296. doi: 10.1073/pnas.0709971104.

Katsila, T., Spyroulias, G. A., Patrinos, G. P., & Matsoukas, M. T., (2016). Computational approaches in target identification and drug discovery. *Computational and Structural Biotechnology Journal, 14*, 177–184.

Kauss, T., Gaubert, A., Boyer, C., Ba, B. B., Manse, M., Massip, S., Léger, J. M., Fawaz, F., Lembege, M., Boiron, J. M., Lafarge, X., Lindegardh, N., White, N. J., Olliaro, P., Millet, P., & Gaudin, K., (2013). Pharmaceutical development and optimization of azithromycin suppository for pediatric use. *International Journal of Pharmaceutics, 441*, 218–226. doi: 10.1016/j.ijpharm.2012.11.040.

Khatri, S., Saini, S., Gurubalaji, S., & Gangawat, K., (2014). Pharmaceutical QbD: Concepts for drug product development. *International Journal of Pharmaceutical Sciences Review and Research.*

Kinders, R., Parchment, R. E., Ji, J., Kummar, S., Murgo, A. J., Gutierrez, M., Collins, J., et al., (2007). Phase 0 clinical trials in cancer drug development: From FDA guidance to clinical practice. *Molecular Interventions*. doi: 10.1124/mi.7.6.9.

Lomenick, B., Hao, R., Jonai, N., Chin, R. M., Aghajan, M., Warburton, S., et al., (2009). Target identification using drug affinity responsive target stability (DARTS). *Proceedings of the National Academy of Sciences*. doi: 10.1073/pnas.0910040106.

Mani, R., Pollard, J., & Dichter, M. A., (2011). Human clinical trials in antiepileptogenesis. *Neuroscience Letters*. doi: 10.1016/j.neulet.2011.03.010.

Mire-Sluis, A., Kutza, J., & Frazier-Jessen, M., (2012). Rapid pharmaceutical product development. In: *BioProcess International* (pp. 12–21).

Narayan, P., (2011). Overview of drug product development. In: Enna, S. J., et al., (eds.), *Current Protocols in Pharmacology / Editorial Board*. Chapter 7, Unit 7.3.1–29. doi: 10.1002/0471141755.ph0703s55.

Niazi, S. K., (2009). *Handbook of Pharmaceutical Manufacturing Formulations* (Vol. 1.) doi:10.1201/9780203489703.pt2.

Organization, W. H., (2002). Guidelines on packaging for pharmaceutical products. *WHO Technical Report Series*. Geneva: World Health Organization.

Pharmaceutical, Q., (2006). Guidance for industry development guidance for industry development. *Quality, 391*, 137–147. doi:10.1016/j.ijpharm.2010.02.031.

Politis, S. N., Colombo, P., Colombo, G., & Rekkas, D. M., (2017). Design of experiments (DoE) in pharmaceutical development. *Drug Development and Industrial Pharmacy, 43*, 889–901. doi: 10.1080/03639045.2017.1291672.

Prašnikar, J., & Škerlj, T., (2006). New product development process and time-to-market in the generic pharmaceutical industry. *Industrial Marketing Management, 35*, 690–702. doi: 10.1016/j.indmarman.2005.06.001.

Program, M., Valerdi, R., Supervisor, T., Development, I., & Hale, P., (2008). Global product development : A framework for organizational diagnosis. *Development, II*, 129.

Proteins, P., & Technology, F., (2015). Biopharmaceutical production: Value creation, product types and biological basics. *Manufacturing of Pharmaceutical Proteins*, 1–32. doi: 10.1002/9783527627691.ch1.

Savjani, K. T., Gajjar, A. K., & Savjani, J. K., (2012). *Drug Solubility: Importance and Enhancement Techniques*. ISRN pharmaceutics.

Schenone, M., Dančík, V., Wagner, B. K., & Clemons, P. A., (2013). Target identification and mechanism of action in chemical biology and drug discovery. *Nature Chemical Biology, 9*, 232. doi: 10.1038/nchembio.1199.

Shah, M. S., & Difalco, R. J., (2016). *Orally Administrable Compositions Comprising Calcium*. Google Patents.

Shin, J. W., Seol, I. C., & Son, C. G., (2010). *Interpretation of Animal Dose and Human Equivalent Dose for Drug Development, 31,* 1–7.

Singh, B., Raza, K., Beg, S., (2013). Developing "Optimized" drug products employing "Designed" experiments. *Chemical Industry Digest.* 23, 70–76.

Singh, H., Khurana, L. K., & Singh, R., (2017). Pharmaceutical development. In: *Pharmaceutical Medicine and Translational Clinical Research* (pp. 33–46). doi: 10.1016/B978–0–12–802103–3.00003–1.

Singh, H., Khurana, L. K., & Singh, R., (2018). Chapter 3—Pharmaceutical development. In: *Pharmaceutical Medicine and Translational Clinical Research* (pp. 33–46). doi: https://doi.org/10.1016/B978–0–12–802103–3.00003–1 (Accessed on 19 November 2019).

Sinha, S., & Vohora, D., (2018). Drug discovery and development. In: *Pharmaceutical Medicine and Translational Clinical Research* (pp. 19–32). doi: 10.1016/B978–0–12–802103–3.00002-X.

Smith, C., (2003). Drug target validation: Hitting the target. *Nature, 422,* 341.

Speck-Planche, A., Kleandrova, V. V., Luan, F., Cordeiro, M. N. D. S., Ma, X. H., Shi, Z., et al., (2017). HHS public access. *Computational and Structural Biotechnology Journal.* doi: 10.1016/j.phrs.2009.12.011. Enabling.

Titov, D. V., & Liu, J. O., (2012). Identification and validation of protein targets of bioactive small molecules. *Bioorganic and Medicinal Chemistry, 20,* 1902–1909. doi: 10.1016/j.bmc.2011.11.070.

Toumazi, A., Comets, E., Alberti, C., Friede, T., Lentz, F., Stallard, N., Zohar, S., & Ursino, M., (2018). DFPK: An R-package for Bayesian dose-finding designs using pharmacokinetics (PK) for phase I clinical trials. *Computer Methods and Programs in Biomedicine.* doi: 10.1016/j.cmpb.2018.01.023.

Tung, H. H., (2013). Industrial perspectives of pharmaceutical crystallization. *Organic Process Research and Development.* doi: 10.1021/op3002323.

U.S. Department of Health and Human Services & Food and Drug Administration, (2009). ICH Q8 (R2) pharmaceutical development. *Workshop: Quality by Design in Pharmaceutical.*

U.S. Department of Health and Human Services, Food and Drug Administration, Center for Drug Evaluation and Research (CDER) (1997). Guidance for industry guidance for industry dissolution testing of immediate release solid oral dosage forms. *Center for Drug Evaluation and Research, 1*–11.

Ursino, M., Zohar, S., Lentz, F., Alberti, C., Friede, T., Stallard, N., & Comets, E., (2017). Dose-finding methods for Phase I clinical trials using pharmacokinetics in small populations. *Biometrical Journal, 59,* 804–825.

Weissman, S. A., & Anderson, N. G., (2015). Design of experiments (DoE) and process optimization: A review of recent publications. *Organic Process Research and Development.* doi: 10.1021/op500169m.

Weng, C., Li, Y., Ryan, P., Zhang, Y., Liu, F., Gao, J., Bigger, J., & Hripcsak, G., (2014). A distribution-based method for assessing the differences between clinical trial target populations and patient populations in electronic health records. *Applied Clinical Informatics, 5,* 463. doi: 10.4338/ACI-2013–12-RA-0105.

Yousefi, N., Mehralian, G., Rasekh, H. R., & Yousefi, M., (2017). New product development in the pharmaceutical industry: Evidence from a generic market. *Iranian Journal of Pharmaceutical Research: IJPR, 16*, 834.

Zhao, C., Hailemariam, L., Jain, A., Joglekar, G., Venkatasubramanian, V., Morris, K., & Reklaitis, G., (2006a). Information modeling for pharmaceutical product development. *Computer Aided Chemical Engineering, 21*, 2147–2152. doi: 10.1016/S1570–7946 (06)80366–4.

Zhao, C., Hailemariam, L., Jain, A., Joglekar, G., Venkatasubramanian, V., Morris, K., & Reklaitis, G., (2006b). Information modeling for pharmaceutical product development. In: *16th European Symposium on Computer Aided Process Engineering and 9th International Symposium on Process Systems Engineering* (pp. 2147–2152). doi: 10.1016/S1570–7946 (06)80366–4.

Zhao, C., Jain, A., Hailemariam, L. M., Joglekar, G., Venkatasubramanian, V., Reklaitis, G. V., Morris, K. R., Hlinak, A., & Basu, P. K., (2005). An informatics framework for pharmaceutical product development. In: *AIChE Annual Meeting, Conference Proceedings* (p. 8279).

CHAPTER 2

Systematic Product and Process Development Tools in Life Cycle Management

MOHAMAD TALEUZZAMAN,[1*] SANJAY CHUHAN,[1]
SADAF JAMAL GILANI,[2] SYED SARIM IMAM,[3] and SARWAR BEG[4]

[1]*Glocal School of Pharmacy, Glocal University, Saharanpur,
Mirzapur Pole, 247121, U.P., India*

[2]*College of Pharmacy, Aljouf University, Aljouf, Sakaka,
Kingdom of Saudi Arabia*

[3]*Department of Pharmaceutics, College of Pharmacy,
King Saud University, Riyadh–11451, Saudi Arabia*

[4]*Department of Pharmaceutics, School of Pharmaceutical Education
and Research, Jamia Hamdard, New Delhi – 110062, India*

*Corresponding author. E-mail: zzaman007@gmail.com

2.1 INTRODUCTION

Pharmaceutical industries are growing in a way quickly to give a service, which is better between customer-centric products, for increasing the revenue the market share and market size refine. It is very important throughout the whole product lifecycle that effective collaboration among customers, developers, suppliers and manufacturers for an advance competitive market. In this study proposed, a collaboration to deliver this requirement a plan work for the product lifecycle. All the trait of these alliance models all over the full product lifecycle are accompanied. In the present study, concentrate on product life cycle alliance, technology to favor collaborative product manufacturing is prefer to developed and executed in this study. The study must have advanced technology for alliance product manufacturing, in product lifecycle management that will leave a frontier basis for further research and development.

In the whole world pharmaceutical manufacturing field are acquiring more challenges of better product quality with precise schedule delivery requirement for the customer, a good profitability shareholders. Currently, world business competition is going up with require on the process, less order, short life cycles, increase suppliers, increase governmental regulation, and as well as also more material and energy costs. Manufacturers begin a more healthy business due to the new business model such as collaborative manufacturing, to friendly collaborate with their customers, suppliers manufacturers and partners for the most modern competitiveness by holding core competencies throughout the entire product lifecycle (Ming et al., 2008).

A new strategic business model has introduced in pharma business *product lifecycle management* (PLM) to support collaborative modeling, management, flow and use of product advantage including data information, knowledge, etc. The all-over enlarged act from concept to end of life-integrating people, process, and technology. The PLM system prominence the management of a case of products, operation, and facility from initial concept, through the plan, engineering, organize, production and use to final allocation. Trade in internal and external, they make a chain and merge products, forecast and process information throughout the whole product value chain among various players. They also goodwill a product–cetric trade solution that unifies product lifecycle by entitling online sharing of product information and business application (Sudarsan et al., 2005; He et al., 2015).

PLM approve manufacturing organizations to get competitive fierce by building better products in very less time, at a lower price and with lesser defects than ever earlier. The product development and revolution research early governed by the design methodologies that schedule the development process research was more concentrated on management and economics. The being product development and upheaval research were dominated by the design methodologies. In the nineteen nineties, the development of exercise research was more focused on management and economics, e.g., Cooper and Kleinschmidt. Since the nineties, the research was focused again on certain development processes of systems and technologies: microsystems and mechatronics.

2.2   LITERATURE SURVEY AND DATA ANALYSIS

In line to recognize the existing unsurpassed practices and current enduring researches, a wide-ranging literature survey was conducted, covering various countries' government official websites, regulatory agencies websites, review articles, industrial and academic approaches to the life cycle management of pharmaceutical products.

Overall different pharmaceutical product life cycle models were examined from various sources and some were included in this study. The majority of references came from industrial research and academic papers. Some important standard regulatory guidelines such as FDA and many more important sources were reviewed.

2.3   PRODUCT LIFECYCLE MODEL

After performing a broad literature survey, some key points can be drawn that in a broad sense we can classify the stages of a product life cycle **(Figure 2.1)** into: (1) beginning of life, (2) median of life, and (3) end of life. But when you go for a microanalysis you will know that a product basically passes with seven stages. These stages can be: (1) requirements, (2) design, (3) manufacturing of hardware and development of software, (4) testing and analysis, (5) distribution, (6) use and maintenance, and (7) disposal or end of life.

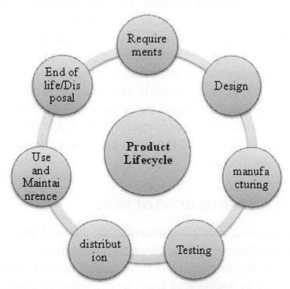

FIGURE 2.1   Schematic diagram showing the lifecycle of a product.

2.3.1 REQUIREMENTS

The initial stage in a product lifecycle is product demand builds on purchaser, industry, market and adviser bodies' viewpoints. The essential stage is fundamentally the determination of demand and identification about the product under progress. This moment is the beginning of the product lifecycle, where they require a new product is identified first when an idea comes into the mind that is not presently available. Not all plans are a good one, so they need screening. In collateral, the first idea to step work is executed explaining the gorgeous of the main practical aspects together with its products. For these processes, many multiple medium are used, including paper to clay models to 3D CAID (computer-aided industrial design software).

2.3.2 DESIGN

Design involves fabricating a substantial track of action for meeting the designation that results from the requirements stage. This stage decides *how* the product will accomplish the provisions (Dennis, 2008). Moving forward to trial product testing, through pilot release to complete product start from this stage the all-inclusive design and development of the products form initiates. The principal tool used for sketch and development is computer-aided design (CAD). It may be elementary 2D drawing/drafting or 3D compile characteristic based solid/surface modeling. These software embrace technology such as cross modeling, back-pedal engineering, knowledge-based engineering (KBE), nondestructive testing (NDT), and assembly construction. Counterfeit, validation, and escalation tasks are passed out using computer-aided engineering (CAE) software additionally incorporated in the CAD package or standalone. Computer-aided quality (CAQ) is used for dimensional tolerance (engineering) analysis tasks.

2.3.3 MANUFACTURE OR DEVELOPMENT

As the product's constituents are outright the method of manufacturing is finalized, the technique of manufacturing is explicate. CAD tasks like as device design, the formation of CNC Machining commandment for the product's parts in insertion to tools to manufacture those parts, using integrated or separate CAM computer-aided manufacturing software. For process simulation for operations like casting, molding, and die press forming it will also engage analysis tools. CPM comes into role as once the manufacturing method has been recognized. This compromise computer-aided production engineering (CAPE) or CAP/CAPP– (production planning) device for the runout company, plant and presentation layout, and production clone.

2.3.4   MANUFACTURE (HARDWARE)

Manufacturing implicates the production and consciousness of the particular depiction and prototypes. Final product units deliberate for conveying to the customer or acquiring agency are made-up and assembled in this stage.

2.3.5   DEVELOPMENT (SOFTWARE)

In the state of affairs to the process of development of coding to generate viable software units that perceive the intended design. Libraries, APIs and software systems from other sources may also be cohesive, if required.

2.3.6   TESTING

Testing is primarily the methodical appraisal of the product to assure its functionality and achievement. The seriousness of testing may oscillate from basic validation to in-depth examination. Evolution mechanisms such as inductive equipment of evaluation software may be received from third party suppliers such as PLM software.

2.3.7   DISTRIBUTION

The distribution stage requires packaging, warehousing, and transportation of the product. The combination of packaging, labeling and alike marketing pledge into the drug development process furnishes a noteworthy business opportunity in the pharmaceutical sector.

2.3.8   USE AND MAINTENANCE

The ending phase of the lifecycle inculpates the organize of in service data. The assuming that shopper and helping engineers with favorable data for restore and its continuity, as well as unwanted management/recycling information. Device like maintenance, repair, and operations management (MRO) software involves.

In another way, we can say that incriminate the operation of the product for its intentional function. Whereas maintenance skirt sustaining and enhancing the capability of the product. This can be ahead isolated into two categories, corrective maintenance, and enhancement. Basically the aim of corrective maintenance to remedy problems and vulnerabilities discovered after the product's delivery. According to customers need enhancement maintenance adapts the product to changes and provides additional functionality.

2.3.9   DISPOSAL

At this stage the final demilitarize and removal of a product at the end of its life.

2.4   PRODUCT LIFE CYCLE MANAGEMENT

In the present scenario, the pharmaceutical industry is cladding downfall in R&D productivity, Healthcare changing with a speedily landscape manner and vicious conflict with inclusive outcome in less growth and profit difference. Still, the pharmaceutical company is concentrating at more integrated approaches to enhance the processes of lead to new products in the market that can give new energy in product development while decreasing its operational costs. Within the pharmaceutical industry, the significant and integrated way to today's current challenges is to focus on product lifecycle management (PLM), which is a business transformation point of view to manage products and related information across the operation (ICH, 2009).

The entire lifecycle of a product from its origination, through design and manufacture, to service and final disposal managing is a phenomenon in Product lifecycle management (PLM). The function of the product lifecycle management is to generate and manages a company's product-related analytical principal beginning from new thought to its final product. In a pharmaceutical company, it advantages through increasing the time period of patent and finance planning. Strengthen patient compliance, profit, increased clinical advantage; price benefits life addendum disconnected and instantly market introduces the important major applications of product lifecycle management (Zhang and Mao, 2017).

2.5   PHARMACEUTICAL LIFE CYCLE MANAGEMENT (PLCM)

Pharmaceutical lifecycle management (PLCM) can be clarified as an activity of regiment the intact lifecycle of a product together with its research, plan, assemble, kindness and up to end of its life (disposal). It's a well-orthodox tool to make the most of deals throughout the product lifecycle and acts as an aggressive frame to provide larger profitability and hold market share as the patent expires. Planning of this will continue to be at the head of the pharmaceutical industry's attempt to tackle a decrease in R&D efficiency, authoritarian compensatory order to and shoot up generic and branded competition.

The key provocation includes pricing pressures, going up development costs, diligent regulatory and atoning policies; decreasing R&D productivity and drug patent cliffs (the immediate fall in sales as the patent gets expires). The important agenda, primarily the productivity gap, push the pharmaceutical companies to reveal to bare generic and biosimilar competition, which can guide to crumbling of a notable percentage of their sales and market share value within a small period of time (Pramod et al., 2016).

The major hurdles in pharmaceutical product lifecycle management can be mentioned as:

1. *Increased Inside and Outside Complication:* While controlling the whole product lifecycle from the product starting point to phase out, most of the pharmaceutical organizations agonize from silos of information across the diverse functional areas leading to different complexities.

2. *Single Data Source for Products and Related Information:* In the case of non-identical authority and deficit of association covering the organization frequently outcome in unlike, unnecessary and unspecific product statistic depending on their practical area.

2.6   RESEARCH AND DEVELOPMENT ENHANCEMENT

The right set of circumstances generally survives in the growing ruthless landscape for evolving pharmaceutical industries who are searching for changing their trade that finally leads to productivity and expansion. Companies who successfully deal with the innovation process to sale with these provocations will notice to enhanced business performance and contrast in the market value.

2.6.1   TRANSFER OF TECHNOLOGY

Till business of the final approved product, Production of a pharmaceutical product is highly demanding and dangerous hence better control must be identified for each lot from scale-up, optimization, and quality assurance. Well-ordered set-up of drug production takes compact across many relevant activities and dependences.

2.6.2   INTEGRATED QUALITY AND RISK MANAGEMENT

Pharmaceutical businesses are influence during regulatory audits quality and risk management, it is found and it continues to be a challenge when problems are filtered out. A supportive deed for quality authority deals with the consolidation and governs of standard starting from the development of the product to trading of that product.

2.6.3   INCLUSIVE PACKAGING

One of the important aspects of trade in worldwide, the packaging is skillfully modulated and this pay notice on the safety of product, probity, and constituents as well as inauspicious event cataloging. For smooth and profitable businesses whole over the world the regulatory and language a necessary condition as well as counterfeit controls by International regulatory bodies direct the pharmaceutical companies to allocate. Whole over the world the business of drugs is highly competitive, to achieve the target a fundamental principle is to apply that manage pricing and maintaining optimum workability. Universal stockroom packaging elements generate for all products, for the convenient purpose of marketing a universal logos and artwork and marketing for that a digital resources uses will get better regulatory integrity.

2.6.4   GLOBAL PRODUCT REGISTRATION

It is a very monotonous; in fixed interval increase in size and creating drug molecule registration authority problem. These causes late in the market introduce and remarkably impact on the anticipate product revenue.

2.6.5   INTELLECTUAL PROPERTY PORTFOLIO

A notable amount of duration under the patent rule of protection for a new drug is typically for the devoured regulatory approval process in a clinical trial. To keep maintain competition in the market, pharmaceutical industries must benefit from the patent-protected period, for this takes a collection of new drugs and drug extensions to market more quickly in a period of time.

2.6.6   MANAGING COMPLEX COLLABORATIVE OUTSOURCING NETWORKS

Pharmaceutical trade presently focuses more strongly on to give opportunity providers to maximize efficiencies, on concentrate interior power and influence the related to all specialization worldwide. Conjoint potentialities gather the grip and adroitness for whole suitable capitals immediately recognize product and process problems and approve changes to interpret the consequences. For better result, the pharmaceutical companies can obscure review and agree to outsource with product development organizations by sharing the portions of products and projects.

2.6.7   CORRECTIVE AND PREVENTIVE ACTION (CAPA) SYSTEM

In worldwide apply to all pharmaceutical industries mandatory to implement additional quality management systems for taking responsibility to deliver a high-quality product. Companies require a unit of section inside the industries to find out standard potential problems, to achieve compliance with CAPA requirements. CAPA procedures online and tightly integrated with interior product information are helpful for cost reduction management. The unnecessary manual documentation are eliminated which reduces the cost to the company and also removes the time taking feedback procedures.

2.6.8   BURDEN OF SYSTEMS VALIDATION

To develop a treaty and validation plan after that the next step is its executing both steps is a time-consuming and costly task. Validate a system over and over again is as much or more than the system itself in respect of time and cost both. Independent third-party, authorize work from granted resistant to finalize a retinue of test plans authorize traders to check and approve an authorization plan, enact the plan of work and deed the outcome so that the decreasing the requirement for costly consulting commitment.

The pharmaceutical companies may adopt to maximize productivity and efficient system operation.

- To extent new drug development, introduction and advertise.
- Allocate R & D resources adequately by improving the ability to remove destitute compounds early and manage new drug.
- Participate efficiently with partners to fasten the innovation, decrease product and process costs and reduce noncompliance risks.
- To allocate effectively the change to products, packaging components, and processes.
- Control of costs and risks across product lines and partners without losing visibility by Outsourcing (Fraser and Kerboul, 2012).

2.7   PRODUCT AND PROCESS LIFECYCLE MANAGEMENT (PPLM)

The basic purpose is to introduce *product and process lifecycle management* (PPLM) is as an alternating type of PLM where the main focus is on the process by which the product is made as to the product itself. The regulatory filing for a new drug application (NDA) is a clue building block that is the step at the back of the manufacture of a compound. The task of the PPLM is to administer the information over the growing of the process in an analogous manner that borderline of PLM discussion about gathering data collection for product development.

A very important parameter of PPLM enactment is *process development execution systems* (PDES). From the initial conception, through the phase of development and into manufacture, they naturally introduce the complete cycle of growth for the manufacturing of high-tech technology developments. The people having different backgrounds like potentially dissimilar legal entities, data, information and knowledge, and business processes and it can be done by merging the people by PDES.

2.7.1   METHODOLOGY

A methodology fundamentally composed of a set of values procedures, techniques belonging to a set of divisions which are basically based on past experiences, goals, and objectives.

In the present scenario, pharmaceutical manufacturing needs a holistic approach based on product and process knowledge that gives companies to preside over data that improves yields, increases confidence and identifies risk to make safer and effective drugs.

Pharmaceutical production high efficient with lower risk, it can be made by the plan of work by PLCM (Figure 2.2). One plan of action supported by PLCM is *quality by design* (QbD) which is a product/process lifecycle that proceeds towards founded on constant growth as mentioned in the FDA.

One of the important proposals given by PLM is QbD, discussed in ICH Q8 Product development quality. ICH Q8 (R2) explains QbD as "a systematic approach to development that starts with earlier defined objectives and spotlight product and process understanding and process control, based on sound science and quality risk management." In this, the product standard is authenticating by understanding and controlling formulation and manufacturing parameters. QbD requires a systematic grip on the relationship of product performance with product credit and process. The fundamental application of QbD in pharmaceutical product development is systematic, joining multivariate experiments deploy *process analytical technology* (PAT) and other may more tests to identify *critical quality*

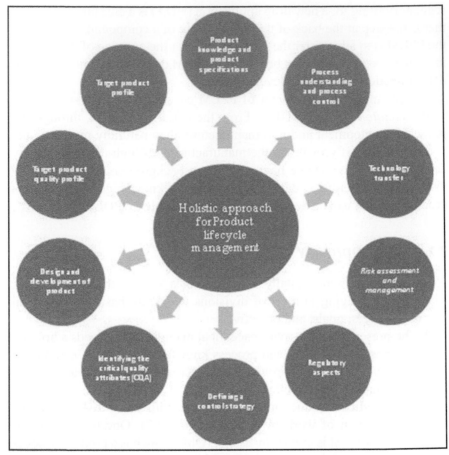

FIGURE 2.2   A holistic approach for product life cycle management.

attributes (CQAs)-based on *risk assessments* (RAs) (Singh et al., 2014, 2015; Beg et al., 2017a,b, 2019). Thus we can say that the QbD starts with predefined objectives and needs to grasp on how formulation and process parameters effect the product quality as depicted in Figure 2.3.

2.7.2 *IMPORTANT STEPS FOR PHARMACEUTICAL QUALITY BY DESIGN IMPLEMENTATION*

1. Describing the desirable presentation of the sample and identifica-tion of the QTPPs.

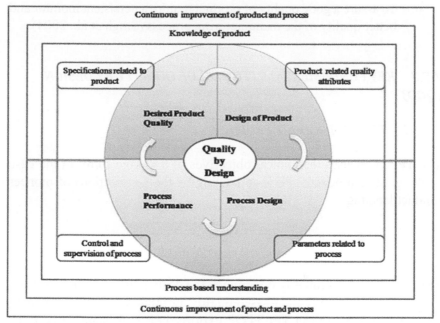

FIGURE 2.3   Schematic diagram showing the overall QbD process.

2. Identification of the CQAs; The important key parameter of product development by QbD are target product profile (TPP), target product quality profile (TPQP), design and development of product, development of the manufacturing process, evaluation and management of the risks connected with the process like, process analytical technology (PAT), design of experiments, identification of the CQA critical material accredit, the establishment of design space, and defining a control plane for a product to stay within the design space. The control plan is fundamentally the knowledge steer from the connection between formulation and manufacturing process parameters that must be controlled in manufacturing a product having accordant quality.

3. Recognition of possible CMAs and CPPs.

4. Framework and implementation of DoE to link CMAs and CPPs to CQAs and get adequate data on how these factors influencing the QTPP. Thereafter, a process outline space should be explained, important to the last product according to QTPP.

5. From the manufacturing process, it must be recognized and control the sources of error of the raw materials.

6.   To assure a good quality of product require a persistent monitor and better quality of the manufacturing process (Singh et al., 2004).

2.7.3   KEY FUNDAMENTALS (TOOLS) OF QUALITY BY DESIGN (QBD)

2.7.3.1   TARGET PRODUCT PROFILE

The TPP condenses the clinical objectives of a dosage form. In the case of the generic product, TPP is appraising by the key portions of pioneer product labeling.

2.7.3.2   TARGET PRODUCT QUALITY PROFILE (TPQP)

This specification primarily determines the design and scope of development. TPQP is the execution-based quality attribute that a product should possess in order to meet TPP.TPQP express TPP into quantitative tests, for example, content uniformity, assay, impurities, dissolution, bioequivalence, stability, etc.

2.7.3.3   DESIGN AND DEVELOPMENT OF PRODUCT

The impartial of the product development schedule using QbD are to fulfill desired patient requirements and to acknowledge attributes that drug product should possess to apply deliberate therapeutic response. The product development must unvarying is systematic, scientific, and risk-based to attain these predefined objectives. A powerful and systematic apprehension of a product and its manufacturing process assists in identifying CQA, which must be controlled to reproducibly produce the desired product.

2.7.4   RISK ASSESSMENTS

In a risk management process, risk assessment can be explained as an orderly step of systematic data to favors take a risk decision. This pharmaceutical industry, identification of threats, the analysis, and estimation of risks added with an exhibit to those hazards. As per guidelines, this step considers as the first mark of quality risk management process; risk review and risk control the other two steps reported. Basically in the risk control step, it includes the decision making to diminish and/or accept risks. The fundamental object of risk control is to reduce the risk to a limit range. The new knowledge and experience, take into account at the final stage. Risk assessments are conveyed through actual use of suitable RA tools like flowcharts, check sheets, process mapping, cause and effect diagrams, etc., are the most commonly used simple methods for RA and management. Finally, there are three components of risk assessment, that is, risk analysis, risk identification, and risk evaluation (Stavros et al., 2017).

2.7.5 PROCESS ANALYTICAL TECHNOLOGY (PAT)

This idea starts from the well of the governor to transfer control of product standard towards a science-based lead that clearly tries to down the risk to patients by scheming the manufacturing based on an understanding of the process. PAT can be defined as "tools and systems that make use of real-time measurements, or rapid measurements during processing, of advance quality and showing credits of in-process materials to impart information to ensure optimal processing to produce final product that again and again conforms to established quality and performance standards." ICH Q8 (Fraser and Kerboul, 2012) identifies the use of PAT to ensure that the process remains within an established design space.

2.7.5.1 PROCESS ANALYTICAL TECHNOLOGY (PAT) STEPS

In the pharmaceutical industry the formulation of the drug is according to PAT three-step-process, designing and optimization both performed mainly by design, analyze and control it also in the manufacturing process. In the first step, the practical is performed to learn what quality allot that are related to the given unit operation and finalize the parameters as well as the raw material quality for the final product. This information gives the knowledge which is used to identify the QTPP, CPP, and CQA, that require to design of an effective PAT based control scheme for the process. In the next step in order to recognize the select standard impute and process framework and the up to date sample characteristic, monitoring of all CQAs and CPPs, require a method computation mechanism orders for real-time (or near real-time), using suitable analytical tools to adopt direct or indirect analytical methods. Lastly, limit plans furnish settlements to defend the control of all critical allot, and build up the grasp of relationships among CQAs, CPPs and QTPPs so as to finalize what activity to take in case the process presentation drift from the most suitable path or product quality from the desired credit.

2.7.5.2   PROCESS ANALYTICAL TECHNOLOGY (PAT) TOOLS

They can be classified into four classes according to the PAT guidance:

1. Process analyzers;
2. Multivariate tools for design, data acquisition, and analysis;
3. Process control tools;
4. Continuous improvement and knowledge management tools.

2.7.5.3   APPLICATION OF PROCESS ANALYTICAL TECHNOLOGY (APAT)

In pharmaceutical industry, the real-time monitoring of the processes is achieved by PAT analytical methods, The instrument used such as *manometric temperature measurement* (MTM), *near infrared spectroscopy* (NIR), *focused beam reflectance measurements* (FBRM), *tunable diode laser absorption spectroscopy* (TDLAS), play important roles in the real-time monitoring of the processes (Stavros et al., 2017).

2.7.5.4   DESIGN OF EXPERIMENTS

The risk assessment should be taken into the function at first, to carry out the design of the experiment. Design of experiments (DOE) is a structured, organized method for determining the relationship between factors affecting a process and the output of that process. It is a valuable tool for choosing experiments efficiently and systematically to give reliable and coherent information. Design of experiments is defined as "a structured, organized method for determining the relationship between factors affecting a process and the output of that process." Design of experiments can be used for comparative experiments, screening experiments, response surface modeling, and regression modeling. It can help identify optimal conditions, CMAs, CPPs, and ultimately, the Design Space (Fraser and Kerboul, 2012; Singh et al., 2013).

2.7.5.5   *CRITICAL QUALITY ATTRIBUTES (CQAS)*

Possible drug product CQAs acquire from the QTPP and/or prior knowledge are used to escort the product and process development and they should be within a suitable limit, range, or distribution to shelter the desired product quality; including physical, chemical, biological, or microbiological properties or characteristics of an output material including finished drug product.

2.7.5.6   *CRITICAL MATERIAL ATTRIBUTES (CMAS)*

CMAs must be within a suitable limit, range, or dispensation to fortify the desired quality of that drug substance, excipient, or in-process material; including chemical-physical, biological, or microbiological properties or characteristics of input material (Bastogne, 2017).

2.8   CONCLUSION

In today's world, the current key challenges within the pharmaceutical industry are to give stress and emphasis on PLM, as it's a trade revolution proceed to deal with products and related information all over the entire company. The problem of the present pharmaceutical trade needs excess well-organized drug development and production. PLM has the chance to make pharmaceutical production more efficacious having lower risk— even in this multifaceted environment. The pharmaceutical companies are glazing at more holistic leads to the development of their processes to bring new products to market that can speed up product development while keeping in mind to lower down the operational costs. Thus we can say that PLM is holistic proceeds to deal with products from early concept through all stages of development and production through to the end of life.

In final wind up of PLM not only gives process management round the whole product lifecycle, but also endorse effective alliance in between networked contributor in product value chain, which differ it from other trade application systems, like enterprise resource planning (ERP), supply chain management (SCM), customer relationship management (CRM), etc.

KEYWORDS

- **corrective and preventive action**
- **critical quality attributes**
- **pharmaceutical life cycle management**
- **process analytical technology**
- **product and process lifecycle management**
- **product life cycle management**
- **product lifecycle model**
- **quality by design**
- **risk assessments**
- **target product quality profile**

REFERENCES

Bastogne, T., (2017). Quality-by-design of nanopharmaceuticals—a state of the art. *Nanomedicine, NBM, 139*(7), 2151–2157.

Beg, S., Rahman, M., Kohli, K., (2019). Quality-by-design approach as a systematic tool for the development of nanopharmaceutical products. *Drug Discovery Today*. 24(3), 717–725.

Beg, S., Akhter, S., Rahman, M., Rahman, Z., (2017a). Perspectives of Quality by Design approach in nanomedicines development. *Current Nanomedicine*, 7, 1–7.

Beg, S., Rahman, M., Panda, S.S., (2017b). Pharmaceutical QbD: Omnipresence in the product development lifecycle. *European Pharmaceutical Review*. 22(1), 2–8.

Dennis, Z. K., (2008). Product lifecycle management: Marketing strategies for the pharmaceutical industry. *J. Med. Marketing.*, 8(4), 293–301.

Fraser, J., & Kerboul, G., (2012). A holistic approach to pharmaceutical manufacturing: Product lifecycle management support for high yield processes to make safe and effective drugs. *Pharmaceutical Eng., 32*(2), 1–5.

He, S. L., et al., (2015). *Model of the Product Development Lifecycle (No. SAND2015–9022)*. Sandia National Lab. (SNL-NM), Albuquerque, NM (United States).

International Conference on Harmonization (ICH), (2009). Guidance for industry: Q8 (R2) pharmaceutical development. *ICH Harmonized Tripartite Guideline, 9*(4).

Ming, X. G., et al., (2008). Collaborative process planning and manufacturing in product lifecycle management. *Computers in Ind., 59*(2&3), 154–166.

Paulo, F., & Santos, L., (2017). Design of experiments for microencapsulation applications: A review. *Materials Sci. and Eng. C, 77,* 1327–1340.

Pramod, K., et al., (2016). Pharmaceutical product development: A quality by design approach. *International J. of Pharma. Investigation, 6*(3), 129–138.

Singh, B., & Beg, S., (2015). Attaining product development excellence and federal compliance employing Quality by Design (QbD) paradigms. *The Pharma Review.* 13(9), 35-44.

Singh, B., & Beg, S., (2014). Product development excellence and federal compliance via QbD. *Chronicle PharmaBiz.* 15(10), 30–35.

Singh, B., Raza, K., Beg, S., (2013). Developing "Optimized" drug products employing "Designed" experiments. *Chemical Industry Digest.* 23, 70–76.

Singh, B., et al., (2004). Optimizing drug delivery systems using systematic "design of experiments." Part I: Fundamental aspects. *Critical Reviews in Therapeutic Drug Carrier Systems, 22*(1), 27–105.

Singh, B., et al., (2005). Optimizing drug delivery systems using systematic "design of experiments." Part II: Retrospect and prospects. *Critical Reviews in Therapeutic Drug Carrier Systems, 22*(3), 215–293.

Singh, B., et al., (2011). Developing oral drug delivery systems using formulation by design: Vital precepts retrospect and prospects. *Expert Opin. Drug Deliv., 8*(10), 1341–1360.

Singh, B., et al., (2017). Systematic development of nano-carriers employing quality by design paradigms. *Nanotechnology-Based Approaches for Targeting and Delivery of Drugs and Genes, Chapter-III,* 111–142.

Stavros, N., et al., (2017). Design of experiments (DoE) in pharmaceutical development. *Drug Development and Industrial Pharmacy, 43*(6), 889–901.

Sudarsan, R. A., et al., (2005). Product information modeling framework for product lifecycle management. *Computer-Aided Design, 37*(13), 1399–1411.

Zhang, L., & Mao, S., (2016). Applications of quality by design (QbD) and its tools in drug delivery. *Asian Journal of Pharmaceutical Sciences II,* 144–145.

Zhang, L., & Mao, S., (2017). Application of quality by design in the current drug development. *Asian Journal of Pharmaceutical Sciences, 12*(1), 1–8.

Recent Advances in the Development of Solid Oral Dosage Forms

MOHAMMED TAHIR ANSARI,[1,4] FARHEEN MOHD SAMI,[1]
MOHAMMAD SAQUIB HASNAIN,[2] SHAHNAZ MAJEED,[1] and
SADAT ALI[3]

[1]*Pharmaceutics Division, Universiti Kuala Lumpur Royal College of Medicine Perak, Ipoh, Malaysia*

[2]*Department of Pharmacy, Shri Venkateshwara University, India*

[3]*Department of Pharmacy, Kanpur Institute of Technology, Kanpur, India*

[4]*School of Pharmacy, University of Nottingham Malaysia, Semenyih, Selangor, Malaysia*

Corresponding author. E-mail: md.a.tahir@gmail.com

3.1 INTRODUCTION

Solid dosage forms are being used since ancient days, tablets and capsules have emerged as the most popular solid oral dosage form. Mostly solid dosage forms are formulated as standard compressed, coated and controlled-release tablets. Recently, the demands in novel therapies for the emerging diseases to show enhanced pharmacological outcomes and increased patient compliance have led to the discovery of innovative technologies in the solid dosage form. Conventional approaches to modify or control the drug release from a solid dosage form include delayed-release through the enteric coating, extended-release or long-acting, microencapsulation and pulsed release solid dosage forms (Ansari et al., 2012; Sant et al., 2011). Alternative or innovative solid dosage formulation technology is expected to significantly improve an existing therapy, minimize the existing adverse effects, optimize the bioavailability, pharmacokinetics and pharmacodynamic properties of the drug, and deliver patient benefits. Further advances in their drug delivery system are by applying nanotechnology in their drug delivery system. Applications of Nanotechnology in drug delivery would further minimize the adverse reaction (Aulton and Taylor, 2017; Helliwell and Taylor, 1993; Mohammed Tahir Ansaria et al., 2018).

Solid dosage forms as oral delivery of drugs are considered by the health industry as one of the most appealing routes of administration. The majority of the recent developments in solid dosage forms have targeted to increase oral bioavailability and drug targeting (Figure 3.1). This has led to the identification and development highly superior solid oral drug delivery system, which has the capacity of delivering consistent delivery of drugs that are not readily absorbed following oral administration (Mrsny, 2012).

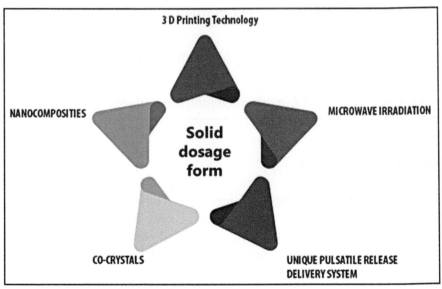

FIGURE 3.1   Advances in solid dosage forms.

It has also been envisaged that excipient-excipient, drug excipient interactions in solid dosage forms may affect the stability of drug formulation. These interactions may lead to major notable organoleptic changes and also retard drug dissolution. Chemical interactions may cause degradation of the active ingredients. Emerging technologies in solid dosage form have also significantly reduced the drug excipient and excipient-excipient interaction thus avoiding stability related issues (Allen, 2014; Lieberman et al., 1989; Narang et al., 2015).

3.1 ADVANCED SOLID DOSAGE FORMULATION TECHNIQUES

3.1.1 ONE STEP DRY COATING (OSDRC®)

One step dry coating (OSDrC®) a patented technique from Sanwa Kagaku Kenkyusho Co. Ltd., Japan. The technique provides dividable, multi-layer, single or multi-core tablets with a practically endless variety of core numbers, shapes, sizes, and placement. The flexible-core capability provides new alternatives in controlled release designs for drug formulators, developers, and marketers in high quality, one-step manufacturing processes. This expands tableting capabilities in many areas that differentiate beyond existing technologies. OSDrC technology employs a double punch action that enables dry coated tablets to be assembled in a single run. OptiMelt® is also a patented technique by Catalent's, the preparation involves hot-melt extrusion with an aim to enhance the solubility of the drug by changing it to a more stable, amorphous solid dispersion. Amorphous solid dispersion is known as an extrudate, which is further processed and changed into a dosage form (Maiti, 2014; Upadhye, 2015).

3.1.2 3-D PRINTED SOLID DOSAGE FORM

Recently, a 3D-printed drug product was approved by the Food and Drug Administration (FDA). 3D printing involves processing drug products using digital designs. Traditionally tablets are manufactured following wet, dry or direct compression techniques. Even though these processes are used for decades but these in this ear it is understood as antique and rigid. 3D printing provides a novel formulation technology that has competitive advantages for complex products, personalized products, and products made on-demand (Figure 3.2). FDA also encourages the manufacturer to adopt technologies such as 3D printing which are advanced and risk-based approaches. It is also a digitally-controlled depositing of materials (layer-by-layer) to create freeform geometries (Goole and Amighi, 2016; Norman et al., 2017).

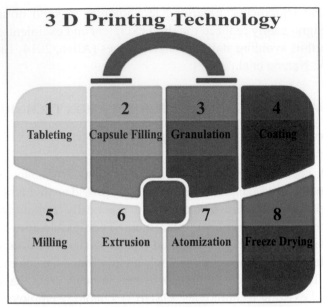

FIGURE 3.2   Application of 3D printing technology.

Guaifenesin was formulated as tablets following 3D printing technique, using Methocel™ K100M, Carbopol (®) 974P NF as a hydrophilic sustained release matrix, Hypromellose (®) was incorporated as a binder, microcrystalline cellulose and sodium starch glycolate were added as disintegratant. Mucinex® was used as standard. The 3D printed tablets exhibited comparable release with commercial guaifenesin tablets. 3D printed tablets also showed that weight variation, friability, hardness, and thickness were within the acceptable range as defined by the international standards stated in the United States Pharmacopoeia (USP). The hydrophilic matrix showed Korsmeyer-Peppas n values between 0.27 and 0.44 indicating Fickian diffusion drug release. (Khaled et al., 2014).

Paracetamol issue of high drug loading was also addressed by the 3D printing technique. The 3D printed tablets exhibited good physical and mechanical properties such as friability, weight variation, breaking force. Disintegration time was measured within the prescribed pharmacopeial limit. PCM tablets were further characterized to confirm the immunity of the pure compound. X-ray powder diffraction (XRPD), attenuated total reflectance Fourier transform infrared spectroscopy (ATR-FTIR), and differential scanning calorimetry (DSC) confirmed the purity of the compound and feasibility of the 3D printed technique. The 3D printed tablets showed a profile characteristic of the immediate release profile releasing most of the drugs in 5 minutes as was desired following the active/excipient ratio used. The study demonstrated that 3D printed tablets can produce tablets with high-dose from approved materials that comply with current USP standards (Khaled et al., 2018).

Wang et al, formulated a device which was loaded with can be loaded with multiple actives ingredients, The design was configured to include a multilayer device, with each layer containing drug, he used PCM and caffeine to form a two-compartment drug-device called as DuoCaplet, The release was tested and it was observed that the device was capable of releasing PCM and Caffeine simultaneously without hindering the solubility or distribution of each. With the innovative DuoCaplet design, it was possible to contrive either rapid drug release or delayed release by selecting the site of incorporation of the drug in the device which would not otherwise be possible using conventional manufacturing methods (Goyanes et al., 2015d). Recently rapid prototype 3D printing technologies such as stereolithographic, powder-based, selective laser sintering, fused deposition modeling, and semi-solid extrusion 3D printing have provided more innovative technology to maneuver the drug release depending on the requirement of the patient (Alhnan et al., 2016).

Stereolithography (SLA) was also used to fabricate modified-release drug formulation for of 4-aminosalicylic acid (4-ASA) and paracetamol (acetaminophen). Polyethylene glycol diacrylate (PEGDA) was used as a monomer and diphenyl (2,4,6-trimethyl benzoyl)phosphine oxide as a photo polymerize monomers. Polyethylene glycol 300 (PEG 300) was added to the printing solution during the process of tablet manufacturing. SLA 3D Printing technology allowed the manufacture of 4A-SA and PCM loaded tablets with specific extended-release profiles (Wang et al., 2016).

Industrial manufacturing of plastic, metallic and ceramic objects utilizes selective laser sintering (SLS) 3-dimensional printing. Fina et al. (2017) used the same to fabricate three different concentration paracetamol (acetaminophen) (5, 20 and 35%) loaded products. They used Kollicoat IR (75% polyvinyl alcohol and 25% polyethylene glycol copolymer) and Eudragit L100-55 (50% methacrylic acid and 50% ethyl acrylate copolymer), with immediate and modified release characteristics respectively. The research concluded that SLS is versatile and a practical 3D printing technology, which can be applied to the pharmaceutical field, for the manufacture of modern medicines.

3D printing (3DP) technology using hot-melt extrusion (HME) and fluid bed coating was used to fabricate modified-release budesonide dosage forms. 9 mg budesonide using a FDM was formulated as capsule-shaped tablets (caplets) and then the caplets were over-coated with an enteric polymer. Commercial Budesonide releases Cortiment® product was delayed and very slow while another commercial Entocort® formulation was rapid in the upper small intestine. The new 3D formulated caplets of budesonide-exhibited release in the mid-small intestine but release continued in a sustained manner throughout the distal intestine and colon. This work has enumerated the advantages of 3D printing techniques over the conventional system. The hot-melt extrusion process used in the designing of 3D printed caplets of budesonide may also improve the powder properties, which may contribute equally in the controlled and extended-release of medicaments (Andrews, 2007; Goyanes et al., 2015b).

FDM based 3D printing was proved as a prudent method to produce and control the dose of extended-release tablets of Prednisolone. The method allowed Skowyra et al to produce digitally controlled patient-tailored medicines. Fused deposition modeling (FDM) based 3D printer was used to design extended-release prednisolone loaded poly (vinyl alcohol) (PVA) filaments tablet. It was evident the designed tablets can extend the *in vitro* drug release up to 24 h. Thermal analysis and XRPD indicated that the majority of prednisolone existed in the amorphous form within the tablets (Skowyra et al., 2015).

Shaban expressed his technique by designing a 3D printing assisted multi-active solid dosage form called polypill. His device represented a cardiovascular treatment regime incorporating an immediate release compartment with aspirin and hydrochlorothiazide and three sustained-release compartments containing pravastatin, atenolol, and Ramipril. The printed polypills showed the intended drug release following the ration of active/excipient ratio used (Khaled et al., 2015).

3D printing also allows tablets of varying geometry. PCM tablets were designed in five different tablet geometries *viz-a-viz* cube, pyramid, cylinder, sphere, and torus. It was confirmed that the technique does not affect the stability of the drug. No difference in the drug release was observed depicting that the shape of the tablets does not influence the drug release (Goyanes et al., 2015c).

Goyanes et al. (2015a) demonstrated FDM 3DP as an efficient and low-cost alternative method of manufacturing individually tailored oral drug dosage, and also for the production of modified-release formulations. The study included two aminosalicylate isomers used in the treatment of inflammatory bowel disease (IBD). The tablets were physically and mechanically strong, and it resulted convinced that FDM 3D printing can be used as an effective process for the manufacture of the drug (Goyanes et al., 2015a).

A miniature, compact, portable, reconfigurable, and automated tablet manufacturing system to manufacture on-demand tablets from drug crystals on a scale of hundreds to thousands per day was designed. This will not only reduce the financial challenges but also the causes of supply chain disruptions (Azad et al., 2018).

3D printing technology has comprehensively allowed to release the formulation of multi-layered disease-based flexible-dose combination. Flexible dose combinations of two anti-hypertensive drugs Enalapril maleate (EM) and hydrochlorothiazide (HCT) in a single bilayer tablet with a range of doses were fabricated using dual fused deposition modeling (FDM) 3D printer. X-ray diffractometer (XRD) and Thermal analysis indicated that the HCT persisted in its crystalline shape whilst EM appeared to be in an amorphous form. The tablet sets provided immediate drug release profiles across all dose combinations. This dynamic dosing system maintained the advantages of FDCs while providing superior flexibility of dosing range, hence offering an optimal clinical solution to hypertension therapy in a patient-centric healthcare service (Sadia et al., 2018).

3.1.3 MICROWAVE IRRADIATED SOLID DOSAGE FORMS

Microwave irradiation cross-linked beads for sulfathiazole were investigated drug dissolution, drug content, drug stability, drug polymorphism, drug–polymer interaction, polymer cross-linkage, and complexation. The beads showed some polymorphic changes without affecting the drug release properties, the influence of microwave irradiation on the drug release properties of alginate which was used as release modifier, alginate–chitosan and chitosan beads was investigated. The release-retarding property of alginate and alginate–chitosan beads was significantly enhanced by subjecting the beads to microwave irradiation. This novel method certainly eludes the use of noxious chemicals and hence reducing the toxicity of dosage form (Wong et al., 2002).

Microwave irradiation may also use to vary the swelling index of polymers used for formulating orally disintegrating tablets (ODTs). Watervapor inside the tablets the wet molded tablets mannitol and silicon dioxide were generated by microwave irradiation. Microwave irradiated tablets showed considerable swelling of a tablet with a high ratio of silicon dioxide and low levels of water volume. The disintegration time was clearly shortened by induction of the swelling, while tablet hardness increased. Thus, it was concluded that this one-step method using microwave irradiation would be a useful method for preparing the ODTs (Sano et al., 2011).

3.2 FIXED-DOSE COMBINATION TABLETS

Nebivolol/valsartan fixed-dose combination exhibited good therapeutic when continued for 52 weeks. The novel dose combination exhibited a significant lowering of blood pressure (BP) than the monotherapy. It was further subsumed that the combination decreased plasma renin and aldosterone levels (Battise et al., 2018).

Hyperuricemia in patients with uncontrolled gout was a recently once-daily combination of lesinurad and allopurinol. It was suggested clinically that the target serum uric acid (SUA) levels in patients which were not achieved by allopurinol alone. The FDC has also approved the combination (Barrett, 2017).

3.3 UNIQUE PULSATILE RELEASE

Pulsatile drug delivery provides spatial that is time-specific drug delivery and temporal that is site-specific drug delivery system. The system is unique as it involves a rapid and transient release of a certain amount of molecules immediately after the lag time period, and also these systems have the ability to deliver the drug rapidly and completely after a lag time period. Pulsatile delivery system is achieved via hydrogel technique, microchip technique or also through implant system. Hydrogels beads can be a good source for solid oral dosage form delivery (Jain et al., 2011; Kikuchi and Okano, 2002; Prescott et al., 2006; Santini et al., 2000).

Time-controlled pulsatile release (PR) formulation to facilitate the management of early morning chronological attacks can be achieved by using a direct compressed prednisone tablet coated in ethylcellulose (EC)-hydroxypropyl methylcellulose (HPMC) excipient blend. The tablet exhibited a lag time of 4-6 hrs by burst release profile under variegated dissolution conditions. The outcome was achieved as desired using the pulsatile system (Patadia et al., 2017).

Decrease in the lag time was observed from HPMC press-coated EC tablets of prednisone. Delay in the lag time was pronounced by the molecule weight of HPMC. It was evident that low MW HPMC was more effective than the high MW of HPMC (Patadia et al., 2016).

Patented technique pulsincap was used to design 5-fluorouracil osmogene filled capsules. The successful circadian rhythm was exhibited to target the drug to colorectal carcinoma according to daily oscillations of rate-limiting metabolizing enzyme dihydropyrimidine dehydrogenase (Patel et al., 2011). Novel diffucaps technology was applied to characterize the pharmacokinetic profiles of oral extended-release methylphenidate products (Yang et al., 2016).

A divisible pharmaceutical tablet comprises two portions: the upper and the lower portion. The upper portion has an upper convex surface bordering at least one dividing notch. Such tablets are characterized by dispensing a pharmaceutical composition to the patients in a measured, predetermined dose (Parikh et al., 2011).

Ketoprofen and ibuprofen pellets fabricated using eudragit and ethyl cellulose demonstrated a chronotherapeutics pattern of drug release extended for 22 h depending on the concentration of ethyl cellulose (Dumpa et al., 2018).

Researchers have successfully demonstrated the pharmaceutical use of cassava starch nanocrystals. The cassava starch nanocrystal could lower the mechanical properties of the ethylcellulose film, and also decreases lag time-sensitivity of the ruptured coating, which provides an excellent pulsatile release system (Charoenthai et al., 2018).

An innovative dual delivery system based on a tablet-in-tablet providing a two-pulse release of rivastigmine with a time difference of 6.5 h between the peaks of the pulses (Penhasi and Gomberg, 2018).

3.4 SOLID SELF EMULSIFYING DRUG DELIVERY SYSTEM

Approximately 40% of new drugs, exhibit poor aqueous solubility and low bioavailability. A novel technique, self-emulsifying drug delivery systems (SEDDS) intended to increase solubility and oral bioavailability of drugs having poor biopharmaceutical properties (Gurudutta et al., 2010).

Conventional SEDDS, however, are mostly prepared in a liquid form, which can produce some disadvantages. Appropriate excipients, solid carriers, and processing parameters must be selected for each solidification technique to enable process-ability and preserve the self-emulsifying ability of the system upon its transformation into the solid formulation (Mandić et al., 2017; Tang et al., 2008).

The solid SEDDS of dexibuprofen powder gave significantly higher AUC and C_{max} than dexibuprofen powder ($P < 0.05$). The results showed that AUC of solid SEDDS was about twofold higher than that of dexibuprofen powder (Balakrishnan et al., 2009).

Liquid lipid-based self-emulsifying drug delivery systems (SEDDS) can be converted into solid dosage forms by adsorbing onto silicates. Probucol was dissolved in liquid SEDDS containing different lipid to surfactant ratios, and the formulations were then adsorbed onto equal weights of silica. The formulation showed the desired release even after 6 months of storage period confirming the viability of SEDDS to be used as a solid dosage form for probucol (Gumaste and Serajuddin, 2017).

Griseofulvin-SEDDS addition to silica was formulated by Agarwal et al. They deduced that special attention should be given to particle size, specific surface area, type and amount of adsorbent since it will affect the drug release characteristics of the active ingredient (Agarwal et al., 2009).

Poorly soluble nitrendipine (NTD) was formulated as the new solid self-emulsifying (SE) spheronized pellets. The SE pellets with 30% liquid SEDDS exhibited uniform size, the oral bioavailability of new SE pellets showed a 1.6-fold increase than the conventional tablets (Wang et al., 2010).

Celastrol, a chemical compound isolated from the root extracts of *Tripterygium wilfordii* which is known to have anti-inflammatory and anti-cancer properties. Oral bioavailability of celastrol is calculated as very low. SEDDS may be a suitable technique to increase the oral bioavailability of celastrol. The optimized formulation of celastrol-SMEDDS dispersible tablets could disperse in the dispersion medium within 3 min with the average particle size of 25.32 ± 3.26 nm. *In vivo* pharmacokinetic experiments on rats, suggest the potential use of SEDDS dispersible tablets for the oral delivery of poorly water-soluble terpenes drugs, such as celastrol (Qi et al., 2014; Zhang et al., 2012).

Studies suggest that adsorption technique, spray-drying process, high-shear granulation, fluid-bed granulation can be used for preparing solid SEDDS powders by using solid carriers. Naproxen SEDDS using different solidification techniques and carriers had considerable influence on the dissolution profile and solubility enhancement of naproxen. It is advised to use appropriate solidification and compression technique to formulate SEDDS tablets (Čerpnjak et al., 2015).

Ibuprofen SEDDS pellets containing Neusilin derivatives were formulated by a fluid bed coating process. Dissolution studies showed that from the formulation composed of 70 wt.% of Neusilin SG2 after 45 min, more than 75% of ibuprofen was dissolved in water and after 30 min, more than 80% of ibuprofen was dissolved in the phosphate buffer (Krupa et al., 2014). Similar trials were done for risperidone, using NSU2. The characterization results showed that NUS2 yield superior flowability of the powder. The SEM revealed that pure risperidone was in irregular crystal shape whereas the drug-loaded solid SEDDS were in smooth regular shape. From the dissolution studies, it was found that solid SEDDS provided significant release profiles (>95%) compared to marketed product risperdal® (Kazi et al., 2017). Dissolution and bioavailability of flurbiprofen were also improved by a solid self-nanoemulsifying drug delivery system (solid SNEDDS) (Kang et al., 2012). Glipizide dissolution improved significantly ($p < 0.001$) from the solid SNEDDS (~100% in 15 min) as compared to the pure drug (18.37%) and commercial product (65.82%) respectively (Dash et al., 2015).

3.5 COCRYSTALS

The pharmaceutical solvates, polymorphs, hydrates, amorphous forms are presented as a one-component system. The two-component system to host drug molecules is called co-crystals (Figure 3.3). These solid forms play a vital role in drug discovery and development in the context of optimization of bioavailability, filing intellectual property rights (Healy et al., 2017; Pankaj Sharma, 2011). The pharmaceutical co-crystals bonded by hydrogen binding helps to optimize physiochemical, pharmaceutical and biological properties of drug molecules (Douroumis et al., 2017; Pindelska et al., 2017; Malamatari et al., 2017). Deep idea of pharmaceutical multicomponent phase design, the intermolecular interactions are desired to formulate co-crystals. These newer systems have the tendency to vary material properties and pharmacokinetics in a patient (Berry and Steed, 2017).

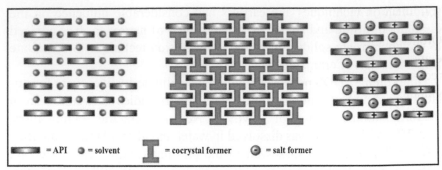

FIGURE 3.3 Schematic diagram of co-crystals (Reprinted with permission from Korotkova and Kratochvíl, 2014. © Elsevier.)

The design of co-crystals was carried out by a CC analysis program, *p*-DISOL-X. Various acid-base combinations of active pharmaceutical ingredients (APIs) and co-formers: (i) carbamazepine cocrystal systems with 4-aminobenzoic acid, cinnamic acid, saccharin, and salicylic acid, (ii) for indomethacin with saccharin, (iii) for nevirapine with maleic acid, saccharin, and salicylic acid, and (iv) for gabapentin with 3-hydroxyben-zoic acid were designed using the system. The carbamazepine-cinnamic acid CC showed a substantial elevation in the API equilibrium concentration above pH 5, consistent with the formation of a complex between carbamazepine and cinnamate anion. The analysis of the gabapentin: 3-hydroxybenzoic acid 1:1 CC system indicated four zones of solid suspensions: coformer (pH < 3.25) and cocrystal eutectic (pH 3.25–4.44), cocrystal (pH 4.44–5.62), and API (pH > 5.62). The general approach allows for testing of many possible equilibrium models, including those comprising drug-coformer complexation (Avdeef, 2017).

Lamotriginenovel cocrystals were designed using 4,4′-bipyridine (2:1) and 2,2′-bipyridine as coformers. Cocrystal was successfully character-ized by X-ray diffraction, thermal and spectroscopic analysis, Raman microscopy, the *in vitro* dissolution rate and the solubility of the two novel cocrystals were significantly improved (Du et al., 2017).

4-aminosalicylic acid (PASA) was crystallized with a number of coformers [pyrazinamide (PYR), nicotinamide (NAM), isonicotinamide (iNAM), isoniazid (INH), caffeine (CAF), and theophylline (TPH)]. The new co-crystallized have exhibited improved solubility and higher stability against the chemical decomposition (Drozd et al., 2017).

3.6 INNOVATIVE ORODISPERSIBLE DOSAGE FORMS

Orodispersible dosage forms based on polymeric matrices have currently demonstrated their prominence in accordance with the actual market requirements and patients' demands. Oral lyophilisates and orodispersible granules, tablets or films have enriched the therapeutic options (Borges et al., 2015); Slavkova and Breitkreutz, 2015; Tahir et al., 2010).

Innovative Flexible oral dispersible system, orally swallowable, orally disintegrating, chewable tablets have certainly increased patient compliance. Pediatric and geriatric patients are preferring novel sprinkle formulations such as pellets, granules packed in capsules or sachets are conveniently used by (Chandrasekaran and Kandasamy, 2018).

Cetirizine, polacrilex ratio of 1:2 to 1:3 showed strong physical strength and an intensely rapid *in vitro* dispersion within 30 s in 2-6 ml of water. Polacrilex resin with taste-masking effect and improved stability exhibited immediate drug release within 30 min in gastric media. This is a novel process of formulating ion exchange resins based on solid oral flexible drug products (Chandrasekaran and Kandasamy, 2017).

Pre-formed resinate of cetirizine HCl cyclodextrin complexes was incorporated into the Zydis® oral lyophilisate technology. It was evident that taste was effectively masked for the designed formulation (Preis et al., 2015).

3.7 GASTRORETENTIVE DRUG DELIVERY SYSTEM

The main aim of the controlled release oral solid dosage forms is to facilitate sustained and continuous, delivery of an active pharmaceutical agent to the upper gastrointestinal tract of a patient. Gastro retentive system confers to the need for such desires of delivering agents on an extended-release basis, to the stomach, duodenum and upper regions of the small intestine, with drug delivery in the lower gastrointestinal tract and colon substantially restricted.

Pregabalin gastroretentive tablets can be formulated as floating once-daily administration. The concentration hydroxypropyl methylcellulose and crospovidone were found to be affecting the drug release and floating properties of the formulated tablets. All the designed formulation showed sustained release and floating ability for over 24 h (Kim et al., 2018).

Hwang et al. (2017) formulated a highly porous floating tablet of cilostazol. The floating properties were realized by compressing granules and excipients with a sublimating agent, followed by sublimation under vacuum. Resultant tablets showed excellent floating tendency and also exhibited higher tensile strengths than conventional tablets of similar porosities. This property certainly qualifies the drug to be classified as a gastroretentive tablet.

Floating gastroretentive tablets of metformin using a camphor as sublimation material and poly ethylene oxide (PEO). Prepared floating gastro retentive tablets floated for over 24 h and had no floating lag time. The pharmacokinetic studies confirmed that the mean plasma concentration of the GR tablets was greater than the concentration of Glucophage XR (Oh et al., 2013).

The short half-life of Gabapentin (GBP), an antiepileptic and anti-neuropathic agent, can be countered by formulating raft-forming systems using gellan gum and pectin. The oral bioavailability of GBP was measured in terms of C_{max}, $AUC_{(0-t)}$, and $AUC_{(0-\infty)}$ and was found to be 1.7 times better than commercially available Neurontin® (Abouelatta et al., 2018).

Bimodal release of Piroxicam hollow/multipolymeric system alginate-based floating gastro-retentive gel-beads was formulated to overcome fluctuations in plasma levels, with sustained release properties It was concluded that *in vivo* anti-inflammatory activity of the floating beads resulted prolonged up to 48 h, compared to standard piroxicam (Auriemma et al., 2018).

Mitiglinide calcium (MTG) microsponge was formulated using Quasi-emulsion solvent diffusion method, employing Eudragit RS100, ethylcellulose, and polyvinyl alcohol. It was shown that the microsponge was highly porous with interconnected pores and good compatibility as confirmed by SEM, DSC, and FTIR analysis. Pharmacokinetic studies showed improvement in C_{max} and $AUC_{0-\infty}$ (1.92- and 20.68-fold, respectively) with marked prolongation in MRT and $t_{1/2}$ (7.22- and 7.97-fold, respectively) than the marketed tablet (Mahmoud et al., 2018).

Long-acting antiretroviral (dolutegravir, rilpivirine, and cabotegravir) enteral system was possible by forming a polymer matrix possible of intervening prophylactically, which could avert hundreds of thousands of new HIV cases (Kirtane et al., 2018).

Antitumor activity of *Brucea javanica* oil (BJO) was highest in the gastroretentive floating bead as showed *in vivo* study (Zhang et al., 2018c).

3.8 NANOCOMPOSITES ORAL DRUG DELIVERY SYSTEM

Hydroxyapatite (HAP) and HAP-based composite nanostructures have shown their effectiveness as a drug carrier agent for different diseases such as bone-related disorders, carriers for antibiotics, anti-inflammatory, carcinogenic drugs, medical imaging, and protein delivery agents (Figure 3.4). The concept should suitably be used for future drug delivery applications (Ahmad et al., 2018; Mondal et al., 2018).

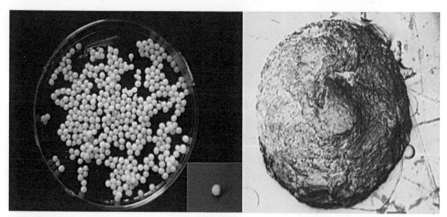

FIGURE 3.4 Alginate based hydroxyapatite nanocomposites for sustained release formulation. (Reprinted with permission from Hasnain et al., 2016. © Elsevier.)

Gold nanorods/mesoporous silica/hydroxyapatite (Au/SiO$_2$/HAP) hybrid nanoparticles exhibiting excellent drug loading capacity can be extended for multi-responsive drug delivery. The hybrid nanoparticles also showed pH-responsive release which may found its application in drug targeting (Majeed et al., 2016a; Majeed et al., 2016b; Song et al., 2018).

Sustained-release Rifampicin (RIF), an anti-tuberculosis drug, were synthesized into a poly (o-anisidine-co-o-toluidine) (PAnis-co-POT) intercalated bentonite nanocomposites. The nanocomposites were found to show zero-order release behavior and hold the potential to be used as an effective anti-tuberculosis drug delivery vehicle (Verma and Riaz, 2018).

Macroporous hydroxyapatite/chitosan foam (HA/CS)-supported polymer micelle (PM/HA/CS) for Candesartan cilexetil (CC) increased the bioavailability of the drug to 1.9 folds (Zhang et al., 2018a).

Insulinconjugated with nano-HAP and PEG showed significantly the *in vivo* absorption of nanoparticles in rat small intestines and lower degradation when administered orally. Overall, HAP may provide a safe, non-toxic, platform for an effective oral insulin delivery system (Zhang et al., 2018b).

Naproxen (NPX)-Cu-cross-linked carboxymethylcellulose/graphene quantum dot nanocomposite hydrogel beads with reduced toxicity and increased effectiveness potentially could be used as an oral drug delivery system (Javanbakht et al., 2018).

Due to biocompatibility of HAP and similarity to biologically formed hydroxyapatite in natural tooth enamel, synthetic hydroxyapatite is a promising biomimetic oral care ingredient that may extend the scope of preventive dentistry (Enax and Epple, 2018).

Recently several active targeting strategies have been designed to target tumors and other diseases. Many methodologies such as liposomes, polymers, micelles, nanoparticles, and antibodies, through passive or active drug targeting to cancer cells, have been reported (Lammers et al., 2012; Mahon et al., 2012). Doxorubicin hydrochloride (DOX) a multifunctional nanoplatform was used for dual-targeted chemo-photothermal therapy (Zhou et al., 2017).

3.9 POLY ELECTROLYTE COMPLEXES AS SOLID DOSAGE FORM

Polyelectrolytes are polymers that have many ionizable functional groups. It has the capacity to form ionized polyelectrolytes in the solution that can form a complex with oppositely charged polyelectrolytes. The role of chitosan has been widely accepted in the formation of polyelectrolyte complexes (PEC) is a good avenue to provide a sustained and controlled release system (Mateescu et al., 2015; Meka et al., 2017).

Oval-shape polyelectrolyte complexes for bovine serum albumin (BSA) were formulated using carboxymethyl starch (CMS), and CS. The PEC BSA exhibited a pH-dependent zero-order controlled release minimizing the undesirable issues such as burst effect and non-sustained release. This also envois a system to control the drug release in specific regions of the gastrointestinal tract (Quadrado and Fajardo, 2018).

Ciprofloxacin-based swellable drug polyelectrolyte matrix (SDPM-CIP) was formulated tablets by the wet granulation method. Human study exhibited urinary excretion of a single oral dose of 500 mg of ciprofloxacin for 36 hrs, the tablet also possesses all other pharmacopeial parameters (Guzmán et al., 2018).

Interpolyelectrolyte complexes (IPEC) using different poly-methacrylate carriers loaded with benznidazole (BZ) were formulated as multiparticulate drug delivery systems (MDDS) with an aim to enhance drug performance. Preclinical studies in a murine model of acute chagas disease of BZ-loaded MDDS exhibited efficacy to reduce parasitemia, while decreasing the levels of liver injury markers in comparison to BZ conventional treatment (García et al., 2018).

Compact polyelectrolyte complexes (CoPECs) of β-cyclodextrin complexed Piroxicam represent a new class of materials, which was able to LPS-induced TNF-α and NO release and moderated the differentiation of LPS-activated macrophages. The success of this system may expand the use of Piroxicam in anti-inflammatory diseases (Hardy et al., 2018).

3.10 NOVEL SOLID DISPERSIONS AND MODIFIED INCLUSION COMPLEXES

The use of newer technologies spray coating on sugar beads with a fluidized bed coating system, hot-melt extrusion, direct capsule filling, electrostatic spinning, surface-active carriers, and supercritical fluid technology in the formulation of solid dispersion have attracted major interest among researchers (Karanth et al., 2006). Electrospun nanofibers composed solid dispersions of has great potential for developing new kinds of functional nanomaterials (Liu et al., 2019).

Complexation efficiency has attracted major interest in reducing the bulk of dosage form (Ansari et al., 2017a, b). The higher affinity of EPI-βCD than βCD for the interaction with TR even in the solid-state, resulting in the formation of completely amorphous products with superior dissolution properties. The addition of hydrophilic polymers failed to effectively promote solid-state interactions between TR and βCD, while their positive influence on drug solubility, observed in phase-solubility studies, was absent in solid TR/βCD/polymer products. Finally, the time-kill analysis, used to evaluate the TR antimicrobial activity against *Streptococcus mutans*, demonstrated the significantly ($p < 0.001$) superior performance of both cyclodextrin complexes than drug alone, and confirmed the higher effectiveness ($p < 0.05$) of TR/EPI-βCD than TR/βCD complex (Jug et al., 2011).

Stable ternary inclusion complex ETD-HP-β-CD-L-Arg was formed, the study led to the conclusion that the ternary complex of ETD-HP-β-CD-L-Arg could be an innovative approach to augment the solubility and dissolution behavior of ETD (Sherje et al., 2017).

The water solubility of neodiosmin was greatly enhanced by forming a neodiosmin/β-cyclodextrin/lysine ternary inclusion complex. The neodiosmin/β-cyclodextrin/lysine ternary inclusion complex showed the highest efficacy, and the bitterness attenuation was statistically significant (Dong et al., 2017).

The complexation efficiency of the ternary bosentan-Arginine-HPβCD system was found to be higher than binary, justifying the addition of ARG as an auxiliary substance to reduce the workable amount of HPβCD during formulation (Jadhav and Pore, 2017).

The effect of different grades of povidone (s) (viz. PVP K-29/32, PVP K-40, plasdone S-630, and polyplasdone XL), organic base (viz. triethanolamine), and metal ion (viz. $MgCl_2 \cdot 6H_2O$) were studies on the complexation efficiency of Gemfibrozil - β-CD inclusion complexes. The study suggested the formation of new solid phases, eliciting strong evidences of ternary inclusion complex formation between GFZ, β-CD, and plasdone S-630, particularly for lyophilized products (Sami et al., 2010). The effect of polymers and amino acids has also been investigated in enhancing the solubility of aceclofenac (Ansari et al., 2017a, b).

3.11 CONCLUSION

A solid dosage form has been one of the most accepted dosage forms. Further innovation like 3D printing, nanocomposites, and polyelectrolyte complexes will increase its efficacy and certainly will reduce the dependence on parenteral. The usage of innovative technology has not been introduced commercially but these newer and advanced technologies have got the potential to enhance the efficacy of the drugs dispensed as traditional tablets and capsules.

KEYWORDS

- advanced solid dosage formulation technique
- cocrystals
- fixed-dose combination tablets
- gastroretentive drug delivery system
- innovative orodispersible dosage forms
- microwave irradiated solid dosage forms
- nanocomposites oral drug delivery system
- polyelectrolyte complexes
- solid oral dosage

REFERENCES

Abouelatta, S. M., Aboelwafa, A. A., & El-Gazayerly, O. N., (2018). Gastro retentive raft liquid delivery system as a new approach to release extension for carrier-mediated drug. *Drug Delivery, 25* (1), 1161–1174.

Agarwal, V., Siddiqui, A., Ali, H., & Nazzal, S., (2009). Dissolution and powder flow characterization of solid self-emulsified drug delivery system (SEDDS). *International Journal of Pharmaceutics, 366* (1), 44–52.

Ahmad, R., Deng, Y., Singh, R., Hussain, M., Shah, M. A. A., Elingarami, S., He, N., & Sun, Y., (2018). Cutting edge protein and carbohydrate-based materials for anticancer drug delivery. *Journal of Biomedical Nanotechnology, 14* (1), 20–43.

Alhnan, M. A., Okwuosa, T. C., Sadia, M., Wan, K. W., Ahmed, W., & Arafat, B., (2016). Emergence of 3D printed dosage forms: Opportunities and challenges. *Pharmaceutical Research, 33*(8), 1817–1832.

Allen, L., (2014). *Ansel's Pharmaceutical Dosage Forms and Drug Delivery Systems.* Wolters Kluwer Health.

Andrews, G. P., (2007). Advances in solid dosage form manufacturing technology. *Philosophical Transactions of the Royal Society A: Mathematical, Physical and Engineering Sciences, 365* (1861), 2935–2949.

Ansari, M. T., Risheshwar, P., & Ali, S., (2017a). Effect of hydroxy acids and organic bases on complexation efficiency of Aceclofenac Beta Cyclodextrin inclusion complex. *European Journal of Biomedical and Pharmaceutical Sciences, 4* (5), 586–589.

Ansari, M. T., Risheshwar, P., & Ali, S., (2017b). Effects of polymers on complexation efficiency of aceclofenac-beta cyclodextrin inclusion complex. *Int. J. Pharm. Bio. Sci., 8* (4).

Ansari, T., Farheen, M., Hoda, M. N., & Nayak, A. K., (2012). Microencapsulation of pharmaceuticals by solvent evaporation technique: A review. *Elixir Pharmacy, 47,* 8821–8827.

Aulton, M. E., & Taylor, K. M. G., (2017). *Aulton's Pharmaceutics E-Book: The Design and Manufacture of Medicines*. Elsevier Health Sciences.

Auriemma, G., Cerciello, A., Sansone, F., Pinto, A., Morello, S., & Aquino, R. P., (2018). Polysaccharides based gastroretentive system to sustain piroxicam release: Development and *in vivo* prolonged anti-inflammatory effect. *International Journal of Biological Macromolecules, 120,* 2303–2312.

Avdeef, A., (2017). Cocrystal solubility product analysis – Dual concentration-pH mass action model not dependent on explicit solubility equations. *European Journal of Pharmaceutical Sciences, 110,* 2–18.

Azad, M. A., Osorio, J. G., Brancazio, D., Hammersmith, G., Klee, D. M., Rapp, K., & Myerson, A., (2018). A compact, portable, re-configurable, and automated system for on-demand pharmaceutical tablet manufacturing. *International Journal of Pharmaceutics, 539* (1), 157–164.

Balakrishnan, P., Lee, B. J., Oh, D. H., Kim, J. O., Hong, M. J., Jee, J. P., Kim, J. A., Yoo, B. K., Woo, J. S., Yong, C. S., & Choi, H. G., (2009). Enhanced oral bioavailability of dexibuprofen by a novel solid Self-emulsifying drug delivery system (SEDDS). *European Journal of Pharmaceutics and Biopharmaceutics, 72* (3), 539–545.

Barrett, J., (2017). FDA approves novel fixed-dose combo treatment for gout. *Pharmacy Times.*

Battise, D., Boland, C. L., & Nuzum, D. S., (2018). Nebivolol/Valsartan: A novel antihypertensive fixed-dose combination tablet. *The Annals of Pharmacotherapy,* 1060028018813575.

Berry, D. J., & Steed, J. W., (2017). Pharmaceutical cocrystals, salts and multicomponent systems, intermolecular interactions and property based design. *Advanced Drug Delivery Reviews, 117,* 3–24.

Borges, A. F., Silva, C., Coelho, J. F. J., & Simões, S., (2015). Oral films: Current status and future perspectives: I—Galenical development and quality attributes. *Journal of Controlled Release, 206,* 1–19.

Čerpnjak, K., Pobirk, A. Z., Vrečer, F., & Gašperlin, M., (2015). Tablets and minitablets prepared from spray-dried SMEDDS containing naproxen. *International Journal of Pharmaceutics, 495* (1), 336–346.

Chandrasekaran, P., & Kandasamy, R., (2017). Development of oral flexible tablet (OFT) formulation for pediatric and geriatric patients: A novel age-appropriate formulation platform. *AAPS Pharm. Sci. Tech., 18* (6), 1972–1986.

Chandrasekaran, P., & Kandasamy, R., (2018). Solid oral flexible formulations for pediatric and geriatric patients: Age-appropriate formulation platforms. *Indian J. Pharm. Sci., 80* (1), 14–25.

Charoenthai, N., Wickramanayaka, A., Sungthongjeen, S., & Puttipipatkhachorn, S., (2018). Use of cassava starch nanocrystals to make a robust rupturable pulsatile release pellet. *Journal of Drug Delivery Science and Technology, 47,* 283–290.

Dash, R. N., Mohammed, H., Humaira, T., & Ramesh, D., (2015). Design, optimization and evaluation of glipizide solid self-nanoemulsifying drug delivery for enhanced solubility and dissolution. *Saudi Pharmaceutical Journal, 23* (5), 528–540.

Dong, Q., Yuan, E., Huang, M., & Zheng, J., (2017). Increased solubility and taste masking of a ternary system of neodiosmin with β-cyclodextrin and lysine. *Starch-Stärke, 69* (5&6), 1600322-n/a.

Douroumis, D., Ross, S. A., & Nokhodchi, A., (2017). Advanced methodologies for cocrystal synthesis. *Advanced Drug Delivery Reviews, 117,* 178–195.

Drozd, K. V., Manin, A. N., Churakov, A. V., & Perlovich, G. L., (2017). Drug-drug cocrystals of antituberculous 4-aminosalicylic acid: Screening, crystal structures, thermochemical and solubility studies. *European Journal of Pharmaceutical Sciences, 99,* 228–239.

Du, S., Wang, Y., Wu, S., Yu, B., Shi, P., Bian, L., Zhang, D., Hou, J., Wang, J., & Gong, J., (2017). Two novel cocrystals of lamotrigine with isomeric bipyridines and in situ monitoring of the cocrystallization. *European Journal of Pharmaceutical Sciences, 110,* 19–25.

Dumpa, N. R., Sarabu, S., Bandari, S., Zhang, F., & Repka, M. A., (2018). Chronotherapeutic drug delivery of ketoprofen and ibuprofen for improved treatment of early morning stiffness in arthritis using hot-melt extrusion technology. *AAPS Pharm. Sci. Tech., 19* (6), 2700–2709.

Enax, J., & Epple, M., (2018). Synthetic hydroxyapatite as a biomimetic oral care agent. *Oral Health and Preventive Dentistry, 16* (1), 7–19.

Fina, F., Goyanes, A., Gaisford, S., & Basit, A. W., (2017). Selective laser sintering (SLS) 3D printing of medicines. *International Journal of Pharmaceutics, 529* (1), 285–293.

García, M. C., Martinelli, M., Ponce, N. E., Sanmarco, L. M., Aoki, M. P., Manzo, R. H., & Jimenez-Kairuz, A. F., (2018). Multi-kinetic release of benznidazole-loaded multiparticulate drug delivery systems based on polymethacrylate interpolyelectrolyte complexes. *European Journal of Pharmaceutical Sciences, 120,* 107–122.

Goole, J., & Amighi, K., (2016). 3D printing in pharmaceutics: A new tool for designing customized drug delivery systems. *International Journal of Pharmaceutics, 499* (1), 376–394.

Goyanes, A., Buanz, A. B. M., Hatton, G. B., Gaisford, S., & Basit, A. W., (2015a). 3D printing of modified-release aminosalicylate (4-ASA and 5-ASA) tablets. *European Journal of Pharmaceutics and Biopharmaceutics, 89,* 157–162.

Goyanes, A., Chang, H., Sedough, D., Hatton, G. B., Wang, J., Buanz, A., Gaisford, S., & Basit, A. W., (2015b). Fabrication of controlled-release budesonide tablets via desktop (FDM) 3D printing. *International Journal of Pharmaceutics, 496* (2), 414–420.

Goyanes, A., Robles, M. P., Buanz, A., Basit, A. W., & Gaisford, S., (2015c). Effect of geometry on drug release from 3D printed tablets. *International Journal of Pharmaceutics, 494* (2), 657–663.

Goyanes, A., Wang, J., Buanz, A., Martínez-Pacheco, R., Telford, R., Gaisford, S., & Basit, A. W., (2015d). 3D printing of medicines: Engineering novel oral devices with unique design and drug release characteristics. *Molecular Pharmaceutics, 12* (11), 4077–4084.

Gumaste, S. G., & Serajuddin, A. T. M., (2017). Development of solid SEDDS, VII: Effect of pore size of silica on drug release from adsorbed self-emulsifying lipid-based formulations. *European Journal of Pharmaceutical Sciences, 110,* 134–147.

Gurudutta, P., Parmar, J. U., Sajid, A. M., & Tahir, A. M., (2010). Self-emulsifying drug delivery systems: An attempt to improve oral absorption of poorly soluble drugs. *Research Journal of Pharmaceutical Dosage Forms and Technology, 2* (3), 206–214.

Guzmán, M. L., Romañuk, C. B., Sanchez, M. F., Luciani, G. L. C., Alarcón-Ramirez, L. P., Battistini, F. D., Alovero, F. L., Jimenez-Kairuz, A. F., Manzo, R. H., & Olivera, M. E., (2018). Urinary excretion of ciprofloxacin after administration of extended release tablets in healthy volunteers. Swellable drug-polyelectrolyte matrix versus bilayer tablets. *Drug Delivery and Translational Research, 8* (1), 123–131.

Hardy, A., Seguin, C., Brion, A., Lavalle, P., Schaaf, P., Fournel, S., Bourel-Bonnet, L., Frisch, B., & De Giorgi, M., (2018). β-cyclodextrin-functionalized chitosan/alginate compact polyelectrolyte complexes (CoPECs) as functional biomaterials with anti-inflammatory properties. *ACS Applied Materials and Interfaces, 10* (35), 29347–29356.

Hasnain, M. S., Nayak, A. K., Singh, M., Tabish, M., Ansari, M. T., & Ara, T. J., (2016). Alginate-based bipolymeric-nanobioceramic composite matrices for sustained drug release. *International Journal of Biological Macromolecules, 83*, 71–77.

Healy, A. M., Worku, Z. A., Kumar, D., & Madi, A. M., (2017). Pharmaceutical solvates, hydrates and amorphous forms: A special emphasis on cocrystals. *Advanced Drug Delivery Reviews, 117*, 25–46.

Helliwell, M., & Taylor, D., (1993). Solid oral dosage forms. *Professional Nurse (London, England), 8* (5), 313–317.

Hwang, K. M., Cho, C. H., Tung, N. T., Kim, J. Y., Rhee, Y. S., & Park, E. S., (2017). Release kinetics of highly porous floating tablets containing cilostazol. *European Journal of Pharmaceutics and Biopharmaceutics, 115*, 39–51.

Jadhav, P., & Pore, Y., (2017). Physicochemical, thermodynamic and analytical studies on binary and ternary inclusion complexes of bosentan with hydroxypropyl-β-cyclodextrin. *Bulletin of Faculty of Pharmacy, Cairo University, 55* (1), 147–154.

Jain, D., Raturi, R., Jain, V., Bansal, P., & Singh, R., (2011). Recent technologies in pulsatile drug delivery systems. *Biomatter, 1* (1), 57–65.

Javanbakht, S., Nazari, N., Rakhshaei, R., & Namazi, H., (2018). Cu-cross-linked carboxymethylcellulose/naproxen/graphene quantum dot nanocomposite hydrogel beads for naproxen oral delivery. *Carbohydrate Polymers, 195*, 453–459.

Jug, M., Kosalec, I., Maestrelli, F., & Mura, P., (2011). Analysis of triclosan inclusion complexes with beta-cyclodextrin and its water-soluble polymeric derivative. *J. Pharm. Biomed. Anal., 54* (5), 1030–1039.

Kang, J. H., Oh, D. H., Oh, Y. K., Yong, C. S., & Choi, H. G., (2012). Effects of solid carriers on the crystalline properties, dissolution and bioavailability of flurbiprofen in solid self-nanoemulsifying drug delivery system (solid SNEDDS). *European Journal of Pharmaceutics and Biopharmaceutics, 80* (2), 289–297.

Karanth, H., Shenoy, V. S., & Murthy, R. R., (2006). Industrially feasible alternative approaches in the manufacture of solid dispersions: A technical report. *AAPS Pharm. Sci. Tech., 7* (4), 87.

Kazi, M., Al-Qarni, H., & Alanazi, F. K., (2017). Development of oral solid self-emulsifying lipid formulations of risperidone with improved *in vitro* dissolution and digestion. *European Journal of Pharmaceutics and Biopharmaceutics, 114*, 239–249.

Khaled, S. A., Alexander, M. R., Wildman, R. D., Wallace, M. J., Sharpe, S., Yoo, J., & Roberts, C. J., (2018). 3D extrusion printing of high drug loading immediate release paracetamol tablets. *International Journal of Pharmaceutics, 538* (1), 223–230.

Khaled, S. A., Burley, J. C., Alexander, M. R., & Roberts, C. J., (2014). Desktop 3D printing of controlled release pharmaceutical bilayer tablets. *Int. J. Pharm., 461* (1&2), 105–111.

Khaled, S. A., Burley, J. C., Alexander, M. R., Yang, J., & Roberts, C. J., (2015). 3D printing of five-in-one dose combination polypill with defined immediate and sustained release profiles. *Journal of Controlled Release, 217*, 308–314.

Kikuchi, A., & Okano, T., (2002). Pulsatile drug release control using hydrogels. *Adv. Drug Deliv. Rev., 54* (1), 53–77.

Kim, S., Hwang, K. M., Park, Y. S., Nguyen, T. T., & Park, E. S., (2018). Preparation and evaluation of non-effervescent gastroretentive tablets containing pregabalin for once-daily administration and dose proportional pharmacokinetics. *International Journal of Pharmaceutics, 550* (1), 160–169.

Kirtane, A. R., Abouzid, O., Minahan, D., Bensel, T., Hill, A. L., Selinger, C., et al., (2018). Development of an oral once-weekly drug delivery system for HIV antiretroviral therapy. *Nature Communications, 9* (1), 2.

Korotkova, E. I., & Kratochvíl, B., (2014). Pharmaceutical cocrystals. *Procedia Chemistry, 10*, 473–476.

Krupa, A., Jachowicz, R., Kurek, M., Figiel, W., & Kwiecień, M., (2014). Preparation of solid self-emulsifying drug delivery systems using magnesium aluminometasilicates and fluid-bed coating process. *Powder Technology, 266*, 329–339.

Lammers, T., Kiessling, F., Hennink, W. E., & Storm, G., (2012). Drug targeting to tumors: Principles, pitfalls and (pre-) clinical progress. *Journal of Controlled Release, 161* (2), 175–187.

Lieberman, H., Lachman, L., & Schwartz, J. B., (1989). *Pharmaceutical Dosage Forms: Tablets (*2nd edn., Vol. 1). Taylor & Francis:.

Liu, X., Yang, Y., Yu, D. G., Zhu, M. J., Zhao, M., & Williams, G. R., (2019). Tunable zero-order drug delivery systems created by modified triaxial electrospinning. *Chemical Engineering Journal, 356*, 886–894.

Mahmoud, D. B. E. D., Shukr, M. H., & ElMeshad, A. N., (2018). Gastroretentive microsponge as a promising tool for prolonging the release of mitiglinide calcium in type-2 diabetes mellitus: Optimization and pharmacokinetics study. *AAPS Pharm. Sci. Tech., 19* (6), 2519–2532.

Mahon, E., Salvati, A., Baldelli, B. F., Lynch, I., & Dawson, K. A., (2012). Designing the nanoparticle-biomolecule interface for "targeting and therapeutic delivery". *Journal of Controlled Release, 161* (2), 164–174.

Maiti, S., (2014). OSDrC: A revolution in drug formulation technology. *Journal of Pharma Sci. Tech., 4* (1), 12–13.

Majeed, S., Bin Abdullah, M. S., Dash, G. K., Ansari, M. T., & Nanda, A., (2016a). Biochemical synthesis of silver nanoprticles using filamentous fungi *Penicillium decumbens* (MTCC-2494) and its efficacy against A-549 lung cancer cell line. *Chinese Journal of Natural Medicines, 14* (8), 615–620.

Majeed, S., Bin Abdullah, M. S., Nanda, A., & Ansari, M. T., (2016b). *In vitro* study of the antibacterial and anticancer activities of silver nanoparticles synthesized from *Penicillium brevicompactum* (MTCC-1999). *Journal of Taibah University for Science, 10* (4), 614–620.

Malamatari, M., Ross, S. A., Douroumis, D., & Velaga, S. P., (2017). Experimental cocrystal screening and solution based scale-up cocrystallization methods. *Advanced Drug Delivery Reviews, 117*, 162–177.

Mandić, J., Zvonar, P. A., Vrečer, F., & Gašperlin, M., (2017). Overview of solidification techniques for self-emulsifying drug delivery systems from industrial perspective. *International Journal of Pharmaceutics, 533* (2), 335–345.

Mateescu, M. A., Ispas-Szabo, P., & Assaad, E., (2015). *4 - Chitosan-Based Polyelectrolyte Complexes as Pharmaceutical Excipients* (pp. 127–161). Woodhead Publishing.

Meka, V. S., Sing, M. K. G., Pichika, M. R., Nali, S. R., Kolapalli, V. R. M., & Kesharwani, P., (2017). A comprehensive review on polyelectrolyte complexes. *Drug Discovery Today, 22* (11), 1697–1706.

Mohammed, T. A., Farheen, S., Fatin, A. K., Mohammad, Z. A., Tengku, A. S., Bin, T. M., Shahnaz, M., Sadath, A., & Hasnain, S., (2018). Medical applications of zinc nanoparticles. *Current Nanomedicine.*

Mondal, S., Dorozhkin, S. V., & Pal, U., (2018). Recent progress on fabrication and drug delivery applications of nanostructured hydroxyapatite. *Wiley Interdisciplinary Reviews: Nanomedicine and Nanobiotechnology, 10* (4), e1504.

Mrsny, R. J., (2012). Oral drug delivery research in Europe. *Journal of Controlled Release, 161* (2), 247–253.

Narang, A. S., Desai, D., & Badawy, S., (2015). Impact of excipient interactions on solid dosage form stability. In: Narang, A. S., & Boddu, S. H. S., (eds.), *Excipient Applications in Formulation Design and Drug Delivery* (pp. 93–137). Springer International Publishing: Cham.

Norman, J., Madurawe, R. D., Moore, C. M., Khan, M. A., & Khairuzzaman, A., (2017). A new chapter in pharmaceutical manufacturing: 3D-printed drug products. *Adv. Drug Deliv. Rev., 108*, 39–50.

Oh, T. O., Kim, J. Y., Ha, J. M., Chi, S. C., Rhee, Y. S., Park, C. W., & Park, E. S., (2013). Preparation of highly porous gastroretentive metformin tablets using a sublimation method. *European Journal of Pharmaceutics and Biopharmaceutics, 83* (3), 460–467.

Pankaj, S. T. A., (2011). Co-crystal: an attractive alternative for solid dosage form. *International Research Journal of Humanities, Engineering and Pharmaceutical Sciences, 1* (1).

Parikh, N. H., Hite, W. C., & Patel, B. R., (2011). *Divisible Tablet and Associated Methods.*

Patadia, R., Vora, C., Mittal, K., & Mashru, R. C., (2017). Quality by design empowered development and optimization of time-controlled pulsatile release platform formulation employing compression coating technology. *AAPS Pharm. Sci. Tech., 18* (4), 1213–1227.

Patadia, R., Vora, C., Mittal, K., & Mashru, R., (2016). Investigating effects of hydroxypropyl methylcellulose (HPMC) molecular weight grades on lag time of press-coated ethylcellulose tablets. *Pharmaceutical Development and Technology, 21* (7), 794–802.

Patel, D. M., Jani, R. H., & Patel, C. N., (2011). Design and evaluation of colon targeted modified pulsincap delivery of 5-fluorouracil according to circadian rhythm. *International Journal of Pharmaceutical Investigation, 1* (3), 172–181.

Penhasi, A., & Gomberg, M., (2018). A specific two-pulse release of rivastigmine using a modified time-controlled delivery system: A proof of concept case study. *Journal of Drug Delivery Science and Technology, 47*, 404–410.

Pindelska, E., Sokal, A., & Kolodziejski, W., (2017). Pharmaceutical cocrystals, salts and polymorphs: Advanced characterization techniques. *Advanced Drug Delivery Reviews, 117*, 111–146.

Preis, M., Grother, L., Axe, P., & Breitkreutz, J., (2015). *In-vitro* and *in-vivo* evaluation of taste-masked cetirizine hydrochloride formulated in oral lyophilisates. *Int. J. Pharm., 491* (1&2), 8–16.

Prescott, J. H., Lipka, S., Baldwin, S., Sheppard, N. F. Jr., Maloney, J. M., Coppeta, J., Yomtov, B., Staples, M. A., & Santini, J. T. Jr., (2006). Chronic, programmed polypeptide delivery from an implanted, multireservoir microchip device. *Nature Biotechnology, 24* (4), 437, 438.

Qi, X., Qin, J., Ma, N., Chou, X., & Wu, Z., (2014). Solid self-microemulsifying dispersible tablets of celastrol: Formulation development, characterization and bioavailability evaluation. *International Journal of Pharmaceutics, 472* (1), 40–47.

Quadrado, R. F. N., & Fajardo, A. R., (2018). Microparticles based on carboxymethyl starch/chitosan polyelectrolyte complex as vehicles for drug delivery systems. *Arabian Journal of Chemistry.*

Sadia, M., Isreb, A., Abbadi, I., Isreb, M., Aziz, D., Selo, A., Timmins, P., & Alhnan, M. A., (2018). From 'fixed dose combinations' to 'a dynamic dose combiner': 3D printed bi-layer antihypertensive tablets. *European Journal of Pharmaceutical Sciences, 123,* 484–494.

Sami, F., Philip, B., & Pathak, K., (2010). Effect of auxiliary substances on complexation efficiency and intrinsic dissolution rate of gemfibrozil-β-CD Complexes. *AAPS Pharm. Sci. Tech., 11* (1), 27–35.

Sano, S., Iwao, Y., Kimura, S., & Itai, S., (2011). Preparation and evaluation of swelling induced-orally disintegrating tablets by microwave irradiation. *International Journal of Pharmaceutics, 416* (1), 252–259.

Sant, S., Swati, S., Awadhesh, K., Sajid, M., Pattnaik, G., Tahir, M., & Farheen, S., (2011). Hydrophilic polymers as release modifiers for primaquine phosphate: Effect of polymeric dispersion. *ARS Pharmaceutica, 52* (3), 19–25.

Santini, J. T. Jr., Richards, A. C., Scheidt, R., Cima, M. J., & Langer, R., (2000). Microchips as controlled drug-delivery devices. *Angewandte Chemie (International edn. in English), 39* (14), 2396–2407.

Sherje, A. P., Kulkarni, V., Murahari, M., Nayak, U. Y., Bhat, P., Suvarna, V., & Dravyakar, B., (2017). Inclusion complexation of etodolac with hydroxypropyl-beta-cyclodextrin and auxiliary agents: Formulation characterization and molecular modeling studies. *Molecular Pharmaceutics, 14* (4), 1231–1242.

Skowyra, J., Pietrzak, K., & Alhnan, M. A., (2015). Fabrication of extended-release patient-tailored prednisolone tablets via fused deposition modeling (FDM) 3D printing. *European Journal of Pharmaceutical Sciences, 68,* 11–17.

Slavkova, M., & Breitkreutz, J., (2015). Orodispersible drug formulations for children and elderly. *European Journal of Pharmaceutical Sciences: Official Journal of the European Federation for Pharmaceutical Sciences, 75,* 2–9.

Song, Z., Liu, Y., Shi, J., Ma, T., Zhang, Z., Ma, H., & Cao, S., (2018). Hydroxyapatite/ mesoporous silica coated gold nanorods with improved degradability as a multi-responsive drug delivery platform. *Materials Science and Engineering: C, 83,* 90–98.

Tahir, M., Awadhesh, K., Swati, S., Sant, S., Sajid, M., & Pattnaik, G., (2010). Optimization of fast disintegrating tablets for diclofenac sodium using isabgol mucilage as super disintegrant. *Int. J. Ph. Sci., 2* (2), 496–501.

Tang, B., Cheng, G., Gu, J. C., & Xu, C. H., (2008). Development of solid self-emulsifying drug delivery systems: Preparation techniques and dosage forms. *Drug Discovery Today, 13* (13), 606–612.

Upadhye, S., (2015). Optimelt® hot melt extrusion-enhance bioavailability of your poorly soluble API which will lead to better treatments for your patients. *Drug Development & Delivery, 15*(7), 62–65.

Urakov, A. L., (2015). The change of physical-chemical factors of the local interaction with the human body as the basis for the creation of materials with new properties. *Építôanyag: Journal of Silicate Based and Composite Materials, 67* (1), 1–6.

Verma, A., & Riaz, U., (2018). Sonolytically intercalated poly (anisidine-co-toluidine)/ bentonite nanocomposites: pH responsive drug release characteristics. *Journal of Drug Delivery Science and Technology, 48*, 49–58.

Wang, J., Goyanes, A., Gaisford, S., & Basit, A. W., (2016). Stereolithographic (SLA) 3D printing of oral modified-release dosage forms. *International Journal of Pharmaceutics, 503* (1), 207–212.

Wang, Z., Sun, J., Wang, Y., Liu, X., Liu, Y., Fu, Q., Meng, P., & He, Z., (2010). Solid self-emulsifying nitrendipine pellets: Preparation and *in vitro/in vivo* evaluation. *International Journal of Pharmaceutics, 383* (1), 1–6.

Wong, T. W., Chan, L. W., Kho, S. B., & SiaHeng, P. W., (2002). Design of controlled-release solid dosage forms of alginate and chitosan using microwave. *Journal of Controlled Release, 84* (3), 99–114.

Yang, X., Duan, J., & Fisher, J., (2016). Application of physiologically based absorption modeling to characterize the pharmacokinetic profiles of oral extended release methylphenidate products in adults. *PloS One, 11* (10), e0164641–e0164641.

Zhang, J., Li, C. Y., Xu, M. J., Wu, T., Chu, J. H., Liu, S. J., & Ju, W. Z., (2012). Oral bioavailability and gender-related pharmacokinetics of celastrol following administration of pure celastrol and its related tablets in rats. *Journal of Ethnopharmacology, 144* (1), 195–200.

Zhang, Y., Dong, K., Wang, F., Wang, H., Wang, J., Jiang, Z., & Diao, S., (2018a). Three dimensional macroporous hydroxyapatite/chitosan foam-supported polymer micelles for enhanced oral delivery of poorly soluble drugs. *Colloids and Surfaces B: Biointerfaces, 170*, 497–504.

Zhang, Y., Zhang, L., Ban, Q., Li, J., Li, C. H., & Guan, Y. Q., (2018b). Preparation and characterization of hydroxyapatite nanoparticles carrying insulin and gallic acid for insulin oral delivery. *Nanomedicine: Nanotechnology, Biology and Medicine, 14* (2), 353–364.

Zhang, Y., Zhang, L., Zhang, Q., Zhang, X., Zhang, T., & Wang, B., (2018c). Enhanced gastric therapeutic effects of Brucea javanica oil and its gastroretentive drug delivery system compared to commercial products in pharmacokinetics study. *Drug Design, Development and Therapy, 12*, 535–544.

Zhou, H., Xu, H., Li, X., Lv, Y., Ma, T., Guo, S., Huang, Z., Wang, X., & Xu, P., (2017). Dual targeting hyaluronic acid - RGD mesoporous silica coated gold nanorods for chemo-photothermal cancer therapy. *Materials Science and Engineering: C, 81*, 261–270.

CHAPTER 4

Recent Advances in the Development of Modified Release Oral Dosage Forms

GOUTAM KUMAR JENA,[1*] CH NIRANJAN PATRA,[1]
MAHFOOZUR RAHMAN,[2] and SARWAR BEG[3]

[1]Department of Pharmaceutics, Roland Institute of Pharmaceutical Sciences, Khodasingi, Berhampur, Odisha – 760010, India

[2]Department of Pharmaceutical Sciences, Faculty of Health Science, Sam Higginbottom University of Agriculture, Technology & Sciences (SHUATS), Allahabad, India

[3]Department of Pharmaceutics, School of Pharmaceutical Education and Research, Jamia Hamdard, New Delhi – 110062, India

*Corresponding author. E-mail: goutam2902@gmail.com

4.1 INTRODUCTION

Oral dosage form always takes the lion's share in pharmaceutical marketing. Gradually the demands for solid oral conventional dosage forms like tablets and capsules, i.e., immediate-release (IR) are plagued due to their untold adverse effects and lack of compliance to patients (Srikonda, Janaki, and Joseph, 2000). In order to minimize the side effects, increase efficacy and make the products patients' friendly and better compliance, oral modified release products are developed. The different pharmaceutical manufacturing companies insisted to develop various novel drug delivery products with MR strategies. Oral MR products are generally administered by oral route and utilized the latest techniques to modify the release of drugs. With the benchmark in pharmaceutical technologies and favored therapeutic benefit, more and more oral MR products including the generic versions of these products are being developed, marketed, and used in the USA (Mohammed and Ali, 2017). Because different types of MR products may exhibit unique drug release modes and specific pharmacokinetic profiles, a better understanding of the regulation and evaluation of these generic MR products can help the development and marketing of generic MR products that are therapeutically equivalent to the corresponding reference product. This chapter emphasizes the general regulatory requirements, rational design of modified release systems, therapeutic challenges, types of modified oral release dosage forms and recent advancement.

Types of MR drug products include delayed-release (e.g., enteric-coated), extended-release (ER), and targeted release and ODT.

The term modified-release drug product is meant for the products that change the timing and/or the rate of release of the drug substance. A modified-release dosage form is a formulation in which the drug-release characteristics of time course and/or location are chosen to accomplish therapeutic or convenience objectives not offered by conventional dosage forms such as solutions, ointments, or promptly dissolving dosage forms. Several types of modified-release oral drug products are recognized:

1. **Extended-release drug products.** The drug products which significantly reduce the dosing frequency to at least twice to that of the conventional dosage forms are called extended-release drug products. These extended-release drug products are exemplified by controlled-release, sustained-release, and long-acting drug products.
2. **Delayed-release drug products.** A dosage form that releases a part or portions of the drug at once other than suddenly after administration. An initial portion may be released promptly after administration. Delayed-release drug products are best exemplified by Enteric-coated dosage forms (e.g., enteric-coated NSAID products).
3. **Targeted-release drug products.** A dosage form that intended to release the drug to the targeted sites. These drug products may have the characteristics of either immediate or extended-release type.
4. **Orally disintegrating tablets (ODT).** ODT are designed to disintegrate promptly in the saliva after oral administration. ODT may be taken without the addition of water. The drug is dispersed in saliva and swallowed with little or no water.

The term controlled-release drug product was previously used to describe various types of oral extended-release-rate dosage forms, including sustained-release, sustained-action, prolonged-action, long-action, slow-release, and programmed drug delivery. The retarded release

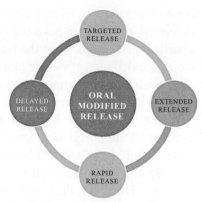

FIGURE 4.1 Different modified release systems.

is an older term for a slow-release drug product. Many of these terms for modified-release drug products were introduced by drug companies to reflect either a special design for an extended-release drug product.

4.2 ADVANTAGES AND DISADVANTAGES OF MODIFIED RELEASE DRUG PRODUCTS

Administration by oral route can render some concerns as the absorption time span is based on the total GI residence time. In addition, certain drugs will only absorb at specific sites within the GI tract, i.e., absorption windows and so total residence time may not represent its timeframe for absorption (Hollinger and Ranade, 2004). The development of gastroretentive drug delivery systems is limited by some physiological factors like gastric pH and gastric motility and also their performance depends on patient compliance and direction for use. For example, the inter-digestive motility cycle and gastric emptying rates are disrupted by feeding and caloric contents of food (Talukder and Fassihi 2004). Generally, the gastric emptying rates for dosage forms taken before meals are a much faster rate than those taken after meals. Wherever sustained drug delivery is desired at the stomach and small intestine, prolonged gastric retention can improve bioavailability, efficacy, targeted therapy, and reduce side effects within the colon and dose size can be reduced (Hoffman et al., 2004). Drugs that prone to degradation and poor alkaline solubility, the therapeutic benefit can be achieved if formulated as a gastro-retentive dosage form (Arora et al., 2005). For high volume formulations, modified enteric delivery systems can be developed which can enhance gastric retention times and can release the drug close to the time when the next dose is delivered, resulting in potential overdose of patients (Colorcon, 2016). Multiparticulate technology in the form of multiple units (capsules or tablets) enables the delivery of two or more coated bead units permitting adjustment of pharmacokinetic variability and improved delivery control (Venkatesh et al., 2015). Based on the nature of such formulations, each bead can possess different release rates. Multiparticulate formulations for colonic delivery have a great advantage over conventional single-unit dosage forms as they are less likely to be affected by food. They also show consistent absorption and capable of uniform distribution of the drug to specific regions of the GI tract. However, there is some uncertainty about the specific location in the GI tract at which the coating may dissolve. In addition, an enteric coating may dissolve unpredictably in different patients with different disease states leading to premature drug release within the small intestine. Alternatively, some enteric coating may fail to dissolve due to certain disease states leading to efficacy implications (Al-Tahami and Singh, 2007). Time-controlled explosion systems are advantageous because the release rate is not dependent on the solubility or dissolution rate of the drug or the complete release of the drug. Furthermore, the release profile is independent of the dissolution medium pH value (Singh, 2007). A push-pull system generally consists of a bilayer tablet with a pull layer with the drug mixed in, and a push layer. The system contains an orifice that is drilled using a laser to provide zero-order drug release. The drug release from this system is generally independent of physiological factors within the GI tract, such as pH, ionic strength and agitation. Several disadvantages of the push-pull systems have been documented including short delay times and slow delivery rates resulting in sub-optimal targeted delivery. As a result, many investigations into the remediation and optimization of such a delivery system have been carried out. Recent formulation developments have therefore aimed to address both issues by improving the composition of delayed-release coatings as well as the rate of drug release in the colon. For example, by modifying the composition of the exterior enteric coat via incorporation of a hydrophobic compound in excess of its solubility, one could prevent the influx of fluids through the coat, particularly during the transit of the dosage form through the stomach (Singh, 2007). Formulations based on azopolymers are relatively stable within the upper GI tract; however, the degradation of such polymers by enterobacteria is slow. In addition, such formulations are not recommended for long-term use given their limitations with regards to toxicity (Singh, 2007).

4.3   RATIONAL DESIGN OF MODIFIED RELEASE SYSTEMS

The larger part of the drug delivery systems for apparent drug absorption modification is generally, based on proprietary or nonproprietary polymeric delivery technologies. The ability to have the desirable in vitro and in vivo performance for a given drug is highly dependent upon several important factors, i.e., the dose, physicochemical, biopharmaceutical, pharmacokinetic, and pharmacodynamic properties of the drug, as well as the proper selection of a formulation approach and formulation design. Each API possesses inherent properties that require considerations specific to both the drug and the delivery system. Thus, successful dosage form development is, in fact, dictated by the properties of a compound in the context of physiological/biological constraints, rather than by the technology platform. This conclusion is supported by the fact that almost all MR products with the expired composition of matter patents have been unable to maintain market exclusivity solely based on delivery technology. There are numerous examples where the performance of the branded products has been matched by their generic counterparts based on similar or different ER technologies.

Leading examples are Procardia XL, Cardizem CD, Concerta, Adalat CC, Wellbutrin XL, Ditropan XL, Glucotrol XL, Glucophage XR, Asacol, and Toprol-XL. Therefore, the first stage in designing an MR delivery system should be to conduct a technical feasibility assessment by integrating a defined clinical rationale with the characteristics of the drug. The second stage is to select an appropriate MR technology based on the desired dosage form characteristics and other development considerations.

More specifically, a rational design process should include the following steps:

1.   Identification of clinical need and target in vivo product performance fixation
2.   Experimental study to be conducted and analyzed to estimate practicability of intestinal absorption, challenges, and risk associated with MR delivery based on

   •   Physicochemical and biopharmaceutical characterization, dose, regional absorption, in vivo disposition and pharmacodynamics of the drug molecule.
   •   Calculation of theoretical drug input rate and its range required to produce the desired plasma concentration-time profile based on in vivo disposition parameters and certain assumptions.

- Determination of physicochemical properties and absorption characteristics of the API in each segment of the GI tract required for drug input within the residence time of the dosage forms.
3. Design and characterize formulations by selecting an appropriate MR technology, associated dosage form, manufacturing process and in vitro test methods.

- Select prototype formulations for testing bioavailability in vivo.
- Identify a formulation with acceptable in vivo performance.
- Explore an in vitro-in vivo relationship (IVIVR) or in vitro-in vivo correlation (IVIVC) if different prototypes exhibit different in vivo performance.

4.4   REQUIREMENTS OF REGULATORY GUIDELINES

CDMOs and CROs give green signals for the regulatory environment for the use of modified-release technologies. Brad Gold, VP of pharmaceutical development at Metrics, says, "Scrutiny by regulatory agencies, such as the FDA or the European Medicines Agency, regarding modified-release dosage forms, has always been higher than for immediate-release counter-parts. The scrutiny arises because modified-release dosage forms typically have more of the API than the immediate-release products do."

Caldwell at Bend Research says that regulatory requirements are increasingly dictating abuse-deterrence mechanisms for certain drug classes. Opioids, combination opioids, and other drugs are often formulated for extended-release, and abusers are manipulating these drugs to get an immediate high. Multiple approaches to formulation involving the use of waxy excipients, gelling agents, and taste modifiers are increasingly being used to deter abuse while achieving the needed extended-release dissolution profiles.

Barman at Integral BioSystems says, "The FDA actually encourages companies to request guidance when creating drugs that use MR technologies. The agency has recognized the medical and other benefits of such systems."

4.5   THERAPEUTIC CHALLENGES

For the management of a product's life cycle or to address the bioavailability profile of a new drug, modified-release techniques will get a closer look as pharma companies pursue more specialized conditions and diseases.

Caldwell at Bend Research sees multiple therapeutic areas related to chronic conditions that can use modified release, including treatment of cardiovascular disease, high blood pressure, diseases of the central nervous system (CNS) and depression, attention-deficit hyperactivity disorder (ADHD), diabetes, and urinary incontinence. In addition to chronic conditions, he sees continued growth for pulsed or sustained release to help in acute areas, such as antibacterials where ideally drugs are delivered locally, and perhaps, without absorption. Also, pulsatile technologies can be helpful for drugs for which developers don't want constant blood concentrations, such as to avoid tolerance buildup for opioids.

Lee at Particle Sciences says that therapeutic areas that require drug delivery over an extended period of time are good candidates for sustained release, particularly for areas where patient compliance or other factors like drug abuse are an issue. The use of sustained-release in drugs treating Alzheimer's disease or providing contraception or HIV prevention can increase patient compliance. Treatment of constant pain and oncology are also good candidates. For oncology, sustained release can provide the highest dose that will kill cancer and not damage tissue. For Parkinson's or other CNS disorders with symptoms that require control long-term, the sustained release is also a good solution.

Barman at Integral biosystems also believes that sustained release provides opportunities for the treatment of urological conditions. She says that menopausal women often have repeated urinary tract infections, and local delivery of a sustained-release antibiotic could allow a drug to focus on the involved cells in the body and tackle bacteria in the bladder and urethra over an extended period to prevent the recurring infections.

Generally, the experts believe that the future is good for modified-release technologies, given that their use can provide a clinical benefit and that the science behind the drugs supports the use of modified release. The challenges around efficacy and LCM make growth likely. The lack of new pharmaceutical compounds in the discovery phase of drug development makes LCM very important, and MR dosage forms should become an important strategy in extending the life of established, high-revenue drugs.

4.6 RECENT ADVANCEMENT IN MODIFIED RELEASE DRUG PRODUCTS

Oral administration is the most popular route due to ease of ingestion, pain avoidance, versatility and, most importantly, patient compliance (Sastry et al., 1997a; Li and Robinson, 1987; Fasano, 1998). Also, solid oral delivery systems do not require sterile conditions and are, therefore, less expensive to manufacture. Several novel technologies for oral delivery have recently become available to address the physicochemical and pharmacokinetic characteristics of drugs, while improving patient compliance. Marketed oral MR products are presented in Table 4.1.

4.6.1   ORAL FAST-DISPERSING DOSAGE FORMS

The novel technology of oral fast-dispersing dosage forms is known as fast dissolve, rapid dissolve, rapid melt, and quick disintegrating tablets. However, the function and concept of all these dosage forms are similar. By definition, a solid dosage form that dissolves or disintegrates quickly in the oral cavity, resulting in solution or suspension without the need of water for the administration, is known as an oral fast-dispersing dosage form. Difficulty in swallowing (dysphasia) is common among all age groups, especially in the elderly, and is also seen in swallowing conventional tablets and capsules (Lindgren and Janzon, 1993). An estimated 35% of the general population, and an additional 30–40% of elderly institutionalized patients and 18–22% of all persons in long-term care facilities, suffer from dysphasia. This disorder is associated with many medical conditions, including stroke, Parkinson's, AIDS, thyroidectomy, head and neck radiation therapy, and other neurological disorders, including cerebral palsy (Avery and Dellarosa, 1994; Gisel, 1994; Anderson et al., 1995; Kahrilas, 1994). One study showed that 26% of 1576 patients experienced difficulty in swallowing tablets. The most common complaint was tablet size, followed by surface, form, and taste. The problem of swallowing tablets was more evident in geriatric and pediatric patients, as well as traveling patients who may not have ready access to water.

The advantages of oral fast-dispersing dosage forms include:

- Administration to patients who cannot swallow, such as the elderly, stroke victims, healthcare facility and bedridden patients; patients who should not swallow, such as those affected by renal failure; and patients who refuse to swallow, such as pediatric, geriatric and psychiatric patients (Wilson et al., 1987; Fix, 1998).
- Rapid drug therapy intervention.

TABLE 4.1   Current Technologies for Modified Release Drug Products

Sl. No.	Names	Keynotes	Release	References
1	Push-Pull OROS™	Multilayer tablet comprising five push-pull units for colonic release	Colonic	Singh, 2007
2	SyncroDose™	A tablet core with a xanthan and locust bean gumerodible dry-coating layer. Lag time is controlled by polysaccharide ratios	All	Marvola et al., 1999
3	The Port® System	Gelatin capsule containing an insoluble plug, a somatically active agent and drug-coated with semi-permeable membrane for pulsatile release	Pulsatile	Gothoskar, Joshi, and Joshi, 2004
4	The Pulsincap® System	Insoluble capsule body housing a drug and hydrogel plug for pulsatile release	Pulsatile	Gothoskar, Joshi, and Joshi, 2004
5	TARGIT® Technology	Enteric polymer, azo-polymer or fermentable sugar-coated starch capsules for colonic release	Colonic	Singh, 2007
6	Time Clock®	Hydrophobic surfactant coated tablet or capsule in order to rapidly release drug after a predetermined lag time for pulsatile release	Pulsatile	Gothoskar, Joshi, and Joshi, 2004
7	COLAL™ Technology	Combinations of a mixture of amorphous amylase and ethyl cellulose in addition to a water-insoluble polymer for colonic release	Colonic	Singh, 2007
8	CODES™ Technology	Core tablet of drug and saccharide(s) with three coating layers for colonic release	Colonic	Singh, 2007
9	WOWTAB®	It is a Japanese patented technology in which taste masking is claimed to offer superior to the mouthfeel due to the patented mouth feel the action.	Immediate	Srikonda, Janaki, and Joseph, 2000
10	FLASHTAB®	This technology is patented by a programpharm laboratory which consists of the preparation of tablets by using API in the form of microcrystals.	Immediate	Srikonda, Janaki, and Joseph, 2000

- More rapid drug absorption, as evident in one bioequivalence study (Selegiline) through pre-gastric absorption from the mouth, pharynx, and esophagus (Virely and Yarwood, 1990).
- Convenience and patient compliance, such as disabled bedridden patients and for traveling and busy people who do not have ready access to water.
- New business opportunities, product differentiation, line extension, and life-cycle management, the exclusivity of product promotion, and patent-life extension.

4.6.2   MODIFIED ENTERIC-RELEASE

Enteric-release products are developed to prevent the release of the drug into the stomach whereas modified enteric-release systems designed to allow for fraction of dose of the drug to be released into the stomach, with the rest of release occurring rapidly upon passage of the dosage form into the small intestine (Marvola et al., 1999). This release pattern is particularly suitable for drugs that have site-specific absorption in the upper part of the gastrointestinal tract or where high-dose drug delivery is required. Such a release pattern can be achieved via hydrophilic pore formers in pH-dependent enteric coatings.

4.6.3   PULSATILE-RELEASE

The pulsatile release pattern of the drug is designed to deliver a burst of the drug at one or more predetermined time intervals after a predetermined lag time. The need for pulsatile-release may include avoidance of drug degradation in the stomach or first-pass metabolism, the ability to administer two different drugs at the same time (released at different sites in the GI tract) or for chronotherapeutic drug delivery. As an example, pulsatile-release can be achieved via coating of multiparticulates with pH-dependent and/or barrier membrane coating systems, followed by blending of the multiparticulates to achieve desired release profiles. In general, such time-controlled systems can be classified as either single-unit (tablets and capsules) or multiple-units (pellets) system (Pozzi et al., 1994).

4.6.4   FLOSS FORMATION TECHNIQUES

The FLASHDOSE® (Fuisz Technologies, Chantilly, VA, USA) dosage form utilizes the Shearform™ technology in association with Ceform TI™ technology as needed, to mask the bitter taste of the medicament. The Shearform technology is employed in the preparation of a matrix known as 'floss', which is made from a combination of excipients, either alone or in combination with drugs. The floss is a fibrous material similar to cotton-candy fibers, commonly made of saccharides such as sucrose, dextrose, lactose and fructose (Cherukuri et al., 1996). For the preparation of sucrose fibers, temperatures ranging from 180–266°F are employed. However, the use of other polysaccharides such as polymalto-dextrins and polydextrose can be transformed into fibers at 30–40% lower temperatures than those used for sucrose fiber production. This modification permits the safe incorporation of thermolabile drugs into the formulation. The manufacturing process can be divided into four steps detailed below.

Step 1. Floss Blending

Initially, approximately 80% sucrose in combination with mannitol or dextrose and approximately 1% surfactant is blended to form the floss mix. The surfactant acts as a crystallization enhancer in maintaining the structure and integrity of the floss fiber. The enhancer also helps in the conversion of amorphous sugar into crystalline sugar, from an outer portion of amorphous Shearform sugar mass, and subsequently converting the remaining portion of the mass to complete crystalline structure. This process helps to retain the dispersed active ingredient in the matrix, thereby minimizing migration out of the mixture (Cherukuri and Fuisz, 1995).

Step 2. Floss Processing

The matrix is produced by subjecting the carrier material to flash heat and flash flow processing in a heat-processing machine. The floss formation machine is similar to a cotton-candy' fabricating type, consisting of a spinning head and heating elements. In the flash heat process, the carrier material is heated sufficiently to create an internal flow condition, followed by its exit through the spinning head that flings the floss by centrifugal forces generated by rotation. The spinning head rotates at approximately 2000–3600 rpm, providing sufficient centrifugal forces. Heating blocks are positioned around the circumference as a series of narrow slots located between the individual heating blocks. A series of grooves, located on the inner circumference of the crown and configured on the outside of the rim of the heaters, narrow the width of the aperture while increasing the path length of the exiting material, resulting in the production of fibers. The material is essentially heated upon contact with heaters, flows through the apertures under centrifugal forces, and draws into long, thin floss fibers. The produced fibers are usually amorphous in nature (Myers et al., 1996, 1999; Cherukuri and Fuisz, 1997).

Step 3. Floss Chopping and Conditioning

The fibers are conditioned to smaller particle size by chopping and rotation action in a high shear mixer-granulator. The conditioning is performed by partial crystallization through an ethanol treatment (1%) sprayed on to the floss that is subsequently evaporated, resulting in floss with improved flow and cohesive properties.

Step 4. Tablet Blending and Compression

The chopped and conditioned floss fibers are blended with active ingredients along with other standard tableting excipients, such as lubricants, flavors, and sweeteners. The resulting mixture is compressed into tablets. The active can also be added to the floss blend before subjecting it to the flash heat process (personal communication: Prior (1999) Fuisz's Flash Dose™ Tablet Technology, 1–9). In one modification to this process, a curing step is added to improve the mechanical strength of the barely molded FLASHDOSE® dosage form in plastic blister package depressions. The curing involves the exposure of the dosage forms to elevated temperature and humidity conditions, such as 40°C and 85% RH for 15 minutes. The curing step is expected to cause crystallization of the floss material that leads to binding and bridging to improve the structural strength. This new class of quick disintegrating oral delivery systems incorporating active ingredients with varying physicochemical characteristics adds value in terms of improved patient compliance as a result of their unique properties.

4.6.5   THREE-DIMENSIONAL PRINTING TECHNOLOGY IN THE PREPARATION OF ORAL DELIVERY SYSTEMS

This novel technology was developed to address several problems associated with drug release mechanisms and release rates. Drug release rates tend to decrease from a matrix system as a function of time-based on the nature and method of preparation of the dosage form (Good and Lee, 1984; Deasy, 1984). Various methods are employed to address these problems through geometric configurations, including the cylindrical rod method and cylindrical donut systems (Sastry et al., 1997b; Hsich et al., 1983). The 3DP method provides several strategies, besides having the advantages mentioned above, including the zero-order drug delivery, patterned diffusion gradient drug release by microstructure diffusion barrier technique, cyclic drug release, and other types of drug release profiles. The technique is often referred to as 'solid free-form fabrication or computer-automated manufacturing or layered manufacturing.' The 3DP method utilizes ink-jet printing technology to create a solid object by printing a binder into selected areas of sequentially deposited layers of powder. Each part is built upon a platform located on a piston-supported pin. The powder bed initially spread over the platform by a powder roller, is selectively printed with the ink-jet printing head by a binder to fuse the powders together in the desired areas. The piston descends to accommodate additional printing layers. The process is repeated until the design is complete. The instructions for each layer are derived from computer aided design (CAD) representation of the component. The 3DP instrument consists of a powder dispersion head driven recipro-cally along the length of the powder bed. An ink-jet print head prints the binder into the powder bed by selectively producing jets of liquid binder material to bind the powdered material at specified regions. This process is repeated to build up the device layer-by-layer (Hull et al., 1995; Cima and Cima, 1996). Activities that dictate the construction and completion of the dosage form using the 3DP technique are detailed below.

4.6.5.1   MATERIAL SELECTION

The processing method dictates the type and form of matrix-forming polymer material for the specific design of the system. The polymer may be in the solution form for stereolithography (SLA) or fine particles for any remaining methods including the 3DP technique. In addition, the SLA polymer should be photo polarizable, and in the later methods, the polymer is preferably in the form of particles and is solidified by the application of heat, solvent, or binder. Commonly used polymers are ethylene vinyl acetate, poly(anhydrides), polyorthoesters, polymers of lactic acid and glycolic acid and proteins such as albumin or collagen, and others including polysaccharides such as lactose (Hull et al., 1995; Cima and Cima, 1996).

4.6.5.2   BINDER SELECTION

Binder function may depend on the end-performance of the binder itself, such as a solvent for the polymer and/or active agent or an adhesive to the polymer particles. The binder function may also depend on the type of release mechanism involved. In the erosion-type devices, the solvent is used either to dissolve the matrix or may contain a second polymer deposited along with the drug. In other applications, the binder is required to harden rapidly upon deposition, and therefore the next layer is not subjected to particle rearrangement from capillary forces (Sachs et al., 1994; Cima et al., 1995).

4.6.5.3   PATTERNS FOR ACTIVE AGENT PRINTING

The active agent can be embedded into the device as either dispersion along with the polymeric matrix or as discrete units in the matrix structure. In the former method, it is mixed with binder polymer and deposited on the matrix, and in the latter type, it is dispersed in a non-solvent to the matrix polymer and deposited. Therefore, through the correct selection of the polymer material and binder system, the drug release mechanisms can be tailored to suit a variety of requirements. The resulting systems can be acid-erosion type, enteric-erosion type, pulsed controlled release, pulsed immediate or controlled release and so on. Novel delivery systems designed by 3DP technology can help to resolve several problems associated with drug release mechanisms and release rates.

4.6.6 ELECTROSTATIC DEPOSITION TECHNOLOGY FOR PHARMACEUTICAL POWDER COATING

In terms of solid dosage form manufacturing, although there have been many developments in raw materials and processes, the fundamental principles have essentially remained unchanged. New technologies involving dry manufacturing processes for the powder coating of active pharmaceutical ingredients onto various surfaces by direct electrostatic deposition have emerged. This revolutionary approach eliminates traditional manufacturing procedures of blending powders, granulation, drying, lubrication, compression and coating in pharmaceutical product development and manufacturing processes (Chrai et al., 1998). The process is less operator-dependent, is continuous and is considerably faster (Grosvenor and Staniforth, 1996).

4.7 CONCLUDING REMARKS

Tremendous advances in drug delivery systems show a continuous boost and development of modified release formulations and drug products for the delivery of the drug. Consequently, the dosing frequency is reduced, patient compliance is improved and the site of drug delivery in the GI tract is controlled successfully. The different brands of modified-release have different release patterns and so it is better to consider each modified-release preparation as a unique formulation. Due to this, the Medicines and Healthcare products Regulatory Agency recommends that all modified-release formulations should be prescribed by their brand name only. It should be kept in mind that modified-release formulations (slow-release, sustained-release, delayed-release, and controlled-release) should only be used where an obvious and clear clinical advantage exists over conventional formulations. In the case of modified-release formulations, it should be noted that the number of doses can be different from conventional and fast-release formulations. Controlled release products on crushing lose their controlled-release behavior resulting in adverse effects and duration of action are shortened. Apart from this, the modified release formulations having pH-dependent polymers, prescribing enteric-coated formulations alongside antacid formulation can enhance the pH of the stomach leading to the drug release in the unwanted region. This kind of information can help non-medical prescribers to reduce errors and enhance patient safety.

Venkatesh, G., Lai, J., Vyas, N. H., et al., (2015). *QD Diffucaps Drug Delivery Systems for Weakly Basic Pharmaceutical Actives*. http://www.adarepharma.com/wp content/uploads/2015/02/Venkatesh_QD_ Diffucaps.pdf (Accessed on 19 November 2019).

Virely, P., & Yarwood, R., (1990). Feb. Zydis – a novel, fast dissolving dosage form. *Manuf. Chem.,* 36–37.

Wilson, C. G., et al., (1987). The behavior of a fast dissolving dosage form (Expidet) followed by g-scintigraphy. *Int. J. Pharm., 40*, 119–123.

CHAPTER 5

Recent Advances in the Development of Parenteral Dosage Forms

ABDUL MUHEEM,[1*] SOBIYA ZAFAR,[1]
MOHAMMED ASADULLAH JAHANGIR,[2] MUSARRAT HUSAIN WARSI,[3]
SYED SARIM IMAM,[2] GAURAV KUMAR JAIN,[1] and
FARHAN JALEES AHMAD[1]

[1]*Nano Research Laboratory, School of Pharmaceutical Education &
Research, Jamia Hamdard, Hamdard Nagar, New Delhi – 110062,
India, Tel.: +91-9704227105*

[2]*School of Pharmacy, Glocal University, Saharanpur–247001, India*

[3]*College of Pharmacy, Taif University, Taif–21431, Saudi Arabia*

Corresponding author. E-mail: muheem.abdul985@gmail.com

5.1 INTRODUCTION

The USP 24/NF19 defines parenteral articles as "those preparations intended for injection through the skin or other external boundary tissue, rather than through alimentary canal, so that the active substances can be administered directly into a blood vessel, organ, tissue, or lesion" (https://www.usp.org/sites). Parenteral route of drug administration generally includes intravenous (IV), subcutaneous (SC), and intramuscular (IM) route, however, lesser-used routes such as intrathecal, intra-arterial, convection-enhanced drug delivery and implants are also included under the broad umbrella of parenterals. The pharmaceutical convention, however, is to use the term parenteral for those medicines that are administered by means of an injection. Parenteral products are the mainstay of treatment for hospitalized patients. This route of drug delivery offers a plethora of advantages for patients who cannot take medications orally or for those who require rapid onset of action. Hospitalized and bedridden patients are dependent on parenteral nutrition like fluids, electrolytes, or nutrients through the parenteral route. The pharmaceutical Parenteral preparations, containing the active pharmaceutical ingredients (API), and other appropriate excipients, can be administered either as a liquid in the form of solutions, emulsions or suspensions or as solid products. Furthermore, novel dosage forms such as biodegradable implants, colloidal drug carriers including polymeric nanoparticles, polymeric micelles, liposomes, and intramuscular depot injections for the sustained, targeted and controlled drug delivery are also administered by the parenteral route (Birrer, Merthy, & Liu, 2001). The advent of biotechnology has further increased the demand for the parenteral route of delivery for biologicals as the biomolecules, peptides, and proteins cannot be readily administered by any other route due to bioavailability and stability issues.

Developing a Parenteral product is endowed with challenges such as drug solubility, product stability (crucial for biopharmaceuticals), drug delivery, and manufacturability. The U.S. Food and Drug Administration (FDA) and Center for Drug Evaluation and Research (CDER) envision modernizing pharmaceutical development and manufacturing so as to enhance product quality. The increased drug recalls and drug shortages, over a span of time, reflect failures in pharmaceutical quality. The major technical and scientific advancements have further challenged the existing regulatory paradigms (Fisher et al., 2016). Pharmaceutical development is aimed to develop a product with the desired quality produced using a defined manufacturing process, i.e., robust and reproducible and consistently delivers the product for the intended usage. The "quality" is built into the pharmaceutical product since the very early research and development (R&D) phase, to ensure that the final product meets the requirements prior to entering the production phase. Pharmaceutical quality by design (QbD) is a systematic, risk-based, and pro-active approach to pharmaceutical development that employs quality-improving scientific methods upstream in the research, development and design phases, to assure that quality is designed into the product at an early stage as possible (Singh et al., 2014 and 2015; Beg et al., 2017a,b and 2019). QbD presents a framework for the understanding and consideration in all pharmaceutical aspects of the drug lifecycle including its development, manufacturing process and the raw materials used therein, distribution, and the inspection and submission/review processes including the pharmacovigilance (Csóka, Pallagi, & Paál, 2018). The QbD approach offers significant benefits to the drug developers; reduced costs, smoother application approval process, and the regulatory relief when changing the

CQAs within the design space post-registration and over-the product life cycle (Politis et al., 2017). Formulation designers seek to optimize the pharmaceutical process so as to assure that the optimal ingredient amounts in the optimal dose are delivered in the right amount, to the right site, at the right rate, at the right time, to obtain a maximum clinical therapeutic effect. It is highly desirable to optimize the pharmaceutical process which establishes the critical process parameters (CPPs) that result in the manufacturing of the acceptable product. However, to evaluate all the possible permutations of process steps and parameters, and raw material is a very tedious task, therefore process optimization can be streamlined using existing data and knowledge, incorporating risk assessment and risk management tools, and applying the statistically designed experiments to identify the acceptable operating ranges for both critical and noncritical process parameters (Hakemeyer et al., 2016). Design of experiments (DoE) is a basic concept in drug development and has found application in all areas of drug development including, active pharmaceutical ingredient synthesis, drug formulation, analytical method optimization, and stability study. DoE has emerged as a very helpful tool in drug formulation optimization and development as it significantly reduces the number of experiments, consumption of time and costs. DoE has evolved into the QbD concept. QbD is adopted by the pharmaceutical legislation as an evidence-based concept for delivering an efficient, safe and effective therapeutic agent of high quality (Savic et al., 2012; Singh et al., 2013). The product and process optimization using QbD will ultimately lead to patient benefit as they will be more likely to get improved access to high-quality affordable and innovative treatment options.

5.2 PROCESS OPTIMIZATION FOR PARENTERAL PRODUCTS USING QUALITY BY DESIGN (QBD)

The primary objective of the process design and optimization is to ensure that manufacturing operations at the initial stages, at phase III clinical trials and also at the commercial level are carried out under optimal conditions confirming the fulfillment of the specifications at the extremes of the limits within the defined design space. This information should be contained in the process design report that includes all the factors such as, facilities and environment, equipment, manufacturing variables, and any material handling requirements (Lawrence, 2008). A process optimization protocol should be developed highlighting all the CPPs that could potentially affect the quality or performance of the drug product. This is intended to establish the working limits within which the process consistently produces a product, which meets the critical quality attributes (CQAs) (Csóka et al., 2018). The definition and concept of "criticality" are of the utmost importance in the pharmaceutical process development. The criticality task team within the ISPE product quality lifecycle implementation (PQLI) initiative has presented a concise, coherent, and universal approach for criticality determination to facilitate the consistent implementation of QbD principles and ICH Q8 (R2) (pharmaceutical development), ICH Q9 (quality risk management), ICH Q10 (pharmaceutical quality systems) and ICH Q11 (development and manufacture of drug substances) guidelines in the pharmaceutical manufacturing processes development (Garcia, Cook, & Nosal, 2008). These documents contain recommendations for the detailed description and explanation of the effects of factors and factor interactions via the consecutive variation of CPPs based on the application of appropriate DoE methods, which enables a reliable determination of the process Design Space (Guideline, 2005, 2008, 2009; Ogilvie, 2017).

QbD has also found its utility in the process validation so that improved process understanding and the design space can be established. FDA "Guideline on General Principles of Process Validation" describes the principles and practices that are acceptable to the FDA and that should be considered when conducting process validation (U. Food & Administration, 1987). The European Agency for the Evaluation of Medicinal Products (EMEA) and the Committee for Proprietary Medicinal Products (CPMP) also issued guidance on process validation to provide requirements for effectively validating pharmaceutical manufacturing processes (EMA/CHMP/CVMP/QWP/70278/2012-Rev1). The process validation ensures that the process will deliver the product of acceptable quality when operated within the design space and the smaller-scale systems used to establish the design space in R&D represent the performance of the commercial production scale process (Hakemeyer et al., 2016). QbD has emerged as a promising tool to comprehend the sources of variability in a product formulation and develop a product with improved characteristics following risk assessment techniques. The QbD concept has replaced the empirical pharmaceutical developments with a risk-based approach comprising of all elements of pharmaceutical development mentioned in ICH guideline Q8 (Guideline, 2009) which includes (a) Defining the Quality Target Product Profile (QTPP) which is a prospective summary of the quality characteristics of a drug product that ensures its safety and efficacy; (b) Determination of CQAs that are the physical, chemical, biological or microbiological characteristics that should be within an appropriate limit, range or distribution to ensure drug product quality and CPPs; (c) Risk assessment that establishes a relationship between material characteristics and process parameters with finished product; (d) Development of multivariate experiments using DoE in order to link the relationships between CPPs and CQAs and establish a Design Space that defines the multidimensional combination and interaction of input variables and process parameters that have been demonstrated to provide assurance of quality. Design space is proposed by the applicant and is subject to regulatory assessment and approval. Working out of the design space is considered as a change and would initiate a regulatory post-approval change process; (e) Designing and implementing a control strategy which involves the set of controls emerged from the current product and process understanding that can include parameters and attributes related to drug substance and drug product materials and components; facility and equipment operating conditions; the in-process controls; finished product specifications; and the associated methods and frequency of monitoring and control; and (e) Product lifecycle management and continuous improvements includes approaches by the company to enable innovations and continuous improvement (Guideline, 2009; Hakemeyer et al., 2016; Sylvester et al., 2018).

The product development process starts with the conduction of preformulation studies to screen the excipients or packaging materials so as to select the ones compatible with the candidate drug, using accelerated stress-testing procedures. The manufacturing process at the R&D stage should closely represent the eventual commercial-scale manufacturing, as any deviation can affect the product performance characteristics and could influence the results of clinical studies. Stability data is finally generated on one or more of the product variants so as to select the best variant. The product and process design and optimization, though being depicted as separate stages in the development framework, but are closely linked practically. For example, while in pack optimization it is important to select a pack that satisfies the demands of a high-speed automated filling line and also that could withstand the stresses of extremes temperature and pressure during autoclaving or freeze-drying (Csóka et al., 2018).

Artificial intelligence (AI) technologies have found great utility in the pharmaceutical field. AI refers to the ability of a machine to learn and "think" for itself from experience and conduct tasks such as solving, reasoning, and process understanding that are normally attributed to human intelligence. AI technologies such as neural networks, neuro-fuzzy logic, and genetic algorithm (GAs) have been developed to assist with the understanding of formulation design and process optimization (Duch, Swaminathan, & Meller, 2007). Artificial neural networks (ANNs) are basically a computer system that is inspired by the human brain, and contains numerous process units (artificial neurons). The ANNs require building up a network of interconnecting processing units or nodes that represent the artificial equivalent of biological neurons. ANN applies the series of mathematical equations to produce information for the biological processes such as recognition, understanding, learning (Sun et al., 2003). Fuzzy logic is a powerful problem-solving technique that generates conclusions from vague, ambiguous, incomplete, and imprecise information (Klement & Slany, 1994). GAs are adaptive search algorithms, which optimize the multivariant systems by identifying and evolving solutions until the desired combination of properties (including the formulation components or process parameters) giving optimum product performance is found. AI technologies are used in situations involving multidimensional tasks and for solving complex nonlinear problems with multiple variables and multiple solutions, for example, studying the underlying relationships between formulation components, manufacturing process conditions, and drug product quality (Rowe & Roberts, 1998; Zhao et al., 2006). Pharmaceutical formulation development is a highly specialized and complex task and to develop a formulation that meets the product specification is generally encountered with several technical issues. To document the knowledge gained during the course of formulation development is tedious and is often passed on by word of mouth from experienced senior formulators to new personnel. However, this irreplaceable knowledge can be lost if the senior formulator retires or is transferred to some other company. Therefore, Formulation "expert systems" that is an advanced computer program have been developed to provide a mechanism of capturing and utilizing this knowledge and expertise. The intent of an expert system is not to replace the human expert but to aid or assist the formulation developer. The interaction between the complex tasks of formulation development can be achieved using a highly structured expert system represented by a series of production rules. An example of a production rule is as follows: IF (condition) THEN (action) UNLESS (exception) BECAUSE (reason). Using a pharmaceutical example, this production rule would read: l IF the drug is insoluble l THEN use a soluble filler l UNLESS the drug is incompatible with the filler l BECAUSE instability will occur. It doesn't require an experimental design with strict rules and can arrive at a conclusion using past or incomplete data. The knowledge within the expert system can be broken down into different types, including, facts, which are the objects and concepts about which expert reasons, and rules and heuristics, which are the expert's rules of thumb. Rules are always true and valid, but the heuristics are the expert's best judgment in a particular situation and therefore may not always be true. Neural networks require less formal statistical training, compared with other statistical analysis methods. Hence neural networks, has recently gained different applications in pharmaceutical fields (Ramani, Patel, & Patel, 1992; Zhao et al., 2006).

5.3 APPLICATIONS OF QBD IN PROCESS OPTIMIZATION FOR PARENTERAL DOSAGE FORMS

Pharmaceutical formulations and their manufacturing processes are quite complex as they involve a large number of manufacturing variables and the formulation variables. The knowledge of statistical tools such as the statistical DoE, optimization and multivariate data analysis is important to study the multi-factorial relationship and interaction between the variables so as to achieve the product with desired QAs (Huang et al., 2009). Pharmaceutical scientists are now almost universally aware of the limitations of traditional "one factor at a time" approach of experimentation and thus have recognized the advantages of a structured statistical approach to product development. DoE, as the main component of the statistical toolbox of QbD, is the strategy for planning, designing and analyzing the experiments as efficiently and precisely as possible in order to obtain the required information. DoE is the systematic approach requiring the implementation of statistical thinking at the initiation of pharmaceutical development in both research and industrial settings. It helps in the development of the newer processes, or enhancing the knowledge of the existing processes and optimizes the processes to achieve desired drug product quality. The potential benefits of DoE based experimentation are- improved process yield and stability, improved process capability, reduced process design, development time and variability, reduced manufacturing costs, increased understanding of the relationship between process parameters and observed responses, increased business profitability by reducing scrap rate. DoE determines the relationships between factors affecting a process and the output of that process through the establishment of mathematical relationships between the process inputs and its outputs (Singh, Kumar, & Ahuja, 2005). A process is a value-adding activity that transforms the series of inputs into outputs, under the influence of several factors, categorized qualitative and quantitative factors. The quantitative factors are set within a range and controlled during the experiment. However, qualitative factors have only discrete values. The choice of DoE is very important in research and industrial settings. Out of the many choices for DoE available, the proper selection is based on the knowledge of process and depends on the following factors, number of factors and interactions to be studied, nature of the problem, the complexity, statistical validity and effectiveness of each design, the ease of understanding and implementation and the time and cost constraints (Singh et al., 2005; Tye, 2004). The different mathematical models of DoE include Plackett–Burman design, Taguchi, mixture, Box–Behnken design (BBD), surface, full factorial, and fractional factorial designs. Mixture designs are applicable when the optimization is required for levels of individual components but the system is constrained by the maximum value for the overall formulation. The formulation of nanoemulsion wherein each component is optimized at a given percentage mass fragment but the sum of all the components of the formulation, including water, must equal 100 %, requires mixture design for optimization (Maher et al., 2011). The full factorial design provides a detailed understanding of the experimental response surface and can be used when the number of variables to be investigated is small (Singh et al., 2005). D-optimal designs are the computer-aided designs generated via computer algorithm and are useful when classical designs do not apply. D-optimal design matrices are usually not orthogonal and effect estimates are correlated (Xu et al., 2012). Screening designs are used for determining the large numbers of CPPs involved in pharmaceutical formulation development. They involve a few experimental runs to identify factors with the main effect. BBD is almost rotatable, which means all design points are equidistant from the center of the design. This property helps creating a response surface plot and the number of runs is given by 2k $(k-1) + C_0$, where k is the number of variables and C_0 is the number of center points (Singh et al., 2005). The various experimental designs with their potential applications in process optimization of a parenteral dosage form are depicted in Figure 5.1.

5.3.1　PROCESS OPTIMIZATION OF LIPID-BASED NANOPARTICLES

Since the discovery of liposomes by Bangham and his colleagues in 1965, scientists have found the application of liposomes in various fields such

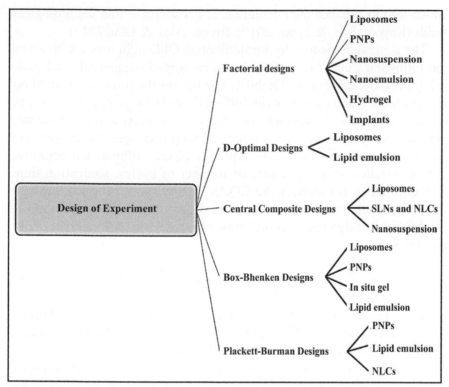

FIGURE 5.1 Flowchart depicting different experimental designs with their application (PNPs – Polymeric nanoparticles; SLNs – Solid Lipid Nanoparticles; NLCs – Nanostructured Lipid Carrier).

as chemistry, physics, biology, and medicine. The structural similarity of liposome bilayers to the cellular membranes has intrigued scientists to explore the liposomes as drug carriers to deliver different therapeutics with different properties to specific regions of the body. The structural versatility of liposomes has made it possible to incorporate lipid-soluble and water-soluble materials into the bilayers and the aqueous compartment of the liposomes, respectively. Lipids constitute the major component of liposomes which has a major influence on the safety and stability of liposomes. Cholesterol and polyethylene glycol (PEG) are the other constituents of liposomes. Cholesterol inhibits the interactions between the lipid chains by intercalating between them, thereby stabilizing the liposome bilayer and PEG imparts stealth characteristics to the liposomes which lead to enhance the circulation of liposomes within the biological fluids (Kapoor, Lee, & Tyner, 2017; Toyota, Asai, & Oku, 2017).

The general procedure for implementing QbD in liposomes involves the following steps; (a) determine the entrapped compounds and their QTPPs (safety, efficacy, and stability); (b) define the formulation method and potential risk parameters (including formulation parameters such as the type and ratio of phospholipids, lipid phase transition temperature, lamellarity, lipid degradation products, drug proportions and the process parameters such as organic to aqueous phase volume, temperature, homogenization speed, pressure or number of cycles, sonication time and amplitude); (c) identify the CQAs (particle size, drug loading and entrapment efficiency, zeta potential, and stability) of the liposomes; (d) establish the design space of the liposomes based on DoE; and (e) apply control strategy in all steps from the formulation design to the manufacturing process. Specifications for the lipid excipient may include but not limited to, source, physicochemical characteristics, and degradants (especially lysophospholipid). The lipid degradants are monitored and controlled based on identification and quantification thresholds defined in ICH Q3B guidelines. The lipid of animal origin necessitates, a transmissible or bovine spongiform encephalopathy (TSE/BSE) statement be provided to demonstrate appropriate control on the risk of potential neurological diseases (Kapoor et al., 2017; Li, Qiao, & Wu, 2017; Xu et al., 2012).

QbD concept was applied for the fabrication of chitosan-coated nanoliposomes (CH-NLPs). A risk assessment study was carried out using Ishikawa fishbone diagrams for selecting the critical processing variables. Three final product QAs selected for the study were particle size, % entrapment efficiency (%EE), and %CE (complexation efficiency). A Plackett–Burman screening design was used to screen the selected CPPs, i.e., concentrations of lipid, cholesterol, drug, and chitosan; the organic phase:aqueous phase ratio; the stirring speed; sonication time; and the temperature. An overlay plot was generated which provided a range within which variations in the value of a CPP will not affect the final response (Pandey et al., 2014). The D-optimal design was computed using JMP software (SAS Institute) 16-run custom design was created to evaluate for two responses namely the SOD %EE and particle size (Xu et al., 2012). The percentage of charged lipid (stearylamine, at 10 mol%) was fixed in all the formulations and the main lipid component percentage was varied according to cholesterol percentage. Based on the risk analysis results, the key variables identified were: total lipid concentration, DPPC% in the main lipid component, % of cholesterol, % SOD and freeze-thaw cycling. Three two-way interactions of the main effects, i.e., X1X2, X1X3, and X2X3 and three second-order terms (X21, X22, X23) of lipid concentration, DPPC%, and cholesterol% were also included. These eleven terms together with the coefficient of the intercept were deemed as "necessary" terms in JMP software and all the other terms (including three third-order terms (X31, X32, X33) were set as "if possible" (Xu et al., 2012). In another report, a three-factor BBD was applied for the development of immunosuppressant, FK506 liposomes. The process parameters were found to influence the responses- particle size, %EE but no changes were observed in zeta potential (Toyota et al., 2017). Application of response surface methodology (RSM) in the formulation of filgrastim (G-CSF) (granulocyte colony-stimulating factor) liposomes was carried out by Kiafar et al., (2016). The responses including particle size and % EE were evaluated using factorial design with dipalmitoylphosphatidylcholine (DPPC) per cholesterol (Chol.) DPPC/Chol molar ratio and hydration time as the two independent factors. Different impacts of influencing parameters including interaction and individual effects were checked employing a mathematical method to obtain desired liposomes. Average percent errors (APEs) were 3.86% and 3.27% for predicting %EE and particle size, respectively, which indicates high model ability in this regard (Kiafar et al., 2016).

QbD concept has been applied to a variety of lipid-based nanoparticles. One such category is solid lipid nanoparticles (SLNs). SLNs are composed of biodegradable and biocompatible lipids with a high melting point including triglycerides and their mixtures, fatty acids, and waxes, as the solid core, coated by nontoxic amphiphilic surfactants as the outer shell. The possibility of controlled drug delivery of the lipophilic therapeutic agent, tolerability and biodegradability, physical stability and possibility of large-scale production are some of the potential benefits of the development of SLNs (Joshi & Müller, 2009; Muller & Keck, 2004). Behbahani et al., (2017) developed and optimized curcumin loaded SLNs using central composite design (CCD) wherein the CMAs and the CPPs were the ratio of lipids, ratio of surfactants, drug/lipid ratio, sonication time and homogenization time optimized for CQAs including particle size and %EE of curcumin (Table 5.1).

TABLE 5.1   Process Optimization of Lipid-Based Nanoparticles Using DOE

Drug	Type of Design	CPPs	Reference
Filgrastim (G-CSF)	3^2 full factorial design.	Dipalmitoylphophatidylcholine (DPPC) per cholesterol (Chol.) molar ratio and hydration time	Kiafar et al., 2016
Superoxide dismutase (SOD)	D-optimal design	Lipid concentration, DPPC% in the main lipid component, cholesterol %, protein concentration, freeze-thaw cycles	Xu et al., 2012
Sirolimus	3^2 full factorial design.	Dipalmitoylphosphatidylcholine (DPPC)/Cholesterol (Chol) molar ratio and Dioleoylphosphoethanolamine (DOPE) /DPPC molar ratio	Ghanbarzadeh, Valizadeh, & Zakeri-Milani, 2013
FK506	Box-Behnken design	PBS volume (mL), Hydration temperature, number of freeze-thaw cycles	Toyota et al., 2017
Influenza peptide GILGFVFTL $(M1_{58-66})$	D-optimal design	Peptide (μg/mL), concentrations of DOPE, DC-Cholesterol, DOTAP, and EPC	Soema, Willems, Jiskoot, Amorij, & Kersten, 2015
Itraconazole (ITZ)	Fractional factorial design	Temperature, rehydration time, sonication type	Ćurić, Reul, Möschwitzer, & Fricker, 2013
	Full factorial design	Lipid concentration and concentration of ITZ	
	Central composite on face design	Lipid concentration and concentration of ITZ	
Curcumin	Central composite design	Ratio of lipids (stearic acid:tripalmitin), ratio of surfactants (tween80:span80), drug/lipid ratio, sonication time and time of homogenization	Behbahani et al., 2017
Quercetin	Central composite design	Compritol concentration and Tween 80 concentration	Dhawan, Kapil, & Singh, 2011

5.3.2   PROCESS OPTIMIZATION OF POLYMERIC NANOPARTICLES (PNPS)

Polymeric nanoparticles can be broadly classified as nanospheres and nanocapsules. Nanosphere is composed of drug molecules embedded polymeric matrix with particle size in the range of 1–100 nm whereas the nanocapsule is a nanoshell made from biodegradable or biocompatible polymers that encapsulates an inner liquid or a semiliquid core at room temperature. The manufacturing processes for the polymeric nanoparticles include: emulsion-solvent evaporation method, double emulsification method, nanoprecipitation method, emulsion-coacervation method, polymer-coating method, and layer-by-layer method. The QbD implementation steps includes the following: (i) Select the preparation method according to therapeutic agent's property and the type of nanoparticles and polymers to be use; (ii) Define the CQAs (particle size, particle size distribution, encapsulation efficiency and drug release) of the formulation and the CPPs (proportion ratio of surfactant, organic phase, and drug concentration, etc.) based on prior knowledge and risk analysis; (iii) establishment of a design space based on DoE; and (iv) verification of the feasibility and robustness of the built design space. The robustness of the design space helps minimize the inter batch and intra batch variation, which is favorable in the manufacturing of polymeric nanoparticles (Li et al., 2017).

With respect to the implementation of QbD in the development of polymeric NPs, Javan et al. (2016) developed poly(3-hydroxybutyrate-co-3-hydroxyvalerateacid) (PHBV)/PLGA NPs for delivering Teriparatide for the treatment of severe osteoporosis. Teriparatide requires administration once a day for over a long period of time of 2 years. This necessitated the development of a long-acting sustained-release system using a blend of polymers, PHBV/PLGA. BBD experimental design was applied for NPs development using three quantitative independent factors: PVA concentration, drug concentration and polymers ratio (PHBV/PLGA), evaluated for particle size, %EE, and Drug loading. The utility of a combined statistical design was investigated for the development of PLGA based linamarin nanoparticles using a double emulsion solvent evaporation method (Hussein, Abdullah, & Fakru'l-razi, 2013). A 2^2 full factorial design was used in the initial steps of formulation optimization to select the most suitable value for the stabilizer, PVA, and polymer, PLGA concentrations. The three independent variables i.e. the values selected from the initial optimization for the PVA and PLGA concentrations and the homogenization speed were then evaluated for three responses- nanoparticles yield, %EE and particle size using BBD to obtain the controlled release of linamarin from optimized PLGA nanoparticles. Critical attributes for establishing a design-space for ovalbumin loaded PLGA nanoparticles was investigated by Sainz et al. (2016). Three levels of full factorial experimental design could assess the impact of three different manufacturing conditions (polymer viscosity, surfactant concentration and amount of model antigen ovalbumin) on the five CQAs (zeta potential, polydispersity index, hydrodynamic diameter, loading capacity, and entrapment efficiency). The satisfactory design-space to meet the product specification was obtained with a polymer viscosity ranging from 0.4 to 0.9 dl/g, surfactant concentration between 8 to 15 % (w/v) and 2.5 % (w/w) of ovalbumin (Sainz et al., 2016) (Table 5.2).

TABLE 5.2   Process Optimization of Polymeric Nanoparticles Using DOE

Drug	Type of Design	CPPs	Reference
Teriparatide	Box–Behnken Design	PVA concentration (%w/v), drug concentration (μg/ml) and polymers ratio (PHBV/PLGA)	Bahari Javan et al., 2016
Linamarin	2^2 full factorial design	PVA concentration and polymer concentration	Hussein et al., 2013
	Box–Behnken design	PVA concentration, polymer concentration, and homogenization speed	
Ovalbumin	3 level full factorial design	Polymer viscosity, surfactant concentration and protein amount	Sainz et al., 2016
Paclitaxel	Plackett–Burman design	Paclitaxel amount (mg), PLGA amount (mg), PLGA molecular weight, PLGA terminal group type, Surfactant type, Surfactant concentration (%), Homogenization rate (rpm), Homogenization time (min)	Yerlikaya et al., 2013
	Box–Behnken design	PLGA amount (mg), Surfactant concentration (%), Homogenization rate (rpm)	
Rivastigmine	3^3 factorial design	Surfactant (Pluronic F127) concentration, polymer (PLGA) concentration and volume of the internal phase	Joshi, Chavhan, & Sawant, 2010
	3^2 factorial design	Surfactant (poloxamer 188) concentration (X1) and monomer (nBCA) concentration	

5.3.3 PROCESS OPTIMIZATION OF NANOSUSPENSIONS

Nanosuspensions are sub-micron sized colloidal dispersions of drug particles stabilized in the presence of polymers, surfactants or both, suspended in aqueous solution for the bioavailability enhancement of drug substances with poor solubility in aqueous and lipid solution (Singare et al., 2010). The two main procedures for the preparation of nanosuspensions are the bottom-up approach and the top-down approach. In the bottom-up techniques, drug nanocrystals are built molecule by molecule, for example, by anti-solvent precipitation techniques or different kinds of liquid atomization-based techniques while in the top-down methods, coarse drug particles are converted to nanoparticles using different techniques such as different kinds of wet milling or high-pressure homogenization (Peltonen, 2018; Singare et al., 2010). Nanomilling is a widely used, commercially available technique for the production of drug nanosuspensions. In the milling process, mechanical energy (specific energy input) is utilized to bring down the size of drug particles to smaller ones. The type and concentration of stabilizer is a crucial formulation parameter in the development of drug nanosuspension. The CPPs having the greatest impact on end-product properties are milling design, time and speed, type and amount of milling medium, bead size and amount of beads. Several process parameters simultaneously affect the development of nanosuspensions, therefore the role of every single parameter should be interpreted and considered appropriately (Peltonen, 2018). QbD emphasizes better product know-how and process understanding that should be based on scientific level research/analysis combined with risk management, throughout the manufacturing chain. QbD can be implemented for the optimization of nanosuspensions using the following steps: (1) determine the preparation method and the stabilizers according to QTPP (microbial quality, efficacy and safety, product performance and stability); (2) define the CQAs (particle size, crystallinity, sterility, isotonicity, test for microbial growth, stability etc.) and CPPs (type and amount of stabilizer) based on prior knowledge and risk assessment; (3) build a design space using DoE and verify its feasibility and robustness (George & Ghosh, 2013; Li et al., 2016, 2017; Verma et al., 2009). Lesteri et al., performed systematic development of nanosuspension of six different APIs (with differing physicochemical properties) using five different surfactant/stabilizer (anionic/cationic, nonionic/nonionic polymeric, polymeric stabilizers) at three different concentrations and three combinations of surfactant with nonionic surfactant or polymeric stabilizer and influence of milling time was observed (Lestari, Müller, & Möschwitzer, 2015). Similarly, CCD based optimization of nanodispersion of β-carotene, a carotenoid with distinguished antioxidant property, was attempted with CPPs as homogenizer speed, evaporation temperature, and rotation speed and CQAs as mean particle size, particle size distribution, and β-carotene amount (Tabar, Anarjan, Ghanbarzadeh, & Hamishehkar, 2016). A novel method, i.e., a combination of freeze-drying with high-pressure homogenization for the production of nanosuspension was attempted by Salazar et al., using DoE (Salazar et al., 2011). The freeze-drying in the initial stages of nanosuspension development produces a brittle, fragile starting material for the subsequent homogenization step. Systematic investigations using two factors, five-level DoE were conducted during freeze-drying to identify optimal process parameters taking drug concentration and organic solvent composition as the independent factors. The product obtained was subsequently homogenized at high pressure (Table 5.3).

TABLE 5.3 Process Optimization of Nanosuspensions Using DOE

Drug	Type of Design	CPPs	Reference
β-Carotene	Central composite design	Homogenizer speed, evaporation temperature, and rotation speed	Rafie Tabar et al., 2016
Glibenclamide	5^2 factorial design	Drug concentration and organic solvent composition (dimethyl sulfoxide (DMSO):tert-butanol (TBA) ratio)	Salazar et al., 2011
Indomethacin	$2^{(5-1)}$ factorial design	Drug concentration, stabilizer type, stabilizer concentration, temperature, milling time, and microfluidization pressure	Verma et al., 2009

5.3.4 PROCESS OPTIMIZATION OF LIPID EMULSION/ NANOEMULSION

Injectable lipid emulsions that provide essential fatty acids and vitamins have been used clinically for decades as an energy source for hospitalized patients. The biocompatible and the biodegradable nature of the lipid-based system has renewed the interest of the scientific community in utilizing lipid emulsions for the delivery of lipid-soluble therapeutic agents, intravenously (Hörmann & Zimmer, 2016). USP chapter 729

"Globule Size Distribution in Lipid Injectable Emulsions" provides the specific particle size requirements for an intravenously applicable emulsion. The mean particle size of the emulsions should be <500 nm with a sufficiently narrow particle size distribution (Gehrmann & Bunjes, 2017). Oil-in-water emulsions, called nanoemulsions, with particle sizes in the range of 20-200 nm, are interesting carriers for the hydrophobic drug molecules. Nanoemulsions are formed by an isotropic mixture consisting of oil, surfactant, co-surfactant, and drug when introduced into the water. Nanoemulsions have special benefits including easy formulation, simple manufacturing processes, thermodynamic stability, and reproducible plasma concentration and drug bioavailability. The methods for nanoemulsions development include the self-nanoemulsion method, the aqueous phase titration method, solvent displacement method, high-pressure homogenization and microfluidization method.

The following steps are involved in the application of QbD for nanoemulsions: (a) define QTPP based on the drug molecules' solubility and administration routes; (b) identify suitable preparation method and specific formulation parameters (type and concentration of oil and emulsifier), and process parameters (pre-emulsion temperature, rate of addition of oil, mixing time and mixer speed, homogenization temperature, operating pressure and no. of cycles); (c) identify CQAs (visual appearance, particle size and size distribution, emulsification rate, viscosity, drug content and drug release) and screen the CPPs based on prior knowledge and risk assessment; (d) conduct DoE to build design spaces; and (e) apply process control strategy in the whole process (Hippalgaonkar, Majumdar, & Kansara, 2010; Li et al., 2017). Control of droplet size is important for the performance of the nanoemulsion product. The concentration of the oil phase affects the size of nanoemulsion droplets as the higher oil phase leads to greater droplet size. An increase in oil phase proportion decreases the emulsifier concentration and results in partial or minimal interfacial surface coverage by the emulsifier that further increases the surface tension and hence the droplet size. For formulation stability, in such cases, an excess amount of emulsifier is required which further increases the viscosity of the system and also the risk of hemolysis (depending on the nature of the surfactant), making intravenous administration painful (Hippalgaonkar et al., 2010).

In exploring QbD application in nanoemulsion, Kelmann et al., (2007) prepared carbamazepine (CBZ) nanoemulsion for intravenous delivery using a spontaneous emulsification method. A 2^2 full factorial experimental design was utilized to study the influence of two independent variables (the type of oil and type of lipophilic emulsifier) on responses such as droplet size, zeta potential, viscosity, drug content and association to oily phase. This optimized formulation with droplet size around 150 nm, drug content around 95% and zeta potential around −40 mV, retained the satisfactory characteristics over the evaluation period of 3 months (Kelmann et al., 2007). Gehrmann developed lipid emulsion of very narrow particle size distribution using an alternative preparation method with low energy input, premix membrane emulsification (ME) method. In the premix, ME, a coarse pre-emulsion (premix), is extruded through a porous membrane resulting in smaller emulsion droplets within the size range of the pore diameter. The desired narrow particle size distribution is achieved by repeating the extrusion step several times. The CPPs applied using DoE were the flow rate, cycle number and type of membrane material (polyester, nylon, cellulose acetate and aluminum oxide with pore sizes of 200 nm) and the formulation parameters were the three different emulsifiers *viz* poloxamer 188, Tween 80 and sucrose laurate. The cycle number and the pore size of the membrane majorly affected the processing of nanoemulsion. For the optimized premix ME process, the most suitable emulsifier, and a favorable cycle number were membrane dependent and should be evaluated separately for the best emulsification result. The very hydrophilic alumina membrane in combination with the emulsifier, sucrose laurate was identified to be the most suitable combination (Gehrmann & Bunjes, 2017). A four factor three-level BBD was utilized to define the CPPs, CQAs and hence the design space for the development of Vitamin E enriched lipid emulsion. The effects of homogenization pressure, number of homogenizing cycles, the viscosity of the oil phase, and oil content on the physical stability (% of vitamin E remaining emulsified after 7 days of storage) and particle size was evaluated (Alayoubi et al., 2015) (Table 5.4).

5.3.5   PROCESS OPTIMIZATION OF IMPLANTABLE DDS

The implantable drug delivery systems (IDDS) are mainly approached for controlled release of therapeutic molecules according to the requirement of the patient and injection of the drug at the required site in the patient body in order to deliver the therapeutic agent for an extended period of time. The other reasons include, decrease the frequency of drug administration, fewer side effects, improved drug stability, protection of rapid metabolization of

TABLE 5.4   Process Optimization of Lipid Emulsion/Nanoemulsion Using DOE

Drug	Type of Design	CPPs	Reference
Vitamin E	Box–Behnken design	Homogenization pressure, Number of homogenizing cycles, Viscosity of the oil phase, and Oil content	Alayoubi et al., 2015
Vitamin E	Plackett–Burman design.	Homogenization pressure, Number of homogenization cycles, % w/w of Primary and secondary emulsifiers (Lipoid® E80 S, Tween®80), Cholesterol %, pre-homogenization temperature, oil loading, and the ratio of vitamin E to medium-chain triglycerides (MCT) in the oil phase	Alayoubi, Nazzal, Sylvester, & Nazzal, 2013
Carbamazepine	2^2 full factorial design	Type of oil and type of lipophilic emulsifier	Kelmann et al., 2007

the drug, a hospital stay may not be required for chronic illnesses. IDDS are generally of two types-drug implants and implantable pumps which can be further subdivided into non-degradable and degradable systems. Insertable DDS, including intraocular, vaginal and intrauterine inserts, that could be inserted into a specific body location and later easily removed when the systems were exhausted, are also included in the broad umbrella of the term IDDS (Kleiner, Wright, & Wang, 2014; Meng & Hoang, 2012).

Another type of biodegradable polymer-based implants, the In situ gelling systems are the stimuli sensitive systems which undergoes a sol-gel transformation when encountered with different stimuli such as temperature change from room to body temperature, pH change from that of the preparation to the biological pH, and also due to precipitation of polymers (soluble in the solvent used in formulation, but insoluble in body fluid). The in situ-gels form drug depots with a prolonged residence time when injected intramuscularly (i.m.) from where the drug is released in a controlled manner over a period of time as the polymer biodegrades. The type, concentration, and molecular weight of the polymer affect drug release from an in-situ gelling system. The in-situ gel of alendronate sodium (ALS) was developed for the treatment of osteoporosis using Box–Behnken experimental design. Three different independent variables; concentration of primary polymer, PLGA, the concentration of copolymer polycaprolactone (PCL) and lipid surfactant Capryol 90 concentration were selected to investigate the gellation character, and drug release. In-situ gels with higher bioavailability, extended-release for more than three months, with the elimination of esophageal side effects of ALS was obtained. PLGA based IDDS has been developed for the delivery of biopharmaceuticals including proteins and peptides. But the lack of easy, fast and effective microencapsulation technologies and the increased risk of protein denaturation, are the major hurdles for the commercialization of proteins-loaded PLGA particulate delivery systems. Within the several microencapsulation methods available for the production of PLGA based particle products, emulsion methods, coacervation, and spray drying have generally reached large-scale production. However, manufacturers still face many problems, such as the significant unanticipated costs in scale-up production, the residual organic solvent, and sterilization. Considering the potential benefits and the limitations of all the available methods of microencapsulation, Spray drying, has attracted lots of interests owing to its scale-up possibility with automatic controlling, cost-effectiveness, commercial availability of different process layouts, and suitability for different types of feeds. Spray drying is a continuous process which involves three steps: (a) atomization of the feed into small droplets via an atomizer; (b) drying of the droplets upon contact with the drying gas and particle formation; and (c) separation of the dried particles from the drying medium. In the spray drying process, the bulk fluid is usually broken into individual droplets through an atomizer. The process controls in the spray drying process include the operating conditions, the rheology of bulk fluids, the channel design of the rotary atomizer, the disc angular velocity and the feed flow rate control the mean droplet size.

Hydrogels, three dimensional, cross-linked water-soluble polymer networks that swell and expand in an aqueous environment, are an upcoming class of polymer-based controlled release drug-delivery systems (Kiene et al., 2018). Natural polymers have shown to exhibit gelation upon temperature change giving a thermosensitive hydrogel. 5-fluorouracil (a widely used anticancer agent) loaded methylcellulose based thermosensitive hydrogels were prepared using a QbD approach utilizing two statistical methods: Quality risk management (QRM) and DoE (Dalwadi & Patel, 2016). The QTPP elements identified were- dosage form, route of administration, drug product QAs, container, and closure system and stability. The CQAs for the intratumorally delivered thermosensitive hydrogel was selected as: appearance, gelling time, gelling temperature, swelling index, drug release, syringebility, dynamic viscoelastic parameters, viscosity, gel strength, and microbial limit. QRM was carried out using the Ishikawa Fish Bone diagram to identify the CMAs and the CPPs, which have the highest influence on the CQAs. The highest risk factors were then subjected to an experimental design study to establish a product or process design space for risk control. The concentration of methylcellulose and trisodium citrate majorly affected the hydrogel development, therefore they were subjected to two-factor three-level full factorial DoE to find the suitable design space to produce the product with desired specification and performance (Dalwadi & Patel, 2016).

Ceramic based IDDS including inorganic bone meal, hydroxy-apatite, aluminum calcium phosphorous oxides, tricalcium phosphate, and ceramic–metal hybrids are the recent advance form of IDDS finding variety of diverse therapeutic applications such as bone infections, intraocular implants for the treatment of glaucoma, nanoporous coatings for DES, and transurethral devices for the treatment of impotence. Hydroxyapatite-ciprofloxacin composites for local antibiotic therapy in osteomyelitis were prepared by the precipitation technique using 2^3 factorial design, with the drug amount added in the process, stirring speed and addition rate of orthophosphoric acid in the synthesis as the critical parameters to be optimized (Nayak, Laha, & Sen, 2011) (Table 5.5).

TABLE 5.5   Process Optimization of Implantable Drug Delivery System

Drug	Type of Design	CPPs	Reference
5-fluorouracil thermosensitive hydrogel	Quality Risk Management (Ishikawa Fishbone Diagram)	Methyl cellulose (MC) concentration, nature of excipient, tri sodium citrate (TSC) concentration, mixing speed and mixing time	Dalwadi & Patel, 2016
	3^2 full factorial design	MC concentration and TSC concentration	
Hydroxyapatite (HAp)-Ciprofloxacin bone-implants	2^3 factorial design	Drug amount, stirring speed and addition rate of orthophosphoric acid in the synthesis	Nayak et al., 2011
Alendronate-sodium in-situ gel	Box–Behnken design	PLGA %, % of polycaprolactone and % of lipid surfactant capryol 90	Hosny & Rizg, 2018

5.4 PACKAGING OF PARENTERAL PRODUCTS

The prime consideration for the packaging of the parenteral products is the maintenance of sterility prior to use and throughout the shelf life of the product. Glass vials with type 1 neutral glass and sealed with rubber stoppers are used for the packaging of SVPs. Blow-fill-seal technology wherein the (plastic) ampoule is molded, aseptically filled, and sealed in a continuous process is being preferred for packaging the parenteral products because of the flexibility in container design, overall product quality, operational output, and low operational costs (Markarian, 2014). For products packaged in vials, a suitable rubber stopper must be selected. For lyophilized products, a stopper with a low moisture absorbing capacity should be selected so as to avoid the moisture absorption autoclaving process, which can be transferred to the product during storage, leading to product deterioration. Teflon coated stoppers and the stoppers containing desiccant are also available now for storing the moisture-sensitive products. Stoppers such as Flurotec1 (Daikyo/ West Pharmaceutical Services, Pennsylvania, U.S.) and Omniflex1 (Helvoet Pharma, Liege, Belgium), siliconized with special silicone polymers have been recently developed to provide lubricity and reduce the potential for formulation and stopper interactions (Rey, 2004).

Sophisticated packages, such as pre-filled syringes, have also been developed for the delivery of parenteral products. These are particularly important for expensive biomolecules as they eliminate the need for over-filling and thus reduce wastage. Needle-free injection technology, including, safety needles, autoinjectors, pens, needle guards, has been in development for many years to try and overcome the issues of needle phobia, needle stick injuries, patient discomfort, and needle safety. Needle-free injectors, without a hypodermic needle, administer liquid medication under sufficient pressure in a fine, high-velocity jet to penetrate the skin tissue. The needle-free technologies do have some disadvantages as well, which includes, causing pain/ bruising and bleeding at the injection site because of the high pressure of the jet, high cost and the challenge to prove bioequivalence between the needle-free device and the needle-based injection. The most established companies providing needle-free devices are Anesiva, Antares, Bioject, Injex, National Medical Products, and The Medical House (Ravi et al., 2015).

Pack selection and optimization involves defining the packaging function, selecting the materials, and then testing the packaging performance to ensure that it will meet all the product design and functional requirements that were identified in the product design report (PDR). The primary container that is in direct contact with the product is more relevant for pack optimization studies. The secondary packaging is the one outside the primary pack and, often includes a carton or a blister that functions to protect the product from light or moisture. Important selection and optimization criteria for the primary packaging include: (a) satisfying the environmental and legislative requirements for worldwide markets; (b) DMF availability; (c) ability to source from more than one supplier/country; (d) consistency of dimensions and pack performance; and (f) ability to meet function/user tests, customer requirements, and specifications.

5.5 REGULATORY ASPECTS

When considering parenterals numbers of guidelines have been published by the FDA and the EMEA. The "Decision Trees for the Selection of Sterilization Methods" document is prescriptive on the selection of a sterilization strategy suitable for the developed parenteral product (Decision Trees for the Selection of Sterilization Methods (CPMP/QWP/155/96)). Similarly, a guidance document entitled "Notes for Guidance on Inclusion of Antioxidants and Antimicrobial Preservatives in Medicinal Products" has been provided which defines the circumstances under which antioxidants and preservatives should be used (Products). The "Guide to Inspection of Lyophilization of Parenterals," provides a useful indication of areas of specific interest to the FDA, which the formulator would be well advised to address during the development program (Food & Administration, 1993). Further, the harmonization of the regulatory requirements among the European Medicines Agency (EMA), US FDA and Japanese Health Agency (MHLW) has been established using the set of guidelines, ICH, International Conference on Harmonization of Technical Requirements for Registration of Pharmaceuticals for Human Use. ICH is also the start of regulatory science that integrates the knowledge of pharmacy, medicine, chemistry, engineering, and operational management. ICH guideline Q8, titled "Pharmaceutical Development," was adopted to predict the product quality in a pharmaceutical development phase, utilizing knowledge management and risk management principles which served as the key elements of scientific-based specifications and manufacturing control within design space (Guideline, 2009). ICH Q8 (R1), the first revision of Q8, extends an annex to the already approved Q8 guideline and demonstrates the practical applicability of concepts and tools outlined in the parent document. It details the pharmaceutical development elements with practical examples for the reliable implementation of the QbD concept and also contains the information required for eCTD submission.

5.6 CONCLUDING REMARKS

This chapter focuses on the optimization of various process and formulation parameters for the development of parenteral dosage form using DOE. The researchers encounter complex technical challenges during formulation development, which makes it imperative to use an effective methodology for formulation development. DOE and statistical analysis are a promising tool for the optimization of different formulation and process variables. The considerable advantage of applying DOE to develop formulations for pharmaceutical products is that it permits all crucial variables to be evaluated systematically and accurately. Once the important variables have been identified, the optimal formulations can be finalized by using accurate DOE to optimize the levels of all critical variables. DoE is the first choice for rational pharmaceutical development for researchers.

KEYWORDS

- **parental dosage**
- **design of expert**
- **process optimization**
- **nanoformulations**

REFERENCES

Alayoubi, A., et al., (2013). "Vitamin E" fortified parenteral lipid emulsions: Plackett-Burman screening of primary process and composition parameters. *Drug Dev. Ind. Pharm., 39* (2), 363–373.

Alayoubi, A., et al., (2015). Effect of lipid viscosity and high-pressure homogenization on the physical stability of "vitamin E" enriched emulsion. *Pharm. Dev. Technol., 20* (5), 555–561.

Bahari, J. N., et al., (2016). Preparation, statistical optimization and *in vitro* characterization of poly (3-hydroxybutyrate-co-3-hydroxyvalerate)/poly (lactic-co-glycolic acid) blend nanoparticles for prolonged delivery of teriparatide. *J. Microencapsul., 33* (5), 460–474.

Beg, S., Rahman, M., Kohli, K., (2019). Quality-by-design approach as a systematic tool for the development of nanopharmaceutical products. *Drug Discovery Today.* 24(3), 717–725.

Beg, S., Akhter, S., Rahman, M., Rahman, Z., (2017a). Perspectives of Quality by Design approach in nanomedicines development. *Current Nanomedicine*, 7, 1–7.

Beg, S., Rahman, M., Panda, S.S., (2017b). Pharmaceutical QbD: Omnipresence in the product development lifecycle. *European Pharmaceutical Review*. 22(1), 2–8.

Behbahani, E. S., et al., (2017). Optimization and characterization of ultrasound-assisted preparation of curcumin-loaded solid lipid nanoparticles: application of central composite design, thermal analysis and x-ray diffraction techniques. *Ultrason. Sonochem., 38*, 271–280.

Birrer, G. A., et al., (2001). Parenteral dosage forms. *Handbook of Modern Pharmaceutical Analysis, 3.*

Csóka, I., et al., (2018). Extension of quality-by-design concept to the early development phase of pharmaceutical R&D processes. *Drug Discov. Today.*

Ćurić, A., et al., (2013). Formulation optimization of itraconazole loaded PEGylated liposomes for parenteral administration by using design of experiments. *Int. J. Pharm., 448* (1), 189–197.

Dalwadi, C., & Patel, G., (2016). Implementation of "quality by design (QbD)" approach for the development of 5-fluorouracil loaded thermosensitive hydrogel. *Curr. Drug Deliv., 13* (4), 512–527.

Decision Trees for the Selection of Sterilization Methods (CPMP/QWP/155/96). From: https://www.ema.europa.eu/documents/scientific-guideline/decision-trees-selection-sterilisation-methods-cpmp/qwp/054/98-annex-note-guidance-development-pharmaceutics-cpmp/qwp/155/96_en.pdf (Accessed on 19 November 2019).

Dhawan, S., et al., (2011). Formulation development and systematic optimization of solid lipid nanoparticles of quercetin for improved brain delivery. *J. Pharm. Pharmacol., 63* (3), 342–351.

Duch, W., et al., (2007). Artificial intelligence approaches for rational drug design and discovery. *Curr. Pharm. Des., 13* (14), 1497–1508.

EMA/CHMP/CVMP/QWP/70278/2012-Rev1.GuidelineonProcessValidation.From:http://www.ema.europa.eu/docs/en_GB/document_library/Scientific_guideline/2012/04/WC500125399.pdf (Accessed on 19 November 2019).

Fisher, A. C., et al., (2016). Advancing pharmaceutical quality: an overview of science and research in the US FDA's office of pharmaceutical quality. *Int. J. Pharm., 515* (1&2), 390–402.

Food, & Administration, D., (1993). *Guide to Inspections of Lyophilization of Parenterals.* FDA.

Food, U., & Administration, D., (1987). *Guideline on General Principles of Process Validation.* US FDA: Rockville, MD.

Garcia, T., Cook, G., & Nosal, R., (2008). PQLI key topics-criticality, design space, and control strategy. *J. Pharm. Innov., 3* (2), 60–68.

Gehrmann, S., & Bunjes, H., (2017). Preparation of nanoemulsions by premix membrane emulsification: Which parameters have a significant influence on the resulting particle size? *J. Pharm. Sci., 106* (8), 2068–2076.

George, M., & Ghosh, I., (2013). Identifying the correlation between drug/stabilizer properties and critical quality attributes (CQAs) of nanosuspension formulation prepared by wet media milling technology. *Eur. J. Pharm. Sci., 48* (1&2), 142–152.

Ghanbarzadeh, S., et al., (2013). Application of response surface methodology in development of sirolimus liposomes prepared by thin film hydration technique. *BioImpacts. BI, 3* (2), 75.

Guideline, I. H. T., (2005). Quality risk management. *Q9, Current Step, 4,* 408.

Guideline, I. H. T., (2008). Pharmaceutical quality system. *Q10, Current Step, 4.*

Guideline, I. H. T., (2009). Pharmaceutical development. *Q8. Current Step, 4.*

Hakemeyer, C., et al., (2016). Process characterization and design space definition. *Biologicals, 44* (5), 306–318.

Hippalgaonkar, K., et al., (2010). Injectable lipid emulsions—advancements, opportunities and challenges. *AAPS Pharm. Sci. Tech., 11* (4), 1526–1540.

Hörmann, K., & Zimmer, A., (2016). Drug delivery and drug targeting with parenteral lipid nanoemulsions—a review. *J. Control Release, 223,* 85–98.

Hosny, K. M., & Rizg, W. Y., (2018). Quality by design approach to optimize the formulation variables influencing the characteristics of biodegradable intramuscular in-situ gel loaded with alendronate sodium for osteoporosis. *PloS One, 13* (6), e0197540.

Huang, J., et al., (2009). Quality by design case study: An integrated multivariate approach to drug product and process development. *Int. J. Pharm., 382* (1&2), 23–32.

Hussein, A. S., et al., (2013). Optimizing the process parameters for encapsulation of linamarin into PLGA nanoparticles using double emulsion solvent evaporation technique. *Adv. Polym. Technol., 32* (S1), E486–E504.

Joshi, M. D., & Müller, R. H., (2009). Lipid nanoparticles for parenteral delivery of actives. *Eur. J. Pharm. Biopharm., 71* (2), 161–172.

Joshi, S. A., et al., (2010). Rivastigmine-loaded PLGA and PBCA nanoparticles: Preparation, optimization, characterization, *in vitro* and pharmacodynamic studies. *Eur. J. Pharm. Biopharm., 76* (2), 189–199.

Kapoor, M., et al., (2017). Liposomal drug product development and quality: Current US experience and perspective. *The AAPS Journal, 19* (3), 632–641.

Kelmann, R. G., et al., (2007). Carbamazepine parenteral nanoemulsions prepared by spontaneous emulsification process. *Int. J. Pharm., 342* (1&2), 231–239.

Kiafar, F., et al., (2016). Filgrastim (G-CSF) loaded liposomes: mathematical modeling and optimization of encapsulation efficiency and particle size. *BioImpacts: BI, 6* (4), 195.

Kiene, K., et al., (2018). Self-assembling chitosan hydrogel: A drug-delivery device enabling the sustained release of proteins. *J. Appl. Polym. Sci., 135* (1), 45638.

Kleiner, L. W., (2014). Evolution of implantable and insertable drug delivery systems. *J. Control. Release, 181,* 1–10.

Klement, E. P., & Slany, W., (1994). Fuzzy logic in artificial intelligence. *Encyclopedia of Computer Science and Technology, 34.*

Lawrence, X. Y., (2008). Pharmaceutical quality by design: Product and process development, understanding, and control. *Pharm. Res., 25* (4), 781–791.

Lestari, M. L., et al., (2015). Systematic screening of different surface modifiers for the production of physically stable nanosuspensions. *J. Pharm. Sci., 104* (3), 1128–1140.

Li, J., et al., (2017). Nanosystem trends in drug delivery using quality-by-design concept. *J. Control. Release, 256,* 9–18.

Li, M., et al., (2016). Nanomilling of drugs for bioavailability enhancement: A holistic formulation-process perspective. *Pharm., 8* (2), 17.

Maher, P. G., et al., (2011). Optimization of β-casein stabilized nanoemulsions using experimental mixture design. *J. Food Sci., 76* (8), C1108–C1117.

Markarian, J., (2014). *Blow-Fill-Seal Technology Advances in Aseptic Filling Applications.* https://www.pharmtech.com/blow-fill-seal-technology-advances-aseptic-filling-applications.

Meng, E., & Hoang, T., (2012). Micro-and nano-fabricated implantable drug-delivery systems. *Ther. Deliv., 3* (12), 1457–1467.

Muller, R. H., & Keck, C. M., (2004). Challenges and solutions for the delivery of biotech drugs—a review of drug nanocrystal technology and lipid nanoparticles. *J. Biotechnol., 113* (1–3), 151–170.

Nayak, A., Laha, B., & Sen, K., (2011). Development of hydroxyapatite-ciprofloxacin bone-implants using» quality by design. *Acta Pharm., 61* (1), 25–36.

Note for Guidance on Inclusion of Antioxidants and Antimicrobial Preservatives in Medicinal Products. From: https://www.ema.europa.eu/documents/scientific-guideline/note-guidance-inclusion-antioxidants-antimicrobial-preservatives-medicinal-products_en.pdf (Accessed on 19 November 2019).

Ogilvie, R., (2017). ICH Q11: Development and manufacture of drug substance. *ICH Quality Guidelines: An Implementation Guide*, 639–665.

Pandey, A. P., et al., (2014). Applying quality by design (QbD) concept for fabrication of chitosan coated nanoliposomes. *J. Liposome Res., 24* (1), 37–52.

Peltonen, L., (2018). Design space and QbD approach for production of drug nanocrystals by wet media milling techniques. *Pharm., 10* (3), 104.

Politis, S. N., et al., (2017). Design of experiments (DoE) in pharmaceutical development. *Drug Dev. Ind. Pharm., 43* (6), 889–901.

Rafie, T. A., et al., (2016). Effect of processing parameters on physicochemical properties of β-carotene nanocrystal: A statistical experimental design analysis. *Iran. J. Pharm. Sci., 12* (4), 77–92.

Ramani, K., Patel, M., & Patel, S., (1992). An expert system for drug preformulation in a pharmaceutical company. *Interfaces, 22* (2), 101–108.

Ravi, A. D., Sadhna, D., Nagpaal, D., & Chawla, L., (2015). Needle free injection technology: A complete insight. *Int. J. Pharm. Investig., 5* (4), 192.

Rey, L. M. J., (2004). *Freeze-Drying/Lyophilization of Pharmaceutical and Biological Products* (2nd edn.). New York: Informa Healthcare.

Rowe, R. C., & Roberts, R. J., (1998). Artificial intelligence in pharmaceutical product formulation: Neural computing and emerging technologies. *Pharm. Sci. Technol. Today, 1* (5), 200–205.

Sainz, V., et al., (2016). Optimization of protein loaded PLGA nanoparticle manufacturing parameters following a quality-by-design approach. *RSC Adv., 6* (106), 104502–104512.

Salazar, J., Heinzerling, O., Müller, R. H., & Möschwitzer, J. P., (2011). Process optimization of a novel production method for nanosuspensions using design of experiments (DoE). *Int. J. Pharm., 420* (2), 395–403.

Savic, I. M., Marinkovic, V. D., Tasic, L., Krajnovic, D., & Savic, I. M., (2012). From experimental design to quality by design in pharmaceutical legislation. *Accreditation and Quality Assurance, 17* (6), 627–633.

Singare, D. S., et al., (2010). Optimization of formulation and process variable of nanosuspension: An industrial perspective. *Int. J. Pharm., 402* (1&2), 213–220.

Singh, B., Kumar, R., & Ahuja, N., (2005). Optimizing drug delivery systems using systematic" design of experiments." Part I: fundamental aspects. *Crit. Revi. Ther. Drug Carrier Syst., 22* (1).

Singh, B., & Beg, S., (2015). Attaining product development excellence and federal compliance employing Quality by Design (QbD) paradigms. *The Pharma Review*. 13(9), 35–44.

Singh, B., & Beg, S., (2014). Product development excellence and federal compliance via QbD. *Chronicle PharmaBiz*. 15(10), 30–35.

Singh, B., Raza, K., Beg, S., (2013). Developing "Optimized" drug products employing "Designed" experiments. *Chemical Industry Digest*. 23, 70–76.

Soema, P. C., et al., (2015). Predicting the influence of liposomal lipid composition on liposome size, zeta potential and liposome-induced dendritic cell maturation using a design of experiments approach. *Eur. J. Pharm. Biopharm., 94*, 427–435.

Sun, Y., Peng, Y., Chen, Y., & Shukla, A. J., (2003). Application of artificial neural networks in the design of controlled release drug delivery systems. *Adv. Drug Deliv. Rev., 55* (9), 1201–1215.

Sylvester, B., et al., (2018). Optimization of prednisolone-loaded long-circulating liposomes via application of quality by design (QbD) approach. *J. Liposome Res., 28* (1), 49–61.

Toyota, H., Asai, T., & Oku, N., (2017). Process optimization by use of design of experiments: Application for liposomalization of FK506. *Eur. J. Pharm. Sci., 102*, 196–202.

Tye, H., (2004). Application of statistical 'design of experiments' methods in drug discovery. *Drug Discov. Today, 9* (11), 485–491.

Verma, S., Lan, Y., Gokhale, R., & Burgess, D. J., (2009). Quality by design approach to understand the process of nanosuspension preparation. *Int. J. Pharm., 377* (1&2), 185–198.

Xu, X., Costa, A. P., Khan, M. A., & Burgess, D. J., (2012). Application of quality by design to formulation and processing of protein liposomes. *Int. J. Pharm., 434* (1&2), 349–359.

Yerlikaya, F., et al., (2013). Development and evaluation of paclitaxel nanoparticles using a quality-by-design approach. *J. Pharm. Sci., 102* (10), 3748–3761.

Zhao, C., et al., (2006). Toward intelligent decision support for pharmaceutical product development. *J. Pharm. Innov., 1* (1), 23–35.

CHAPTER 6

Recent Advances in the Development of Semisolid Dosage Forms

RABINARAYAN PARHI

Department of Pharmaceutical Sciences, Susruta School of Medical and Paramedical Sciences, Assam University (A Central University), Silchar, Assam

*Corresponding author. E-mail: rabi59bls623@gmail.com

ABSTRACT

Dosage forms are defined as the systems comprised of one or more active ingredients in association with inert excipients (additives) that constitute the vehicle or formulation matrix. These additives are usually incorporated in the formulation to enhance physical appearance (aesthetic value), facilitate handling, improve stability and potentially influence the absorption and/or bioavailability of the active ingredients. In this context, pharmaceutical semisolid dosage forms including ointment, cream and gels contain one or more medicaments dissolved in or dispersed in a suitable base and appropriate excipients such as emulsifier, gelling agent, viscosity modifiers, antimicrobial agents, antioxidants and or stabilizing agents. These conventional forms of semisolids are meant for delivering drugs into skin and body cavities. But, the recent development in semisolid dosage forms is mainly oriented towards the systemic circulation and more particularly site-specific delivery of drug in an amount, which can elicit therapeutic action. Therefore, this chapter focuses on recent advances in semisolid dosage forms to enhance their aesthetic value and to increase the drug permeation across the skin without impacting their stability, including micro- and nanoemulsion (NE) systems, bioadhesive/mucoadhesive gel, in situ gels (e.g., thermal gel), in situ injectable gels, semisolid containing vesicular systems (e.g., liposomes, ethosomes, niosomes, proniosomes, ethosomesand transfersomes, and particulate systems (such as polymeric micro- and nanoparticles, lipid-based particles), cryogels, and pluronic lecithin organogels (PLO). This article also discusses the theory of semisolids, new tools available for the evaluation of semisolids. Furthermore, regulatory requirements for the semisolid dosage forms are also described in this chapter.

6.1   INTRODUCTION

Pharmaceutical products applied topically are generally categorized into two classes, those applied with the intention to exert local action and those applied to produce the systemic action. Transdermal patches are exclusively belongs to latter category, whereas semisolids such as ointments, creams, and gels can belong to either category as they can be used to target either skin tissues (intradermal) for local action or can be used to help the drug to cross skin barriers to exert systemic effects (transdermal) (Ueda et al., 2009). Therefore, pharmaceutical semisolid preparations are refereed to topical products intended for the application on the skin or accessible mucous membranes to provide basically localized action at the site of application and occasionally systemic effects.

Traditional semisolids comprised of ointments, creams, and gels. Ointments are the semisolid dosage forms intended for the application to the skin or mucous membrane. They generally composed of higher than 50% hydrocarbons, waxes or polyols as vehicles and less than 20% of water. Creams are semisolid dosage forms that contain one or more drug substances dissolved or dispersed in a suitable base. They are either oil-in-water (o/w) or water-in-oil (w/o) types. Gels are semisolid preparations that composed of either suspension of small organic particles or large organic molecules interpenetrated by a liquid. Thus, in the gel system, a liquid phase is constrained within a rigid three-dimensional polymeric network. Among the three types of semisolids, gels usually have higher patient acceptability due to their transparent characteristics and contain a high ratio of solvent to the gelling agent (Vintiloiu and Leroux, 2008; Kumar and Verma, 2010; Parhi, 2017).

Semisolid dosage forms have certain advantages over orally administers dosage forms, including less amount of drug required to treat local ailments (e.g., dermatitis, inflammation) as there is no requirement of drug distribution across the body, rapid onset of action as they are applied locally, less or no side effects as they are applied at the site where the action is desired, first-pass effect can be avoided as the drug molecules are not subjected to degradation by enzymes present in GI tract and lover, and no toxic effect due to higher dose administration as it offers drug termination in any time after application. Furthermore, semisolids not only serve as carriers for drugs to be delivered to the skin but also to various body cavities such as rectum, nose, eye, vagina, buccal cavity, external ear and urethral membrane (Idson and Lazarus, 1991). Compared to parenteral administration semisolids increase patient compliance and acceptance as self-administration is possible, there are no pain and infection at the administered site, avoids stress for the patient due to invasiveness of injection, and there is no requirement of frequent outpatient visits and qualified medical staff for the administration (Hajdukiewicz et al., 2013). Similarly, transdermal patches due to its occlusive nature produce local skin problems such as irritation, redness, blistering and microbial proliferation thereby reducing patient compliance and acceptance (Valenzuela and Simon, 2012; Yapar and Inal, 2014; Lopez et al., 2011). Furthermore, to prepare multicomponent systems such as patch and to avoid the drug crystallization problem on storage has always been a challenge (Parhi and Swain, 2018). In addition, specific types of semisolids such as bioadhesive and *in-situ* forming gel can provide sustained drug effects resulting in the reduction of dosing frequency.

Despite all above advantages, traditional semi-solid dosage forms suffers due to inherent problems such as dosage inaccuracy, instability as the bases in semisolids can be easily oxidized, possibility of their removal from the applied skin surface due to contact, wetting and body movement and finally to achieve desired concentration of drug in the plasma limits the use of number of drug for systemic action (Kumar and Verma, 2010; Maqbool et al., 2017).

To circumvent the above limitations various improvements are imminent. This includes adhering the dosage forms on the skin or mucous membrane for prolong period of time with bioadhesive or mucoadhesive gel systems, *in-situ* gelling systems, delivering the amount of drug sufficient enough to produce desired systemic effect with semisolids incorporated with nanoparticles (polymeric as well as solid lipid nanoparticles) and vesicular systems (liposomes, niosomes, transfersomes, etc.), releasing the incorporated drug in a controlled manner with the use of nanocomposite systems and avoiding any possibility of local skin problems with lecithin organogels are employed. Semisolids are continued to be a significant proportion of pharmaceutical dosage forms. The worldwide research on semisolids can be reflected in the ever-increasing number of publications throughout the years. Figure 6.1 demonstrated the number of Scopus indexed publications from 1998 to October 2018 pertaining to research on semisolids.

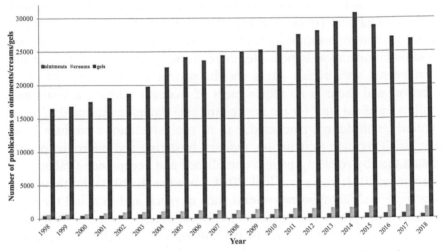

FIGURE 6.1 Scopus indexed publications related to semisolids such as ointments, creams, and gels.

Therefore, this chapter discussed various advancements in the semisolids in recent times including bioadhesive/mucoadhesive systems, *in-situ* gelling systems, nano-semisolids, cryogel, a gel containing vesicular systems, nanocomposite gel systems. In addition, advancement in the evaluation is discussed along with regulatory requirements for semisolid.

6.2 COMPOSITION AND CLASSIFICATION

Semisolid dosage forms are generally complex formulations consisting of complex structural elements. The basic composition of the semisolid dosage form is unique to its particular need, but usually contains active ingredients, solubilizers, antioxidants, and preservatives. Bases are the major components of an ointment. Creams are generally composed of two phases namely: oil and water. Between two phases, one phase is a discontinuous phase (internal phase), which is dispersed uniformly across a continuous phase (external phase) to produce either o/w or w/o types of creams. However, the gel is composed of a gelator molecule disperses in an appropriate solvent (Figure 6.2). The active ingredient is generally is dissolved in the base (ointment), either in the phases (cream) or insolvent (gel). The physical properties and the release of the incorporated drug depends on various factors, including interfacial tension between the phases, the particle size of the dispersed phase, drug's portioning ability between the phases and finally the rheology of the resulted product (Lieberman et al., 1989).

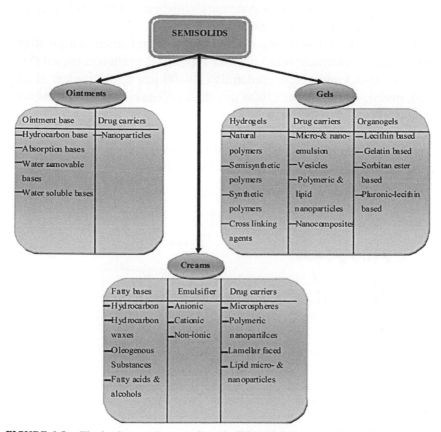

FIGURE 6.2   The basic constituents of semisolids with incorporated novel carriers.

6.3   THEORY OF SEMISOLID DOSAGE FORMS

Semisolids are the drug products intended to deliver the drug in the skin or in the body cavities for local action or into the bloodstream for systemic action. Semisolids incorporate drug classes such as non-steroidal anti-inflammatory agents (NSAIDs) to treat deeper tissues such as muscles and sunscreens and anti-infective for surface action. In the case of systemic action, the drugs have to cross the different skin layers to reach systemic circulation in the desired concentration. Therefore, the former is termed as intra-dermal drug delivery and later is termed as percutaneous/systemic/transdermal drug delivery (TDD) (Kumar and Katare, 2005; Mills and Cross, 2006). However, a small fraction of these drugs present in a topical product intended for skin target may unintentionally reach to the systemic circulation, but in sub-therapeutic concentrations and does not produce any effects.

The human skin is consisting of three physically and functionally distinct layers namely: outermost skin layer has superficial stratum corneum (SC, 10–20 μm thick) and viable epidermis (50-100 μm thick) (Selzer et al., 2013), middle dermis layer (2000 μm thick) contains blood vessels and nerves (Bal et al., 2010), and subcutaneous layer composed of adipocytes. Apart from three major layers, the skin also has appendages on its surface, including hair follicles associated with sebaceous gland (pilosebaceous gland) and sweat glands such as eccrine and apocrine (Figure 6.3).

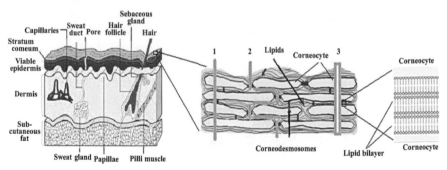

FIGURE 6.3 Representation of cross-section of human skin (left). Brick and mortar model (middle) with penetration pathways: 1 – transcellular, 2 – intercellular, and 3 – transappendageal routes. Arrangement of lipid layer (right).

Whether the target is skin or systemic circulation, the drug present in the semisolids formulations has to cross SC, the main barrier in drug transport into or across the skin. SC composed of corneocytes (made of keratin protein) distributed in a continuous matrix of bilipid layer in a special type of arrangements called "bricks and mortar" structure (Selzer et al., 2013). Here, bricks referred to corneocytes which provide a high degree of tortuosity to the path of drug molecules, whereas mortar corresponds to organized lamellar bilipid structure that imparts a tight barrier property to the already tortuous route of drug permeation (Meno, 2002).

Basically, there are two potential routes through which drug molecules can cross SC and reach either to adjacent layers of skin or to the systemic circulation, including the transepidermal route and transappendageal route. The drug pathway across the brick and mortar structure is considered as a transepidermal route, which may be though the corneocytes (transcellular) or between the corneocytes and across the bilipid layer (intercellular). Transcellular penetration is less likely to happen because the drug molecules have to partition repeatedly between the lipophilic layer and the hydrophilic layer consisting of corneocytes. Therefore, penetration of drug molecules across SC is usually achieved through the intercellular route (Menon and Ghadially, 1997). In transappendageal route, the movements of drug molecules occur through either the eccrine-sweat glands or hair follicles (Mills and Cross, 2006). The advantage of drug delivery via transappendageal route is that very high molecular weight molecules and substances such as nanoparticles and vesicular systems can be delivered in the desire amount. In addition, this route contributed to the rapid diffusion of drug molecules much before the steady-state. However, the presence of 0.1% of the total surface area of human skin limits the use of transappendageal route for drug delivery (Lane, 2013).

Drug permeation/absorption into the skin is usually occurred by passive diffusion and the permeation rate across the SC follows Fick's law of diffusion (Alkilani et al., 2015). The rate of drug permeation, dQ/dt, across SC in the steady-state is expressed in Eq. (6.1) as:

$$\frac{dQ}{dt} = P_s \ (C_d - C_r) \tag{6.1}$$

where, dQ/dt is the steady-state flux across SC, Cd, and Cr are the concentration of drug on the skin surface (in the donor compartment) and in the skin (receptor compartment), respectively, Ps is overall permeability coefficient of the skin tissue to the penetrant and expressed in Eq. (6.2) as:

$$Ps = \frac{KsDs}{hs} \tag{6.2}$$

where, Ks is the partition coefficient of the penetrant molecule from formulation to SC surface, Dss is apparent diffusivity for the steady-state diffusion of the penetrant across the thickness of skin, hs. Under the sink condition C_d is greater than C_r, therefore (Cd–Cr) is reduced to Cd. Inserting the value of Ps in the final Eq. (3) is:

$$\frac{dQ}{dt} = \frac{KsDsCd}{hs} \tag{3}$$

Ps can be measured from the slope obtained by plotting cumulative permeation of permeant on the y-axis and time on the x-axis, which are obtained from an experimental study.

From the typical permeation plot Figure 6.4, it can be concluded that the initial portion indicates a non-steady state of diffusion and later portion demonstrates the steady state of diffusion. Diffusion of the drug across SC is influenced by characteristics of the permeant, the properties of the medium in which the permeant is either dissolved or dispersed and other ingredients present in the formulations. Whereas percutaneous absorption based on two steps: the first step is epidermal diffusion, and the second step is the clearance of permeant from the dermis to systemic circulation which influenced by interstitial fluid moment, blood flow and other factors associated with dermal constituents.

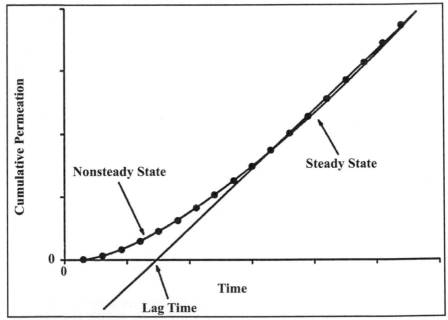

FIGURE 6.4 A typical plot of permeation study (Reprinted with permission from Alkilani et al., 2015. Copyright © 2015 by the authors; licensee MDPI, Basel, Switzerland. https://creativecommons.org/licenses/by/4.0/)

6.4 RECENT ADVANCES

Novel semisolids should possess characteristics such as nongreasy, less irritant, excellent emollient effect, and better spreadability. Non-greasy property and higher emollient effect can be achieved by using water washable bases and incorporation of microspheres and nanoparticles, respectively. In addition, the incorporation of particulate systems in semisolids facilitates the spreading ability of semisolids on the skin surface.

6.4.1 OINTMENTS

The novelty in the case of ointments can be achieved by incorporating a base that will absorb excess water and promote drug permeation across or into the skin. In addition, the applied ointment should form an occlusive film that prevents moisture evaporation from the skin and should not produce any type of discomfort to the skin after application. The recent advancement in ointments is the use of novel hot-melt extrusion (HME) method to prepare ointments, nanoparticles in ointments and gene delivery.

6.4.1.1 HOT-MELT EXTRUSION METHOD

Fusion and levigation are the general methods used to prepare ointments. In the fusion method, ointments are being manufactured by melting oil and aqueous phase in two different jacketed vessels with mixing elements such as agitators. Then, both phases are transferred into the main ointment vessel and mixed thoroughly. Most often, non-uniform distribution of drugs in base and formation of agglomerates are the main limitations of the above methods due to improper design and insufficient mixing. These problems augmented if dead spots are present in the vessels (http://www.pharmaceuticalmachinery.in/ointment_section.htm). Therefore, a novel, robust and limitations free method called HME. The arrangement has a modified screw design along with an optimized feeding rate, barrel temperature and screw speed were in place to produce uniform products (Bhagurkar et al., 2016). Figure 6.5 represents the preparation of ointment based on polyethylene glycol (PG) base containing lidocaine as a model drug using HME technique.

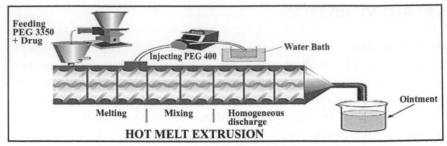

FIGURE 6.5   Schematic diagram of hot-melt extrusion technology used to prepare ointment (Reprinted by permission from Bhagurkar et al., 2016. © Springer Nature.)

6.4.1.2   OINTMENTS CONTAINING NANOPARTICLES

Nanoparticles are also incorporated into ointments in order to improve their ability as DDS. Recently, a novel ointment composed of silver chloride nanoparticles stabilized with chitosan oligomer (AgCl-CHI-NPs) was developed to investigate its potential as an antibacterial on burn wound healing in the rat model. The burn treated with AgCl-CHI-NPs based ointments demonstrated complete healing in 14 treatment days because of the highest regenerated collagen density compared to Vaseline and chitosan ointments treated animal groups (Kang et al., 2016). In another study, Ag-NPs based ointment showed better wound healing properties in the rabbit model and therefore could be used as an alternative to antibiotic cream whenever there is any chance of antibiotic resistance (Ponnaian et al., 2015).

6.4.1.3   GENE THERAPY

In the present time the use of gene therapy to stimulates skin angiogenesis is of great interest in the health care sector as this gene therapy stimulates the formation of new blood vessels in the skin and develop a new avenue in the treatment of various diseases dependent on angiogenesis, including cancer, diabetes, and psoriasis (Małecki et al., 2005). Presently, gene therapy clinical trials are mainly performed with injection preparation which has its own limitations, such as their clinical availability and other parenteral disadvantages (Hajdukiewicz et al., 2013). To circumvent above limitations, gene therapy using both viral and non-viral vectors are applied on the skin in ointment based on cholesterol and the number of a blood vessel formed in the mouse skin was counted using Sidky and Auerbach suggested method. Compared to injection therapy, ointment application formed 3–4 times weaker blood vessels in the skin. Between viral and non-viral vectors, the former strongly stimulate new vessel formation in the mouse skin (Hajdukiewicz et al., 2013).

6.4.2 CREAMS

Compared to ointments there are more advancement happened in the form of creams containing microspheres and lipid micro- and nanoparticles, and lamellar faced creams.

6.4.2.1 CREAMS CONTAINING MICROSPHERES

Microspheres are small spherical, free-flowing particles with an average diameter of particles in the micrometer range (1 μm to 1000 μm) consisting of polymers or proteins (Hussain et al., 1983; Patel et al., 2011). Microspheres are also referred to as microparticles and micro-beads. Microspheres containing therapeutic agents incorporated in creams basically to control the drug release. For instance, urea is encapsulated in poly (D, L-lactic-co-glycolic acid) (PLGA)-based microparticles of size ranging from 1 to 5 μm and then loaded in o/w and w/o creams in order to avoid stability issues with urea. Both the creams containing microparticles showed the slower release of urea compared to a cream containing urea. The w/o creams containing microparticles demonstrated zero-order release profile, whereas o/w creams exhibited Higuchi kinetics (Haddadi et al., 2008).

Microspheres in cosmetic cream formulations are widely studied because these formulations can improve feel, optical blurring, better drug absorption, and to stabilize the incorporated drugs. In one study, albumin microspheres (222±25 μm) incorporated with Vitamin-A was developed and then dispersed in a cream base. *In-vivo* study on a group of six human volunteers showed retention in the skin for a long period of time; thereby release vitamin A for an extended period (Bharat et al., 2011). In another study, to improve the effectiveness of sunscreen agents and photostability, ethylhexyl methoxycinnamate (EHM) is loaded in polymethylmethacrylate (PMMA) based microspheres. The water-removable cream-based formulations containing EHM microspheres exhibited better sun protection factor (SPF) (>16.0) and photostability in comparison to a cream containing 3% free EHM (Gogna et al., 2007).

6.4.2.2   CREAMS CONTAINING NANOPARTICLES

Creams containing nanoparticles also termed as nano-cream or semi-solid emulsion is having advantages over normal cream formulations, including the smooth and uniform spreading of deposition on the skin and enhanced release of active ingredients on or into the skin (Bouchemal et al., 2004; Rajalakshmi et al., 2011). Like cream containing microspheres, nano-creams are also very widely used in cosmetics and personal care.

Due to poor aqueous solubility and short half-life, the administration of dacarbazine (DZ) in the oral route is limited. Therefore, dacarbazine nanoparticles were prepared and then laden into the cream base. The obtained nanoparticles size was 16.9±7.8 nm and the cytotoxicity was found to decrease compared to the pure drug (Hafeez and Kazmi, 2017). Likewise, solubility and absorption of curcumin were increased by converting it into nanoparticles and then incorporating it into the cream. The resulted cream containing curcumin nanoparticles was found to be effective against human bacterial pathogens, including *E. Coli, Staphylococcus aureus* and *Pseudomonas aeruginosa* (Pandit et al., 2015). Creams containing morin-NPs (90.6nm) demonstrated excellent sun protection factor (≈ 40) and showed higher deposition in the skin. The optimized sunscreen creams exhibited exceptional anti-oxidant property and UV radiation protection along with excellent dermal safety (Shetty et al., 2015). Both hydrocortisone (HC) and hydroxytyrosol (HT) were loaded in chitosan-based nanoparticles. The cream containing above nanoparticles showed good stability at 25°C and there was no indication of local redness, irritation, and toxicity (Siddique et al., 2017).

6.4.2.3   LAMELLAR FACED CREAMS

Lamellar faced creams, an o/w emulsion, composed of fatty alcohol, water along with cationic surfactant, generally cetrimide. The cationic surfactant demonstrated phenomenal swelling in water due to electrostatic repulsion (Patel et al., 2013; Bharat et al., 2011). Another technology called derma membrane structure (DMS), which stands for the lamellar cream base has been developed for the treatment of barrier disorders in the skin due to its water- and sweat proof properties along with structural similarity with skin structure. They are composed of soy phosphatidylcholine, sebum compatible medium-chain triglycerides, phytosterols, and squalane. In one investigation, skin-whitening ingredients such as 3-O-ethyl-ascorbic acid (EA) and potassium 4-methoxysalicylate (4-MSK) were incorporated into lamellar liquid crystalline cream (LLC) in order to improve their the skin retention as shown in Figure 6.6. LLC cream demonstrated a significant increase in the skin retention of the ingredients compared to simple o/w emulsion cream (Li et al., 2016).

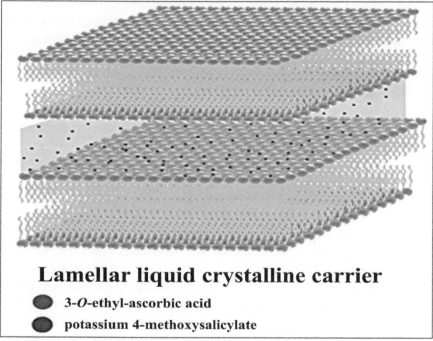

Lamellar liquid crystalline carrier

● **3-O-ethyl-ascorbic acid**

● **potassium 4-methoxysalicylate**

FIGURE 6.6 Schematic representation of the LLC system loaded with EA and 4-MSK (Reprinted with permission from Li et al., 2016 . © Springer Nature.)

6.4.2.4 CREAM CONTAINING LIPID MICRO- AND NANOPARTICLES

Occlusivity is an important criterion for any semisolid preparations. In the case of creams, occlusivity increases the penetration of drugs into the skin by reducing water loss from the skin surface and thereby increasing skin hydration. This can be achieved by using oils and fats (liquid and semisolid paraffin) in large quantities in cream preparation. However, these creams resulted in providing poor cosmetic properties including greasy feel and glossy appearance. To circumvent these limitations, solid paraffin particles with a mean size of 200 nm can be used to form nanodispersion creams. These nanodispersion showed rough texture when applied to the skin. Therefore, lipid micro- or nanoparticles are incorporated in the aqueous phase of water in oil cream, wherein the external oil phase played a key role as a lubricant (Farboud et al., 2011; Patel et al., 2013). Other advantages of lipid particulate systems are discussed in a later section of this chapter.

The stability of butyl methoxydibenzollmethane (avobenzone) was found to be significantly improved when solid lipid microparticles (SLM) of the actives were incorporated in cream. Furthermore, SLM prepared by the spray congealing method showed the better results in terms of avobenzone stability compared to SLM prepared by melt dispersion method, when both were incorporated in cream (Albertini et al., 2009). Coenzyme Q10 (CoQ10) loaded solid lipid nanoparticles (SLN) cream exhibited prolonged release with biphasic release pattern of actives compared to simple cream. In addition, *in-vivo* skin hydration and elasticity studies demonstrated a good dermal penetration and needed activity of Q10 on the skin (Farboud et al., 2011). SLN of 6-methyl-3-phenethyle-3, 4dihydro-1H-quinazoline-2-thione (JSH18), a depigmentation agent, of particle size ranging from 59.8 to 919.6 nm were developed and then incorporated in cream. The optimized SLM cream-containing 4 μM of JSH18 showed a quick recovery of UV irradiated rat skin to normal compared to SLN creams without active ingredients (So et al., 2010). Water removable cream base formulation containing SLN of sunscreen agent oxybenzone (5%) demonstrated controlled drug release and higher SPF (>25) compared to cream base without SLN. Confocal Laser Scanning Microscopy indicated SLN containing cream showed the better distribution and prolonged retention of SLNs in the SC compared to simple cream (Gulbake et al., 2010).

6.4.3   GELS

6.4.3.1   MUCOADHESIVE/BIOADHESIVE GELS

Adhesion is the process of formation of attractive bonds between a pressure-sensitive adhesive and a surface that resists separation. Alternatively, it can be defined as the state in which two surfaces are held together by interfacial forces involving either valence forces or interlocking action or both (Kinloch, 1982; Jimenez-Castellanos et al., 1993). The adhesion could be strong if both the surfaces have the ability to form covalent, ionic or metallic bonds along with weaker forces, including van der Waals interaction, dipole-dipole and hydrogen bonding (Bhushan, 2003). Bioadhesion is a specific case of adhesion involving two substrates, at least one biological in nature, are held together for an extended period of time due to interfacial forces. It can also be defined as the ability of a material (natural/synthetic) to adhere to a biological tissue for a considerable period of time (Jimenez-Castellanos et al., 1993). In addition, bioadhesion is particularly referred to as mucoadhesion if the biological tissue or adherent surface is a mucosal surface (Park and Robinson, 1984; Andrews et al., 2009). From the drug delivery perspective, the bioadhesion implies the attachment of a drug delivery carrier to a specific location. Bioadhesive polymers as a whole and mucoadhesive polymer as particular has been widely used to improve the delivery of therapeutic agents from different semi-solid dosage forms such as gels, creams, and ointments due to their potential advantages. Among many, the increase in residence time of dosage forms at the site of application due to interaction between biological tissue and mucoadhesive dosage forms leading to higher bioavailability, localized drug delivery in the desired regions such as skin and various body cavities, modification of permeability of mucosal tissue or membranes resulted in enhanced adsorption of micro- and macromolecules, and providing sustained or controlled release of therapeutic agents, thereby reducing frequency of application and patient compliance (Khutoryanskiy, 2011).

Bioadhesion/mucoadhesion is a complex process and several theories have been proposed to understand the mechanism of adhesion (Yu et al., 2014; Donnelly and Wolfson, 2013). The theories are: (1) the wetting theory is a measure of spreadability of a semisolids over the biological substrate and involves interfacial tension and intermolecular interaction between formulation and biological tissue (Gu et al., 1988; Shaikh et al., 2011); (2) the electronic theory based on the transfer of electrons between bioadhesive platform and mucous leading to formation of electrical double layer at the interface and generating attractive forces all along the double layer (Carvalho et al., 2010; Dodou et al., 2005); (3) adsorption theory depends on surface interactions, such as permanent interaction involving primary chemical bonds e.g., ionic and covalent bond and semi-permanent interactions due to secondary chemical bonds including van der Waals forces, hydrogen bonding and hydrophobic interactions (Jimenez-Castellanos et al., 1993; Ahagon and Gent, 1975); (4) the diffusion theory involves the interpenetration and entanglement between the polymeric chain and mucous (Vasir et al., 2003); (5) fracture theory is the measure of the force required (adhesive/fracture strength) to separate mucoadhesive system and mucous surface (Gu et al., 1988; Jimenez-Castellanos et al., 1993); and (6) the mechanical interlocking theory relates to the adhesion between a rough surface or surface having pores and mucoadhesive systems (Carvalho et al., 2010). There are various factors influencing the bioadhesion, including polymer related factors such as molecular weight polymer, the concentration of active polymer, the flexibility of polymer chains and spatial conformations, and environmental factors such as pH, initially applied strength, contact time, swelling and selection of model substrate (Donnelly and Wolfson, 2013). There are many bioadhesive polymers used in the pharmaceutical field are listed elsewhere in the literature (Dasari et al., 2007).

Chitosan-based bioadhesive gel containing insulin was developed for nasal delivery. The optimized gel was found to compose of 2% LMW chitosan with EDTA and showed zero-order kinetics in insulin release. The optimized gel in the nasal route demonstrated increased insulin absorption and a decrease in glucose level by as much as 46% of IV administration (Varshosaz et al., 2006).

6.4.3.2   IN-SITU GELS

In-situ gels are polymeric solutions that are in sol form in the container, i.e., before application, but change to gel forms under various physiological conditions. The gelation or sol-gel transition is triggered by one or a combination of different stimuli. *The in-situ* gel is considered to possess both the diffusive transport characteristics of liquids and cohesive properties of solids due to the presence of a swollen network of polymer (Abdel-Mottaleb et al., 2007). These novel semisolid dosage forms are having many advantages: (i) compared to hydrogel, these gels adhere well to skin or mucous membrane or secreting fluid from the body; (ii) improve contact time and retention, especially for ophthalmic delivery of *in-situ* gel, compared to eye drops having short residence time due to lachrymation, solution drainage and non-productive absorption by conjunctiva; (iii) prolonged and sustained action of drug; (iv) ease of application due to their minimum viscosity and reduced frequency of administration;

(v) protection of drug from external environment; (vi) both natural and synthetic polymers can be used; and (vi) potentially can be used in all most all drug delivery routes, including oral, buccal, rectal, vaginal, ocular, parenteral and intraperitoneal routes (Kouchak et al., 2014). Various natural and synthetic polymers used in the preparation of *in-situ* gel are summarized in Table 6.1. There are various approaches in the preparation of *in-situ* gel DDS, including physiological stimuli, physical changes in biomaterial and chemical reactions as described in Table 6.2.

TABLE 6.1 List of Polymers Used in the Preparation of *In-Situ* Gels (Kumbhar et al., 2013)

Polymers	Examples
Natural	Alginic acid, Chitosan, Pectin, Dextran, Gellan gum, Xyloglucan
Synthetic	Poly(lactic acid), Poly(glycolic acid), Poly(D,L-lactide)-PEG-poly((D,L-lactide), Poly-ε-caprolactone, Poly (N-isopropyl acrylamide)

6.4.3.2.1 *Thermogel*

Thermogel is also called thermal gel or temperature-sensitive gel. These are class of gel which undergoes phase transition i.e., sol to gel and vice versa or swelling/shrinking in response to the change in temperature. These gels are of two types based on the temperature of sol-gel transition such as negative and positive temperature-sensitive systems. A negative temperature system gel has a lower critical transition temperature (LCTT) and became gel or shrink at a temperature above LCTT. Conversely, a positive temperature-sensitive hydrogel has an upper critical transition temperature (UCTT). Thus, these hydrogels contract upon cooling below the UCST (Mahalingam et al., 2008). A list of polymers with their LCTT and UCTT are presented in Table 6.3. POL (Pluronic®) is a group of polymers that forms a thermosensitive gel in aqueous solutions and showed LCTS. In fact, POL exhibits thermoreversible gel property, i.e., at refrigerated condition (at 4°C) the POL in water present in the form of solution and become gel at body/room temperature. Reversible gels are those which have the ability to make, break or modify the bonds accountable for holding the polymeric network together (Escobar-Chávez et al., 2006; Dumortier et al., 2006).

TABLE 6.2 Various Approaches with Their Mechanisms and Examples of Polymer (Kumbharet al., 2013; Mahalingam et al., 2008; Jain et al., 2007; Murdan, 2003; Nirmal et al., 2010; Davis et al., 2003)

Approaches	Triggering factors	Mechanism	Example of polymers
Physiological stimuli	pH	The polymers containing pendant acidic or basic groups which either accept or release protons in response to changes in environmental pH. Accordingly, the polymers with a higher number of ionizable groups are called polyelectrolytes. External pH increases in the case of weakly acidic (anionic) groups resulting in swelling of the hydrogel, whereas weakly basic (cationic) groups, decrease swelling.	Carbopol, polyvinylacetal diethyl aminoacetate (AEA), poly (acrylic acid) (PAA)
	Temperature	Thermally-induced sol-gel transition based on the concept of conversion of a polymeric solution containing the drug in to gel due to change in temperature upon application into the body and form the implant system due to change in temperature. (Detail discussion are made in Section 6.4.3.2.1).	Poly(N-isopropyl acrylamide (PNIPAAM), Poloxamer (POL)
Physical changes in biomaterials	Solvent exchange/ Diffusion	This method involves the diffusion of solvent from polymer solution into surrounding tissue and results in precipitation or solidification of the polymer matrix.	N-methyl pyrrolidone (NMP).
	Swelling	Swelling mechanism is based on the absorption of water from surrounding environment and subsequently, expands in desired space.	Myverol 18-99 (glycerol mono-oleate)

TABLE 6.2 *(Continued)*

Approaches	Triggering factors	Mechanism	Example of polymers
Chemical reactions	Enzymatic	This approach based on the conversion of sol to gel upon the catalyzed reaction of available enzymes at the site of application such as body cavities.	Cationic pH-sensitive polymers containing immobilized insulin and glucose oxidase.
	Ionic	Polymers may undergo phase transition in the presence of various ions. Some of the the polysaccharides fall into the class of ion-sensitive ones.	(i) k-carrageenan forms rigid, brittle gels in reply of a small amount of K^+. (ii) Gellan gum (Gelrite®) forms gel with Ca^{2+}, Mg^{2+}, K^+, and Na^+. (iii) Low-methoxy pectin forms gel with Ca^{2+}
	Photo-initiated polymerization	When the solution of monomer or macromer molecules and photosensitive initiators are exposed to light (e.g., UV light), the monomers or micromeres form network by rapid cross-linking thereby entrap incorporated drug inside and releases them at a predetermined rate.	PEG- olgoglycolylacrylates and PEG-PLA.

TABLE 6.3   Examples of Polymers with Their Phase Transition Temperature (Kumbharet al., 2013)

Polymers with LCTT behavior	Phase transition temperature (°C) in aqueous solution
POL	20–85
Poly(N,N-diethyl acrylamide)	32–34
PNIPAM	30–34
Poly(methyl vinyl ether)	37
Poly(N-vinyl caprolactam)	30–35
Poly(GVGVP)	28–30
Polymers with UCTT behavior	
PAAm/PAAc	25

POL is a tri-block polymer consisting of hydrophobic polypropylene oxide (PPO) blocks at the center and hydrophilic polyethylene oxide (PEO) blocks on either side. The gelation phenomenon of POL in the aqueous solution not only depends on temperature but also on concentration POL in an aqueous medium (Escobar-Chávez et al., 2006). The gelation of an aqueous solution of POL has two steps, namely: micellization and gelation. In the micellization step, spherical micelles are formed due to aggregation of POL monomers at an increased temperature called a critical micellar temperature. Further increase in temperature packs the micelles in an orderly manner to form a gel as shown in Figure 6.7. POL molecules are present in monomer forms at very low concentrations in aqueous solutions. By increasing the concentration of POL up to 10^4 to 10^5 % (w/w) resulted in the formation of spherical micelles due to the attainment of critical micellar concentration. Further increase in concentration leads to a tightly packed system with gel consistency (Antunes et al., 2011; Hemelrijck and Muller-Goymann, 2012). Therefore, POL 407 showed the thermoreversible property at the concentration range of 20-30% in aqueous solution (Parhi, 2016a).

6.4.3.3   CRYOGEL

Cryogels are a class of physically cross-linked hydrogel formed by one or more freezing and thawing cycles (F-T cycle). These are consisting of a water-swellable cross-linked polymer and exhibit both liquid and

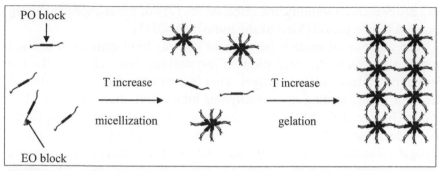

FIGURE 6.7   Schematic representation of the gelation mechanism of POL 407 in water (Reprinted with permission from Dumortier et al., 2006. © Springer Nature.)

solid-state characteristics (Werys et al., 2015). This physical cross-linking method to prepare gel has advantages such as non-toxic, non-carcinogenic, better biocompatibility and enhanced elasticity compared to gel formed by chemically cross-linked gel (Chhatri et al., 2011). Polyvinyl alcohol (PVA) is such as a polymer which forms cryogel.

A standing solution of PVA in water can only form a weak gel at room temperature due to the formation of less number H-bond between adjacent -OH groups. But, F-T cycle leads to the formation of crystallites that plays a crucial role in the cross-linking of PVA chains by strong inter-chain H-bonding. The crystals formed by this method have a two-molecule monoclinic unit cell with -OH groups randomly placed on either side of both polymer chains. It has been assumed that in the first F-T cycle freezing of water leading to expansion which resulted in the increased concentration of polymer in the unfrozen zone. Crystallization can then occur within the polymer-rich macrophages (McGuinness et al., 2015).

Processing parameters, including the number of thermal cycles, thawing rate, and concentration polymers affect the mechanical behavior of cryogel. It was reported that the increase in the number of thermal cycles resulted in the formation of cryogel with higher mechanical strength due to the increase in intermolecular H-bonding and thereby molecular chain aggregates. In addition, there was no change in elastic properties of the above gel by increasing the thawing rate from 0.333C/min to 0.067C/min (Pazos et al., 2009). In another study, four F-T cycles were found to be optimum in the preparation of composite cryogel of metronidazole using PVA and carboxymethyl tamarind kernel polysaccharide. Above cryogel had better thermal stability and released 75.77% of the encapsulated drug over a 6 h time period (Meenakshi and Ahuja, 2015).

The addition of another polymer to PVA to form composite cryogel negatively affects the formation of crystallites and subsequently the formation of less ordered cryogel. This is attributed to the formation of junction points leading to interpolymer interaction after a series of F-T cycles (Berger et al., 2004). The strength and thermal stability were found to be decreased when chitosan was added to PVA to form composite cryogel (Bhattarai et al., 2010). In contrast, the strength of composite cryogel increased with the increase in microcrystalline cellulose content from 0 to 50% wt (Paduraru et al., 2012).

6.4.3.4   INJECTABLE IN-SITU GEL

Initial burst release is one of the major disadvantages pertaining to *in-situ* gel (ISG). This is due to the rapid distribution of the administered drug during the sol-gel transition process leading to an initial high drug release rate and subsequently higher plasma drug concentration (Ahmed et al., 2012; Ahmed et al., 2014). In these cases, biodegradable injectable ISG forming DDS seems to be an attractive alternative. In addition to that, injectable ISG can be a better alternative to liposomes, microspheres, and emulsion as parenteral depot systems. This is because liposomes preparation involves high-cost production and stability issues. Similarly, the microemulsion (ME) formulations suffer due to stability issues. Microspheres manufacturing process is complex. *In-situ* injectable gel has many advantages compared to conventional method of drug administrations, including (i) administration of accurate dose; (ii) ease of administration; (iii) decreased dosing frequency; (iv) maintaining constant plasma drug concentration for prolonged period of time; (v) improved patient compliance and acceptance; and (vi) less complex production process with low manufacturing cost (Nirmal et al., 2010).

There are four approaches to form injectable ISG forming DDS namely: (i) photo cross-linking; (ii) thermally induced sol-gel transition; (iii) pH-dependent; and (iv) solidifying organogels. First, three approaches already discussed in the previous section and solidifying organogels are discussed elsewhere inside the manuscript. ISG forming injectable solutions are different from only ISG as the former must be composed of biodegradable and biocompatible so that it will not produce any remaining residue in the body and at the same time any type of immunological reaction produced inside the body, respectively. There are certain common problems associated with *in-situ* injectable DDS: the shrinkage and brittleness of the polymer due to high cross-linking and *vice versa* may happen in photo cross-linked gels, burst release may be the disadvantage in case of both thermally induced sol-gel transition as well as pH-dependent gels, and lack of toxicity data and phase separations are the limitations of organogels (Kumbhar et al., 2013).

6.4.3.5 GEL CONTAINING MICRO- OR NANOEMULSION

MEs are monophasic, clear, thermodynamically stable, and an isotropic mixture of water, oil, and surfactant, most cases having a co-surfactant, in which either water globules dispersed in oil (W/O) or oil globules dispersed in water (O/W). On the other hand, NEs are thermodynamically stable and require expensive and high-energy input during manufacturing. Micro- or nano-emulsions have many potential advantages such as the ability to solubilize high drug amount, providing long term stability, ease and low cost of preparation (Zhang and Michniak-Kohn, 2011; Kogan and Garti, 2006). The use of ME and NE to deliver the drug in dermal and transdermal routes are widely explored as they can successfully deliver both hydrophilic and lipophilic drugs. Additionally, they deliver drugs across the skin better than any conventional semisolid dosage forms (Fouad et al., 2013). This is possible due to different proposed mechanisms to deliver the drugs into and across the skin as they; (i) have high drug loading capacity resulting in higher thermodynamic activity towards the skin and subsequently higher drug partitioning; (ii) act as strong penetration enhancers; (iii) increased solubility of drugs inside skin by allowing its monomer to enter into the skin; and (iv) allowing to form supersaturated system with a high thermodynamic activity (Hathout and Nasr, 2013). They are relatively more stable at room temperature compared to liposomes (Kweon et al., 2004).

One of the major disadvantages of ME is their low viscosity resulting in poor retention at the affected body surface. Thus, their viscosity needed to be increased by mixing the ME in the plain gel. However, to maintain the globule size is always a challenge to the formulators as it may change upon the incorporation of micro- or nano-emulsion into a gel. In such a case ME of Diclofenac Epolamine was developed using capryol® as oil phase, a mixture of Labrasol® surfactant and Transcutol® as co-solvent in the different ratios (Smix) and water as aqueous phases and then dispersed in gel made up of POL (25%) at 1:2 w/w ratio (ME to gel) in order to have ME in gel formulation with maximum amount of oil and minimum globule size. Compared to only POL gel and commercial Flector® gel, the optimized ME gel showed highest cumulative drug permeated across skin after 8 h of study and the release of drug was continued even after the removal of gel from the skin surface due to the formation of an in-skin depot (Shahinaze et al., 2013). In another case, ME composed of isopropyl myristate (IPM), water, Tween 80 and Labrasol was developed as a transdermal therapeutic system for poorly soluble and lipophilic drugs Lacidipine. The optimized ME gel exhibited higher bioavailability compared to oral suspension of the drug with non-irritant and non-erythema potential upon transdermal administration (Gannu et al., 2010). Similarly, optimized ME of terbinafine based on oleic acid as oil phase (5.75%), Smix (Labrasol at 26.87% and transcutol P at 26.87%) and water (40.5%) was converted into gel form employing 0.75% w/w of carbopol 934P. The globule size and solubility of optimized formulation were found to be 18.14 nm and 43.71 mg/ml, respectively and the cumulative amount of terbinafine permeated across human cadaver skin after 12 h was 244.65 ± 18.43 µg/cm^2 which was 3-fold higher than the selected commercial cream. The optimized ME-based gel showed higher activity against microorganisms such as *Candida albicans* and *Trichophyton rubrum* (Barot et al., 2012). In another study, optimized ME of clobetasol propionate composed of IPM (3%), cremophor EL (15%), IPA (30%), and water (50%) was developed and converted into gel form using carbopol 934P and found to show better retention and less skin irritation potential compared to marketed formulation. The ex vivo permeation study exhibited that the gel containing ME had higher cumulative amount of drug release at 8 h, which was attributed to the interaction between the components of emulsion and skin structure (Patel et al., 2013).

NEs of ropinirole comprised of Capryol 90 as the internal phase, water as an external phase. The highest flux of 51.81 ± 5.03 µg/cm^2/h was observed for the NE formulation containing 0.5% w/w of ropinirole, 5% w/w of Capryol 90, 23.33% w/w of Tween 20, 11.66% w/w of Carbitol and remaining 59.5% w/w of water. This optimized NE was incorporated in carbopol gel employing Box-Behnken design to investigate the effect of oil and polymer concentrations, and drug content. Oil and polymer concentrations showed a negative influence on permeation, whereas drug content had a positive impact on the permeation. In addition, the NE gel demonstrated 7.5 times increase in skin permeation rate compared to the normal gel (Azeem et al., 2009).

6.4.3.6   GEL CONTAINING VESICULAR SYSTEMS

Various approaches have been employed to overcome the percutaneous permeation problem associated with topically applied formulations. Among all the use of the vesicular system is one of the better approaches to breach the barrier property of SC of skin (Chaudhary et al., 2013). Out of different vesicular systems, liposomes, niosomes, proniosomes, ethosomes, and transfersomes are widely used. However, the low viscosity of almost all types of vesicular systems limits their applications as topical formulations either for intradermal or TDD. Therefore, biocompatible gels made up of gelling agent having weak or no interaction with the components of vesicular components can be explored to modify their viscosity so that they can be applied topically.

Liposomes are microscopic vesicular structures with an enclosed aqueous core surrounded by a bilipid layer of amphiphilic molecules such as phospholipids and cholesterol. The sizes of liposomes are greatly varied, but most are ≤400 nm. Liposomes with vesicles in the nanometer range are recognized as nanoliposomes (Mudshinge et al., 2011). Liposomes have the ability to encapsulate both hydrophilic (in the aqueous core) and lipophilic drugs (in the bilipid layer). Unlike nanoparticles and emulsion, liposomes promotes/enhances the drug release in the skin due to their adherence to corneocytes of the skin leading to diffusion or fusion of bilipid layer of liposomes with the cell membrane (Mudshinge et al., 2011). In addition above adherence not only fix the active ingredients in contact with skin but also delays the removal by washing out (Cevc, 1997). Furthermore, liposomes can be used to enhance their targeting capability by modifying their surface compared to other nanoparticles and ME (Goyal et al., 2005). If the phospholipids are of natural origin can prevent undesirable side effects on the skin. Not only that, both phospholipids and liposomes maintains moisture level which helps in restoring the barrier function of the skin (Niemiec et al., 1995).

Liposomal formulations of both naproxen and nimesulide were developed with phospholipon and cholesterol at different ratios and then incorporated into aloe vera-based gel containing carbopol934 as a gelling agent. The permeability coefficient and *in-vivo* efficacy were found to be better in nimesulide based liposomal gel compared to commercial nimesulide gel and aloe vera gel alone (Venkataharshaet al., 2015). In another study, liposomes of prednisolone with dipalmitoyl phosphatidylserine (DPPS), soya lecithin and cholesterol were developed and then dispersed in carbopol 940P based gel. The resulted liposomal gel showed better stability at freezing temperature, higher permeation and deposition in skin compared to control (Varde et al., 2013). Liposomal gel of diflurasone diacetate was developed by incorporating liposomes, prepared with soya and egg phospholipids, of the drug in carbopol based gel (2%). The obtained gel exhibited excellent sustained release of the drug along with better ex vivo permeation leading to more efficient treatment of psoriasis (Umalkar and Rajesh, 2013).

The major drawback of liposomes is its lack of chemical and physical stability. Physical stability is attributed to oxidation and hydrolysis of phospholipids that limits the use of liposomes as DDS (Wang et al., 2015). On the other way, physical instability of liposomes occurs due to aggregation or fusion and sedimentation upon storage. On the contrary, niosomes, a class of molecular clusters developed by the self-association of non-ionic surfactants in an aqueous phase, are chemically stable which resulted in long storage time. In addition, unlike phospholipids, there are no requirements for special precautions and conditions to handle surfactants. Furthermore, niosomes are water-based suspension leading to better patient compliance (Moghassemi and Hadjizadeh, 2014). Niosomes are biocompatible vesicles, less irritating compared to other colloidal vesicle carriers and can improve the penetration of encapsulated actives across the skin (Marianecci et al., 2014; Yapar, 2017).

In one study, niosomes of piroxicam were developed with span 20 and 60 as surfactant along with cholesterol. Thereafter, these niosomes were dispersed in different gels composed of various gelling agents. The niosomal gels demonstrated that the types of a gelling agent influences the viscosity and thereby the permeation of drug across the skin. The best niosomal gel was found to be composed of MC (4%) as a gelling agent which may be due to lower viscosity allowing higher drug release on the skin surface (Ahmed et al., 2014). Lyotropic liquid crystals (LLCs) are self-assembled nanomaterials formed from one/more surfactants and water. Depending on the concentration of different components and temperature used in the preparation, their phase sequence may be off cubic, hexagonal and lamellar. The lamellar phase is widely used in TDD due to their structural similarity with the skin (Kossena et al., 2004). This novel approach was used to develop LLC-niosomal formulations of sulfadiazine sodium, propranolol HCl and tyrosol with sodium bis(2-ethylhexyl) sulfosuccinate (AOT) and pluronic L64 as anionic and non-ionic surfactant, respectively. The niosomal gel showed higher drug permeation compared to the free drug solution and is affected by the chemical structure of drugs (Tavano et al., 2013).

Proniosomes are niosomal hybrid and used as stable precursors for the instant conversion into niosomal carrier systems upon hydration with water (Mokhtar et al., 2008). When applied topically, proniosomes should be hydrated with water accumulated over the skin under occlusion (Alsarra et al., 2005). As a precursor of niosomes, proniosomes avoid physical stability problems of niosomes including aggregation, fusion, and leakage during storage (Ammar et al., 2011).

Oral administration of NSAID tenoxicam leads to severe side effects in the GIT. Therefore, the transdermal route with proniosomal gel as the formulation is most effective for its systemic action. Among various compositions, tween 20 and cholesterol in 9:1 ratio showed high drug entrapment, better release characteristics, and stability. These proniosomes were mixed with carbopol gel (1%) in a 1:1 ratio to obtain proteasomal gel. The resulted proniosomalgel demonstrated significantly higher anti-inflammatory and analgesic activities compared to commercial tenoxicam tablets (Ammar et al., 2011).

Ethosomes are the modified version of liposomes with the exception of the presence of high ethanol content (20-45%) (Chandrababu et al., 2013). These are soft, deformable vesicles and can enhance skin permeation of a large number of drugs. Ethanol is a known penetration enhancer, hence when present in higher concentration causes disorders in the lipid bilayer of SC to a greater extent which resulted in the higher penetration of ethosomes (Ceve, 2004).

In order to avoid side effects such as GI irritation, edema, ulcerative colitis and peptic ulcer upon oral administration of piroxicam, alternative transdermal route, and better dosage form transethosomal gel was employed. Soya phosphatidylcholine (Soya PC) at 2-4% w/v and ethanol in the range of 0-40% v/v found to influence the drug entrapment, drug retention, permeation, and vesicular size. The optimized transethosomal gel formulation of piroxicam demonstrated higher drug entrapment, drug retention and permeation, highest elasticity and improved stability compared to other vesicular systems, including liposomes, ethosomes, and transfersomes (Garg et al., 2017).

More recently, a new type of vesicular carrier system called transfersome has been used as topical preparations for TDD of both low and high molecular weight drugs. Transfersomes are defined as ultra-flexible lipid vesicles composed of at least one aqueous compartment at the center which is surrounded by bilipid layer having a special tailored characteristics owning to the presence of edge activator (Zheng et al., 2012). The presence of edge activator (single chain surfactant having high radius of curvature) make the transfersomes flexible or deformable by decreasing the stiffness of phospholipids (Shuwaili et al., 2016). As a result transfersomes can squeeze through the pores in the SC less than $1/10^{th}$ of their diameter when applied topically under non-occlusive condition. Thus, a size of around 200-300nm can easily penetrate through the SC (Gupta et al., 2012). The hydrostatic pressure difference across the skin is responsible for the passage of intact transfersome through the SC either through transcelluar or intracellular route (Dubey et al., 2006; Chaudhary et al., 2013).

Transfersomes of celecoxib were prepared using soya PC and sodium deoxycholate and then converted into transfersomal gel by dispersing above vesicles in carbopol 940 based dermal gel. Compared to simple celecoxib gel, tranfersomal gel demonstrated better skin permeation ability and stability which may be due to simultaneous presence of stabilizing phospholipids and destabilizing surfactant molecules leading to redistribution of drug in bilayers of transfersomes (Preeti and Kumar, 2013). Another drug sertraline was incorporated in soya lecithin and span 80 based transfersomes in order to circumvent the poor soluble property and troubles associated in oral routes. Tranfersomal gel was prepared using carbopol 940 as gelling agent. The gel composed of 1.6% of the drug and 20% of span 80 was found to be optimized formulation, which demonstrated significantly higher cumulative amount of drug permeation and flux with lower lag time compared to drug solution and simple gel of drug. In addition, tranfersomal gel showed better antidepressant activity than the control gel of drug (Gupta et al., 2012).

6.4.3.7 GEL CONTAINING POLYMERIC NANOPARTICLES

Nanoparticles are generally defined as solid, colloidal drug carriers with diameter ranges from 10 to 1000 nm that may or may not be biodegradable. Previously, non-biodegradable polymers including polyacrylamide, polystyrene and poly(methyl methacrylate) (PMMA) were used to develop nanoparticles. However, later it was found that nanoparticles based on non-biodegradable polymer showed tissue and immunological responses due to chronic toxicity. Therefore, these polymers are replaced with biodegradable polymers such as poly lactic-co-glycolic acid (PLGA), poly (dl-lactic acid) (PLA), poly (caprolactone) (PCL) and poly (butyl cyanoacrylate) as synthetic and chitosan as natural polymers (Mishra et al., 2010). Moreover, these polymers are approved by the U.S. Food and Drug Administration (FDA) (Mudshinge et al., 2011). The major advantages of nanoparticles are: (i) enhancement of bioavailability due to the improvement of aqueous solubility of encapsulated drugs; (ii) increase in half life drug in the body by increasing resistance towards clearance resulting into low dose requirement and reduction in frequency in administration; and (iii) target-specific delivery of drugs in the body, thereby reduces the toxicity by protecting non target tissue and cells from side effects (Mudshinge et al., 2011). Polymeric nanoparticles may be of two types: (i) nanocapsules, having a drug reservoir entrapped inside a solid material shell; and (ii) nanospheres are matrix particles where the drug is uniformly distributed throughout a polymeric matrix (Rao and Geckeler, 2011).

Aceclofenac nanoparticles based on a combination of aceclofenac and egg-albumin were prepared and subsequently characterized and incorporated into carbopol 940 based gels. The gel of optimized nanoparticles (200 mg of chitosan, 500 mg of egg albumin and had the size of 352.90 nm) showed sustained ex-vivo permeation of drug over 8 h across excised mouse skin and also exhibited better anti-inflammatory activity compared to commercial aceclofenac gel (Jana et al., 2014). Polymeric nanoparticles based gels are also used in cosmetic active delivery into the skin. In one such case, nanoparticles loaded with vitamin A and E derivatives are incorporated into gel formulations. The resulted nanogel was found to show increased skin humidity upon the application on skin surface. In addition, the above nanoparticles were capable of penetrating the upper layer of SC and fused with skin lipids resulting in the release of the cosmetic actives (Agrawal et al., 2016).

6.4.3.8   GEL CONTAINING LIPID NANOPARTICLES

Solid lipid nanoparticles (SLN) are submicronic particulate carriers, which composed of lipids that are solid at room temperature such as highly purified triglycerides (e.g., trimyristin, tripalmitin), fatty acids (e.g., stearic acid) and waxes (e.g., cetyl palmitate), emulsifier (e.g., POL, polysorbates), suitable solvents (e.g., ethanol, acetone), and drugs of either hydrophilic and lipophilic characteristics (Mehnert and Mader, 2001). In case of nanostructured lipid carriers (NLC), solid lipid is partially replaced with liquid lipids such as Miglyol 812 to improve drug loading and prevent/minimize the expulsion of drug during manufacturing and storage by inducing great degree of imperfection in the crystal lattice of lipids present within nanoparticles (Date et al., 2007; Jenning et al., 2000; Jenning and Gohla, 2001). These lipid-based nanoparticles combined advantages of liposomes, emulsion and polymeric nanoparticles including the ability to encapsulate both hydrophilic and lipophilic drugs, drug targeting, biocompatibility, biodegradability, enhanced drug loading, increased drug stability and bioavailability, easy scale-up, controlled drug release, prolonging residence time of some actives such as sunscreens in the SC and targeting drug to the upper layer of skin (Nair et al., 2011; Souto and Müller, 2010; Schäfer-Korting et al., 2007; Montenegro, 2017; Almeidaa et al., 2014; Jenning et al., 2000).

Moreover, they have a wide spectrum of applications like oral, intravenous and topical. However, these are prepared in dispersion form which possesses low viscosity approximately 100 mPa.s with yield value of practically zero. Therefore, these lipid-based nanodispersions have to be incorporated in convenient topical dosage forms such as gel or creams to provide desired semisolid consistency (Lippacher and Mäder, 2001). When applied topically, they display benefits such as skin moisturizing effect through occlusion and better suited to be used in case of damaged or inflamed skin because of their non-irritant and non-toxic properties (Gönüllü et al., 2015).

There are many drugs incorporated in either SLN or NLC and then dispersed in gel vehicles to make them suitable for topical applications. Meloxicam loaded SLN-gel was developed and found to show controlled drug release ability. The gel has the capability of the fluidizing the lipid bilayer of SC which was attributed to the interaction of the gel with the skin. Moreover, nano-gel demonstrated significant ant-inflammatory activity and excellent skin tolerability (Khurana et al., 2013). Irritant contact dermatitis (ICD) is generally treated in a long-term basis using topical corticosteroids. However, it can induce skin atrophy, hypopigmentation, and increase in transepidermal water loss. Therefore, resveratrol incorporated SLN with Precirol ATO 5 as lipid and tween 20 as a surfactant was developed and then incorporated in carbopol gel. The resulted nano-gel demonstrated improved skin barrier properties by providing occlusive properties and also improved the drug permeation across the SC with minimum systemic absorption (Shrotriya et al., 2017).

Docetaxel (DTX) belongs to the toxoid family and is used in the treatment of skin tumors and inflammation (Kilfoyle et al., 2012). However, higher molecular weight and poor water solubility limit DTX permeation across the SC (Zahedi et al., 2011). Therefore, being hydrophilic in nature and the ability to co-crystallizing many active ingredients, nicotinamide was used to form complex with DTX to enhance its transdermal penetration. NLC of the complex was developed and dispersed in carbomer 940 based gels. The complex of DTX with nicotinamide in gel vehicle showed better permeability across the skin compared to a gel containing only DTX (Fan et al., 2013). NLC and monoolein aqueous dispersion (MAD) of clotrimazole were prepared and diluted in POL 407 and carbomer based gel. Both the preparation exhibited superimposable diffusion and exhibited higher activity against *Candida albicans* with respect to the pure drug (Esposito et al., 2013). A comparison was made between rosemary oil (RO)-based gel and RO loaded NLC. RO-loaded NLC demonstrated higher skin hydration and elasticity compared to RO loaded gel (Montenegroet al., 2017).

Flurbiprofen based SLN and NLC were prepared and subsequently incorporated into freshly prepared hydrogel prepared with four different gelling agents such as chitosan, carbopol 934, hydroxypropyl cellulose (HPC) and xanthan gum. NLC gel showed C_{max} and AUC values of 1.8-fold and 2.5-fold higher than SLN gel and bioavailability of flurbiprofen was 4.4 times with reference to oral administration. In addition, anti-inflammatory effects were better for SLN and NLC gel compared to oral administration and both the formulations were stable for three months (Bhaskaret al., 2009). SLN, NLC and NE of lornixicam was prepared using Campritol® 888 ATO as solid lipid, Lane e®O and oleic acid as liquid lipids. The highest rate of drug release was achieved with NE followed by NLC, SLN and a gel formulation. Similarly, all nanoformulations significantly improved drug permeation across the rat skin compared to gel (Gönüllü et al., 2015).

6.4.3.9 NANOCOMPOSITE GEL

Nanocomposites are the matrix, which incorporates either a single entity or multiple nanoscale material to improve mechanical, thermal, electrical, electrochemical and optical properties of finished dosage forms (Parhi, 2018; Gilani et al., 2018; Pina et al., 2015; Mariano et al., 2014). Thus, nanocomposites are composed of two components: (i) continuous phase called matrix; and (ii) discontinuous phase or reinforcing phase or nano-fillers dispersed in the matrix as the continuous phase. Based on the nature of the matrix, nanocomposites are broadly classified in to three classes: (i) ceramic; (ii) metallic; and (iii) polymeric nanocomposites (Camargo et al., 2009). Among the three matrix materials, polymeric matrix is widely used in the pharmaceutical field to deliver different therapeutic agents because of many advantages such as better processibility, available in different forms and nature, easy tailoring to different forms and long term stability (Jeon and Baek, 2010). Polymers covering all classes can be used to prepare matrix, including thermoplastics, thermosets, elstomers, and more importantly, specially designed biodegradable and biocompatible polymers have been used for a while (Camargo et al., 2009). The nano-fillers that are used in the development of polymeric nanocomposites may include metals (such as iron, gold, and silver), clays, silica or carbon-based namely graphene oxide, fullerenes, and carbon nanotubes (Krolowet al., 2013). A typical structure of the polymeric matrix nanocomposite is illustrated in Figure 6.8.

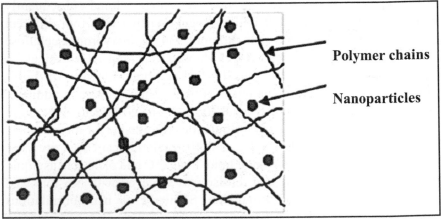

FIGURE 6.8   Typical structure of polymer nanocomposite (Reprinted with permission from Parhi, 2017. © Elsevier.)

A nanocomposite hydrogel of diclofenac sodium was developed with carboxymethyl guar gum (CGG) and nanosilica as polymer and nanofillers, respectively. Out of different concentrations (0.5 to 5 wt%) of nanosilica, 1 wt% showed better uniform dispersion and the same concentration exhibited slowest release but steady transdermal release. The release mechanism was non-Fickian that indicated its ability to encapsulate the drug efficiently. In addition, the above gel demonstrated higher thermal stability (up to 270°C) because of better adhesion between polymer and nanofiller (Giri et al., 2012). The same group of researchershas developed nanocomposite hydrogel of diclofenac sodium by incorporating multi-walled carbon nanotubes (MWCNT) at 0.5, 1 and 3 wt% in CGG.A strong interaction between CGG and MWCNT was observed leading to slow release of drug. In addition the drug encapsulation was increased with the addition of MWCNT and the maximum entrapment and slowest but steady drug release was observed for the gel containing 1wt% of MWCNT (Giri et al., 2011).

6.4.3.9.1   Intelligent Nanocomposite Hydrogel

Intelligent hydrogels are those which exhibit alteration in their structure, property and/or shape with respect to internal or external stimuli (Qiu and Park, 2012). If any nanofillers are incorporated in to the above gel that can respond to particular stimuli are termed as intelligent nanocomposite hydrogel (Figure 6.9). The stimuli that can bring about the changes in gel include electric field, ionic strength, pH, temperature, enzyme and magnetic field (Hoffman, 2013). The important feature of intelligent nanocomposite gel is that the selection of stimuli solely depends on nano-fillers (Merino et al., 2015). The alteration in the hydrogel can control the drug release by virtue of dissolution, erosion and/or swelling. Electro-responsive hydrogel is an example of intelligent nanocomposite hydrogel, which controls the drug release by swelling the gel. An electro-responsive hydrogel composed of PVA and MWCNT was developed for the trans-dermal delivery of Coomassie brilliant blue R-250 (CBB). In response to applied voltage above hydrogel swelled and demonstrated bigger pore diameter. The increase in MWCNT concentration and voltage further increased the pore diameter. This resulted in higher drug release (Kim et al., 2010). Both temperature and pH-responsive nanocomposite hydrogel of CBB with PVA/poly(acrylic acid) (PAA) and PAA/poly(N-isopropylacrylamide) (PNIPAAm) as polymers and MWCNT as nano-fillers was developed. Incorporation of MWCNT had enhanced the thermal and mechanical properties of gel and the release of drug from the gel depends on the amount of MWCNT present in the gel (Jung et al., 2012). Amoxicillin release was sustained from polyacrylamide (PAAm) based hydrogel containing polyaniline nanofibers in response to the application of electric stimulus. Further, the gel showed "ON and OFF" pattern of drug release with the alternate stimulation and removal of electrical potential (Pérez-Martínez et al., 2016).

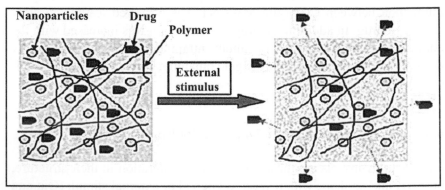

FIGURE 6.9   A typical intelligent nanocomposite hydrogel releasing drug upon stimulated externally (Reprinted with permission from Parhi, 2017. © Elsevier.)

6.4.3.10   PLURONIC LECITHIN ORGANOGELS

Lecithin organogels additionally containing pluronic is termed as pluronic lecithin organogels (PLO) or POL organogels or pluronic organogels or PLO gel. From the application point of view it is recognized as cream owing to is smoother feel when applied on the skin surface. PLOs are composed of lecithin as phospholipid, organic solvents (commonly IPM or IPP), POL and polar solvent, generally water. It is also called as ME based gel as organic solvent containing lecithin dispersed in aqueous solvent containing pluronic (Kumar and Katare, 2005; Franckum et al., 2004). These are widely used as topical and transdermal semisolid dosage form because of it is viscoelastic, thermodynamically stable, biocompatible, and has the ability to incorporate both hydrophilic and lipophilic drugs (Agrawal et al., 2010; Belgamwar et al., 2008). Additionally, it can improve the penetration of drugs across the skin either by increasing diffusivity of incorporated drug due to the presence of IPM/IPP or by disorganizing structure of skin due to the presence of lecithin (Limpongsa and Umprayn, 2008; Parhi et al., 2016b).

Preparation of PLO involves the mixing of oil phase with a chilled aqueous phase employing a high shear mixing method. The oil phase is prepared by mixing lecithin in either IPM or IPP and allowing the resultant mixture to stand overnight for complete dissolution. The aqueous phase is prepared by adding POL to ice-cold water (at 4°C) and keeping it in the refrigerator with intermittent mixing for complete dissolution. PLOs are prone to microbial attack because of presence of aqueous phase as well as lecithin. Therefore, sorbic acid (0.2wt%) is used as preservatives and added both of the phases before preparing the final PLOs (Belgamwar et al., 2008; Murdan, 2005). The organic solvent IPM/IPP can partially or fully replaced with other solvents such as PG and terpenes. Organogels were successfully developed using PG as organic solvent. In addition terpenes such as limonene, cineole and linalool were also added to organic phase to enhance drug permeation (Fung et al., 2006; Fung et al., 2008). When terpenes are used as organic solvent the organogels is called terpene gel. We have prepared PLOs of diltiazem HCl with IPM, a mixture of IPM with PG, terpenes such as DMSO and limonene, and limonene alone (Parhi et al., 2016b).

Depending on the solubility, the drugs are added to either organic phase of aqueous phase i.e., if drug is hydrophilic such as diltiazem HCl (Parhi et al., 2016b), sumatriptan (Agrawal et al., 2010), ondansetron (Giordano et al., 1998), they are usually mixed with aqueous phase and if the drug is lipophilic such as tamoxifen (Bhatia et al., 2013), ketamine (Flores and Crowley, 1998), ketoprofen (Berti and Lipskys, 1995), diclofenac (Burnham et al., 1998), and fluoxetine (Ciribassi et al., 2003), they are mixed with oil phase.

In the development and stability of PLO the weight ratio of organic phase to aqueous phase plays an important role. Bhatia et al., (2009) used different ratios of organic phase to aqueous phase ratios (1:1 to 1:5 and 2:1) to develop PLOs of tamoxifen and found that at and above 1:2 ratio of organic:aqueous phase PLO formation was possible. They also concluded that at higher concentration of lecithin in organic phase yield PLOs even if at lower concentration of pluronic in aqueous phase. This may be attributed to the formation of extensive network-like structure with very high viscosity, thereby preventing the separation of phases (Bhatia et al., 2013). In addition, this extensive network formation due to higher concentration of lecithin might decrease the release rate of entrapped drug inside the PLO (Pandey et al., 2009).

6.4.3.9.1   Small Molecule Gelling Agents (SMGA) Gel

Small molecule gelling agents (SMGA) or low mass gelling agents (LMGA) based gel is a type of organogels consisting of gelators of molecular weight less than 3000 Da and can form supramolecular networks to immobilize water or organic solvents. Unlike polymeric gel, SMGA gels are formed through non-covalent interaction where nanosized fibers organized to form three-dimensional fibrous network structured. Due to non-covalent interaction SMGA gels are thermoreversible. The SMGA can be used as gelling agents for all most all types of polar and non-polar liquids. In such a case SMGA gels loaded with haloperidol using gelator, N-lauroyl-l-glutamic acid di-n-butylamide (GP1) in isostearyl alcohol (ISA) and PG was developed. Based on factorial design the composition of optimized formulation was: drug 3mg/ml, GP-1 and farnesol (penetration enhancer) each at 5% (w/v). This optimized formulation showed slow release of drug which was attributed to the three-dimensional network structure of GP-1 and demonstrated good potential for topical and TDD (Kanga et al., 2005).

6.4.3.11   EMULGEL

In spite of number of advantages of gels, the main disadvantage is their inability to deliver hydrophobic drugs. To circumvent this limitation, emulgels are developed in which an emulsion, either o/w or w/o type, is gelled by mixing with a gelling agents. Thus, presence of a gelling agent in aqueous phase converts either type of classical emulsions to emulgel (Mohamed, 2004a; Kapoor et al., 2014). Emulgel combines the advantages of both emulsions and gels. Emulsions provide high degree of elegance, easy washability and higher ability to penetrate the skin (Mohamed, 2004b). Moreover, a formulator can easily control the viscosity, degree of greasiness and appearance. The w/o emulsions exert emollient action, therefore widely used for the treatment of dry skin, whereas o/w emulsion are generally used for water-washable drug base and cosmetic purpose.

The gels have several favorable properties for dermatological applications including, greaseless, thixotropic, easily removable, easily spreadable, emollient and non-staining, water-soluble, transparent, longer half-life and compatible with several excipients. Moreover, the addition of gelling agent into emulsion enhances the stability of emulsion by reducing the surface and interfacial tension and simultaneously increasing the viscosity (Gupta et al., 2010). Therefore, emulgels have high patient acceptability and capable of delivering both hydrophilic and lipophillic drugs. They are also termed as gel cream, quassi emulsion and gelled emulsion as well (Joshi et al., 2012). There are many drugs successfully incorporated in emulgel formulation, including valdecoxib (Bansal et al., 2008), metronidazole (Rao et al., 2013), mefenamic acid (Khullar et al., 2012), clarithromycin (Joshi et al., 2012), diclofenac (Pakhare et al., 2017), and calcipotriol (Varma et al., 2014).

6.4.4   MISCELLANEOUS

6.4.4.1. NANO-GEL OINTMENTS

A novel nanogel ointment was developed with combination of 3% of ketoprofen, 0.5% of MC and 3% of carbopol 934. Compared to micro gel ointment, nano-based gel ointment showed significantly higher *in-vivo* percutaneous absorption and better attenuated enhancement of paw edema in rats (Nagai et al., 2015). In another study, in order to avoid poor aqueous solubility, photodegradation and systemic side effects, tranilist (an antiallergic agent) in nanoparticle form was incorporated in gel ointment composed of sodium docusate, 2-hydroxypropyl-β-cyclodextrin (2-HP-βCD), MC and carbopol 934. The penetration rate, the penetration coefficient across the skin and drug concentration in the skin tissue and plasma of rats was found to be higher in the case of tranilast-based nanogel ointment compared to microgel-based ointment (Nagai and Ito, 2014).

6.4.4.2   NANO-GEL CREAMS

In an attempt, emulsion cream (O/W) containing SLN of acyclovir was prepared by high-pressure homogenization technique and then 0.3% of carbopol was added to form gel creams. It was observed that the amount of acyclovir present in the epidermis of rat skin was 2-times compared to marketed acyclovir gel cream (Gide et al., 2013). Examples of different types of semisolids with their composition and applications are presented in Table 6.4.

6.5   EVALUATION OF SEMISOLID DOSAGE FORMS

General quality tests for the semisolid dosage forms including identification, content uniformity, impurities, water content, assay, microbial limits, antimicrobial and antioxidant preservative limits and sterility, especially for injectables and ophthalmic semisolids, should be performed. Apart from that, specific tests for topical semisolids should be performed such as quality tests (rheological behavior, gel-strength), and performance tests (*in-vitro* release studies).

6.5.1   RHEOLOGICAL PROPERTIES

Rheological properties such as viscosity of semisolid dosage forms not only affect its application to treatment site like pourability and spreadability, but also the diffusion rate of drug at the microstructural level (Ramachandran et al., 1999). In addition, viscosity has a great influence on the adhering duration at the application site and thus the sustained release characteristics. Particularly, gels as semisolid systems demonstrate viscoelastic behavior. The viscous and elastic properties of gel were due to chain entanglement and intermolecular aggregation/association of monomers, respectively. Therefore, to maintain the reproducibility of products flow behavior at the time of application and drug release is primary important parameters, especially for semisolids (Kulkarni and Shaw, 2016).

When sheared, most of the semisolids exhibit non-Newtonian behavior such as shear thinning and thixotropy. Moreover, the viscosity of semisolid dosage form is influenced by many factors, including product-sampling technique, inherent physical structure of the product, container size and shape, specific methodology employed for the measurement and finally, sample temperature for viscosity measurement. Therefore, for the measurement of viscosity, the properties of the products at rest (in its container) as well as it sheared during application must be taken into consideration. This is because the former can effects the self-life of product and the later can influence its spreadability affecting its safety and efficacy of the drug product. As mentioned, temperature of the sample must be precisely maintained. There

TABLE 6.4 Examples of Different Types of Semisolids with Their Composition and Application

Semisolid types	Drug	Polymer	Application	Reference
Ointments				
Hot-melt extrusion method	Lidocaine	PG	Local anesthesia	Bhagurkar et al., 2016
Ointments containing nanoparticles	AgCl	Chitosan	Burn wound	Kang et al., 2016
	Ag	Starch	Burn wound	Ponnaian et al., 2015
Gene therapy	Viral & non-viral vectors	Cholesterol	Skin angiogenesis	Hajdukiewicz et al., 2013
Creams				
Creams containing microspheres	Vitamin-A	Albumin	Extended release & stability	Bharat et al., 2011
	EHM	PMMA	Photostability & sunscreen	Gogna et al., 2007
Creams containing nanoparticles	Dacarbazine	Stearic acid	Melanoma	Hafeez and Kazmi, 2017
	Curcumin	—	Bacterial disease	Pandit et al., 2015
	Morin	PLGA	Antioxidant & sunscreen	Shetty et al., 2015
	Hydrocortisone (HC) & hydroxytyrosol (HT)	Chitosan	Atopic dermatitis	Siddique et al., 2017
Lamellar faced creams	EA & 4MSK	Oils (Floremac, Florasum, DIA & DISM ester)	Skin whitening	Li et al., 2016
Cream containing lipid micro and nanoparticles	Avobenzone	Carnauba wax	Sunscreen	Albertini et al., 2009
	CoQ10	Cetyl palmitate or stearic acid	Antiwrinkle	Farboud et al., 2011
	JSH18	—	Skin whitening	So et al., 2010
	Oxybenzone	—	Sunscreen	Gulbake et al., 2010

TABLE 6.4 *(Continued)*

Semisolid types	Drug	Polymer	Application	Reference
Gels				
Mucoadhesive/ bioadhesive gels	Insulin	Chitosan	Diabetes	Varshosaz et al., 2006
In situ gels	Proteins	PEG-PLA	—	Nirmal et al., 2010
	Metoprolol succinate	Poloxamer & HPMC	Hypertension	Parhi, 2016a
	Metronidazole	PVA & carboxy methyl tamarind kernel polysaccharide	Metronidazole	
Injectable in situ gel				
Gel containing micro or nanoemulsion	Diclofenac epolamine	Smix & poloxamer	Soft tissue injuries	Shahinaze et al., 2013
	Terbinafine	Oleic acid, Smix & carbopol 934P	Onychomycosis	Barot et al., 2012
	Clobetasol propionate	IPM, cremophor EL, IPA, & carbopol 934P	Vitilogo	Patel et al., 2013
	Ropinirole	Capryol 90, carbitol & carbopol	Enhance skin permeation (Parkinson's disease)	Azeem et al., 2009
Gel containing vesicular systems				
Liposomes	Naproxen & nimesulide	Phospholipon, cholesterol, Aleo vera & carbopol 934	Inflammation	Venkataharsha et al., 2015
	Prednisolone	DPPS, soya lecithin, cholesterol & carbopol 940P	Enhance skin permeation & stability	Varde et al., 2013
			Inflammation & auto-immune disease	

TABLE 6.4 (Continued)

Semisolid types	Drug	Polymer	Application	Reference
	Diflurasone diacetate	Soya & egg phospholipids	Sustained-release (Psoriasis) & carbopol	Umalkar and Rajesh, 2013
Niosomes	Piroxicam	Span 20 and 60, cholesterol, HPMC, CMC, sodium alginate, & xanthan gum	Inflammation	Ahmed et al., 2014
	Sulfadiazine sodium, propranolol HCl & tyrosol	AOT & pluronic L64	Enhance skin permeation	Tavano et al., 2013
Proniosomes	Tenoxicam	Tween 20 & cholesterol	Inflammation & pain	Ammar et al., 2011
Ethosomes	Piroxicam	Soya PC	Enhance skin permeation	Garg et al., 2017
Transferosomes	Celecoxib	Soya PC, sodium deoxycholate & carbopol 940	Stability & enhance skin permeation	Preeti and Kumar, 2013
	Sertraline	Soya lecithin, span 80 & carbopol 940	Depression	Gupta et al., 2012
Gel containing polymeric **Nanoparticles**	Aceclofenac	Egg-albumin, chitosan & carbopol 940	Inflammation	Jana et al., 2014
	Vitamin A and E		Enhance skin permeation & retention	Agrawal et al., 2016
Gel containing lipid Nanoparticles	Meloxicam		Inflammation	Khurana et al., 2013
	Resveratrol	Precirol ATO 5, tween 20 & carbopol	ICD	Shrotriya et al., 2017
	Docetaxel & nicotinamide	Egg lecithin glycerin mono-stearate triglyceride & carbopol	Better skin permeation (Skin, capric tumor & inflammation)	Fan et al., 2013

TABLE 6.4 (Continued)

Semisolid types	Drug	Polymer	Application	Reference
	Clotrimazole	Dynasan®116, Miglyol®812, Tyloxapol, poloxamer 407 & carbomer	Bacterial	Esposito et al., 2013
	Flurbiprofen	Dynasan 114, phosphatidyl-choline, Captex-355, chitosan, carbopol 934, HPC & xanthan gum	Inflammation	Bhaskar et al., 2009
	Lornixicam	Campritol® 888 ATO, Lane e®O, oleic acid	Inflammation	Gönüllü et al., 2015
Nanocmposite gel	Diclofenac sodium	CGG & nanosilica	Slow release & thermal stability	Giri et al., 2012
	Diclofenac sodium	CGG & MWCNT	Sustained release	Giri et al., 2011
	Coomassie brilliant blue R-250 (CBB)	PVA & MWCNT	Higher rate release	Kim et al., 2010
	CBB	PVA, PNIPAAm & MWCNT	Modulated release	Jung et al., 2012
	Amoxicillin	PAAm & Polyaniline nanofibers	ON & OFF pattern release	Pérez-Martínez et al., 2016
Pluronic lecithin organogels (PLO)	Diltiazem HCl	Soya lecithin, poloxamer 407, d-limonen, IPM, & PG.	Higher skin permeation (hypertension)	Parhi et al., 2016b
	Sumatriptan succinate	Soya lecithin & Pluronic F 127	Drug stability (Migraine)	Agrawal et al., 2010; Bhatia et al., 2013
	Tamoxifen	Lecithin, Pluronic F 68, 127, 108 & span 40, 60,80	Drug stability (Breast cancer)	
	Haloperidol	GP-1, PG	Psychosis	Kanga et al., 2005

TABLE 6.4 *(Continued)*

Semisolid types	Drug	Polymer	Application	Reference
Emulgel	Valdecoxib	Ethyl oleate, PG & tween-80	Stability inflammation & arthritis)	Bansal et al., 2008
	Metronidazole	Capmul 908 P, Acconon MC8-2, & PG	Topical infections	Rao et al., 2013
	Mefenamic acid	Carbapol940, Liquid paraffin, Tween 20, Span 20 & PG	Inflammation & pain	Khullar et al., 2012
	Calcipotriol	Carbopol, Kollicream 3C, Kolliphor CS, Liquid paraffin, PG, PEG& IPA	Enhanced skin permeation (psoriasis)	Varma et al., 2014
	Diclofenac	Carbopol-940 & PG	Stability (inflammation)	Pakhare et al., 2017
Miscellaneous				
Nanogel ointment	Tranilast	Sodium docusate, 2-HP- βCD, & carbopol 934	Allergy	Nagai and Ito, 2014
Nano-gel creams	Acyclovir	Miglyol 810, Lipoid S 100, Pluronic-F68 & carbopol	Higher dermal retention (herpes virus simplex infection)	Gide et al., 2013

is no hard and fast rule for it, but temperature of sample during viscosity measurement should be according to the intended use of the product like skin temperature for topical application (Kulkarni and Shaw, 2016).

The viscosity of semisolid dosage forms can be determined in variety of methods, including viscometry and rheometry. Between two, rotational methods are widely used for their versatility and precise results. In rotational methods, the sample semisolid is continuously sheared between two surfaces, one or both of which are rotating. Furthermore, the sample can be sheared for an unlimited period of time. Thus, an equilibrium or transient-state behavior can be monitored under a controlled condition. The rotational viscometer determines the torque required to rotate and immersed spindle in a semisolid at a fixed rate. Finally, conversion factors are required to calculate viscosity from the obtained torque and the values varies depend on specific geometries of spindle. On the other handrotational rheometers are high-precision and continuously variable shear instruments, wherein the sample is sheared either using rotating cylinders and cones and plates, under controlled stress or controlled rate conditions. As a result of this, there are at least three modes of measurement of semisolids, including (i) flow, in this the response of sample material is measured by subjecting it to increased shear stress followed by decreasing it in a controlled manner; (ii) creep, in which a constant stress is applied for a long period of time and the displacement response is measured; and (iii) oscillation, in which a small sinusoidal stress is applied and the obtained sinusoidal strain is measured. Out of various parts in the rheometer, measuring geometry played a major role as its selection is based on the characteristics of the material being evaluated and the type of rheological information desired. Like, concentric cylinders and spindles typically are employed for less viscous, more flowable semisolid dosage forms and cone-plate more particularly used for more viscous and less flowable or sample size is small (Kulkarni and Shaw, 2016).

6.5.2   GEL-STRENGTH MEASUREMENT

Like viscosity, strength of gel plays a major role in determining the amount of drug release from semisolid matrix. Recently, advancement has occurred in the apparatus used in the measurement of gel strength. The proposed apparatus (Ferrari et al., 1994) comprised of a sample holder placed on an electronic microbalance and a probe connected to a computer. The probe is lowered into the sample by means of a motor equipped with a speed transformer and the force required to penetrate the gel is measured. The displacement covered by the probe as a function of time is measured and used to calculate the gel-strength or mechanical resistance of the gel system

6.5.3 IN-VITRO RELEASE STUDY

The release of the encapsulated drug from the semisolid dosage forms is one of the important quality control tools. To date, for the measurement of *in-vitro* drug release from semisolid dosage forms, there is no single device has been universally accepted. This is because currently no compendia *in-vitro* release test methodology is described for semisolid dosage forms, although the FDA includes general methodology descriptions pertaining to diffusion systems (Markovich, 2001; FDA-SUPAC-SS, 1998). However, US pharmacopeia described transdermal dosage form release apparatus such as apparatus 5 (paddle over disc), apparatus 6 (cylinder) and apparatus 7 (reciprocating disc). Among various devices, diffusion cells are by far more frequently used with many modifications in it. Moreover, the diffusion cells are classified into two categories, namely static and flow-through cells. In the case of static types, all the components such as a receptor, donor compartments and in between membrane may be either vertically arranged as in Franz diffusion cell (Barry, 1983) or horizontally as in Bronaugh cell (Lu et al., 1992) (Figure 6.10). Flows through cells are usually similar to the upright Franz diffusion cells but with certain modifications that allow the continuous replacement of the receptor solution with the aid of a pump (Selzer et al., 2013). However, a serious limitation using vertical Franz diffusion cell is the formation of air bubbles underneath the membrane, which can be noticed easily. Therefore, failure to remove these air bubbles can have a serious impact on the accuracy, precision, and reproducibility of the resulted data (Kanferet al., 2017). The recent development of devices is based on the automated operations, better instrument controls and minimal variable related to the instrument.

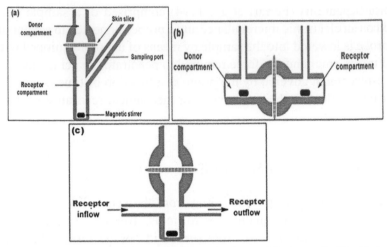

FIGURE 6.10   Schematic diagram of: (a) static Franz diffusion cell, (b) side-by-side diffusion cell, and (c) flow-through Franz diffusion cell. The receptor compartment of a) may be maintained at a given temperature by placing the cells in a water bath or by an additional water jacket surrounding the cell body (not shown) (Reprinted with permission from Selzer et al., 2013. © Elsevier.)

6.5.3.1   MODIFIED USP TYPE II DISSOLUTION APPARATUS

It is comprised of an Enhancer cell (VanKel, Cary, NC) made up of PTFE, 2.5 ×1.5 cm paddle and 200ml of vessel. Enhancer cell is an alternative device developed for the Franz-type diffusion cell. This cell consists of a donor chamber with adjustable sample reservoir, a washer for controlling the exposure of the surface area, and an open screw-on cap to secure the washer and a sample membrane to cover the semisolids. Filled cells were placed in the bottom of the vessels, and the paddles were positioned 1 cm above the sample surface. The 200 ml capacity vessels are filled with 50ml of dissolution media and maintained at 37°C (Fares and Zatz, 1995; Gupta and Garg, 2002).

6.5.3.2   PLEXIGLAS FLOW-THROUGH CELLS

Plexiglas flow-through cells are recent development to carry out auto-mated *in-vitro* drug release from semisolid dosage forms (Figure 6.11). The cell system usually consists of six parts: base plate, sample reservoir, semi-permeable membrane, receptor fluid reservoir, and block seal for the receptor fluid reservoir. The sample reservoir is supported by a base plate and then a receptor-fluid reservoir is placed above it. The semi-permeable membrane is placed between the sample reservoir and receptor fluid reservoir. Further the receptor fluid reservoir is divided into two equal sections wherein one section carrying the inlet and the other section carrying the outlet for the receptor fluid. A solid plexiglass block seals the top of the receptor-fluid reservoir. The entire cell is immersed in a constant temperature water bath and is computer-controlled by connecting it to a pump for the receptor fluid, a medium splitter, and a fraction collector. This device is particularly useful for the measurement of the influences of variables including membrane type, the flow rate of a receptor fluid and release rates at different temperatures (Chattaraj et al., 1995; Kanfer et al., 2017).

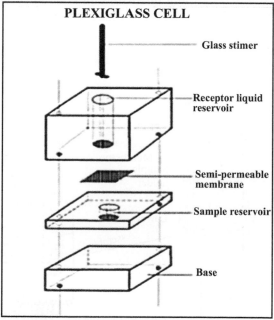

FIGURE 6.11   Diagrammatic representation of Plexiglass cell (Reprinted with permission from Chattaraj et al., 1995. © Elsevier.)

6.5.3.3   INSERTION CELL

The intention of the development of the insertion cell is to avoid the entrapment of air bubbles at the membrane-receptor liquid interface, a common problem associated with Franz diffusion cell. This method is similar to the

USP paddle over-disc method (USP 37–NF 32, 2014) but, in this case, an additional membrane is used in the immersion cell (Rege et al., 1998). The insertion cell (Figure 6.12) consists of an oblong Plexiglas upper block with 9 mm circle cut out of it. The middle section also has similar 9 mm diameter cut out area, matching with the upper Plexiglas block that acts as the sample holder. A membrane is placed between the upper block and sample holder. The lower part is a solid Plexiglas block. All the three parts are tightly screwed together. A stainless steel spring is used to supports the cell for the turbulent-flow mode and a layer of glass beads in the conical section to support the cell for the laminar flow mode. The insertion cell is positioned in such a way that its distance from the conical section of the insertion cell is 10 mm when it is used with the spring support. It is recommended to be used in a downward orientation with direction of fluid flow from top to bottom. Like Plexiglas flow-through cell, the entire assembly is automated (Chattaraj and Kanfer, 1996; Gupta and Garg, 2002; Liebenberg et al., 2003).

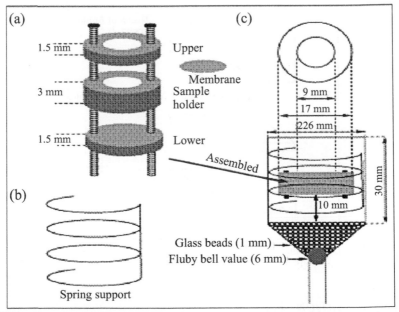

FIGURE 6.12   Schematic representation of flow through cell (compendia): (a) insertion cell; (b) spring support used during turbulent-flow experiments; (c) insertion placed inside compendial flow-through cell (Reprinted with permission from Chattaraj et al., 1996. © Elsevier.)

6.6   REGULATORY REQUIREMENTS FOR SEMISOLIDS

FDA has set forth guidelines for various aspects of semisolid dosage forms that serve as the primary reference for the development of dosage forms in order to facilitate their regulatory approval (Flynn et al., 1999). In fact Center for Drug Evaluation and Research (CDER), one section of FDA established guidelines to ascertain the main requisite such as identity, quality, strength, efficacy and safety of semisolid drug products. Various pharmaceutical activities are undertaken to fulfill above requirements including: (i) manufacturer needs to comply with above requisite at the time of filling investigational new drug (IND), abbreviated new drug application (ANDA), or abbreviated antibiotic application (AADA); (ii) all dermatological products should have standard chemistry, manufacturing and chemistry (CMC) tests; (iii) additional information on particle size distribution, polymorphic form and other characteristics are needed to be submitted along with NDA; (iv) likewise, the manufacturer should meet the standards of compendial requirements if available and match the important characteristics such as *in-vitro* and *in-vivo* characteristics of the reference listed drug (RLD), appropriate *in-vitro* release methods are submitted to ensure batch-to-batch consistency if such informations are not available; and (v) if any changes are made for an approved semisolid product in the later stages pertaining to its components, composition, process, equipment manufacturing site, batch size, and process, it is the prerogatory of the formulator to submit necessary details to the regulatory agency.

The above guidelines includes various aspects such as *in-vitro* release, *in-vivo* bioavailability, bioequivalence, scale-up and post-approval changes (SUPAC), skin irritation and skin sensitization tests of generic semisolid transdermal drug products (http://www.fda). Such a typical guideline based on the type and levels of SUPAC is outlined in Table 6.5. Based on the SUPAC, it is essential for manufacturer to submit application and compendial product release requirements, identification, and assay for new preservative, test for preservative effectiveness, executed batch records, long-term and accelerated stability data, validation methods to support absence of interference of preservatives with other tests, *in-vitro* release test, and *in-vivo* bioequivalence data to the FDA. Bioequivalence studies are recommended if changes are made pertaining to the quality and quantity of excipients or crystallinity of drugs. Furthermore, derma-topharmacokinetic studies and pharmacodynamic or comparative clinical trials are recommended to establish bioequivalence of topical products as routine pharmacokinetic studies is not the correct indicative of drug in blood, plasma, urine and other biological fluids. In addition, *in-vitro* release data are used to evaluate the *in-vivo* bioequivalence of a lower strength product in case bioavailability or bioequivalence data of a highest strength product are already available. Specific requirements for different SUPAC levels are presented in Table 6.5 (US-FDA, 1997).

TABLE 6.5   SUPAC Guidelines Description for Nonsterile Semisolid Dosage Forms

Type of change	Level	Description	Requirements [a]
Change in component and composition	1	(i) Partial deletion or deletion of color, fragrance, or flavor; (ii) up to 5% change in approved amount with total excipient changes $\leq$ 5%; (iii) change in supplier for structure forming or any technical-grade excipient.	A & C
	2	(i) Excipient changes between>5% and $\leq$10% with total excipient changes $\leq$10%; (ii) change in supplier for structure forming excipient that is not covered under level 1; (iii) change in technical grade of a structure forming excipients; (iv) if drug is in suspension, then its change in particle size distribution.	A, B, D & G
	3	(i) any quantitative and qualitative changes in an excipient beyond the specified ranges in levels 1 and 2; (ii) if the drug is in suspension, then its change in crystallinity.	A, B, E, G & H
Changes in components and composition of preservatives	1	$\leq$ 10% quantitative change in preservative	A & I
	2	> 10% and $\leq$20% quantitative change in preservatives	A & I
	3	> 20% quantitative changes in preservative, deletion or inclusion of a different preservative	A, B, D, I & J
Change in manufacturing process	1	(i) Changes in process within approved application ranges; (ii) addition of excipients	A
	2	(i) Changes in process outside approved application ranges; (ii) process of combined phases	A, B, F & G

TABLE 6.5 *(Continued)*

Type of change	Level	Description	Requirements [a]
Change in manufacturing equipment	1	(i) Changes to automated or mechanical equipment for the transfer of ingredients; (ii) use of alternative equipment of same design and operating principle	A & C
	2	(i) Use of alternative equipment of a different design and operating principle; (ii) change in type of mixing equipment.	A, B, F & G
Change in batch size	1	Batch size changes ≤ 10 times of pivotal clinical	Trial/biobatch.
	2	Batch size changes > 10 times of pivotal clinical trial/biobatch.	A, B & D
Change in manufacturing Site	1	Changes within existing facility	A
	2	Changes within same contiguous campus/ facilities in adjacent city blocks	A, B, C & K
	3	(i) Changes to different campus; (ii) changes to contract manufacturer	A, B, E, G & K

[a]Only those written with capital letters:

A: Application/compendia product release requirement.

B: Executed batch records.

C: Long term data for first production batch.

D: Accelerated stability data for 3-month for first batch and long term data for first production batch.

E: Accelerated stability data for 3-month for first batch and long term data for first three production batches if significant information is available or accelerated stability data for three batches and long term data for first three production batches if significant information is not available.

F: Accelerated stability data for 3-month for first batch and long term data for first production batch if significant information is available or accelerated stability data for three batches and long-term data for first three production batches if significant information is not available.

G: In vitro release test.

H: In vivo bioequivalence.

I: Test for preservative effectiveness at the lowest specified preservative level.

J: Identification and assay for new preservatives; validation methods to support the absence of interference with other tests.

K: Location of the new site.

6.7 CONCLUSIONS

Previously, people used to think that semisolid dosage forms are the traditional one that exerts only local action. However, since the last decade or so it has been the subject of extensive research, particularly in TDD. This research on semisolids orientated toward the improvement of the performance of these systems, including the cosmetic acceptability and therapeutic efficacy. As a result, the novel semisolid dosage forms posses many ideal cosmetic properties such as non-greasy, non-hygroscopic, non-staining, non-hydrating, smooth texture and elegant appearance. In addition, extreme care has been taken during formulation so that these novel systems are free from causing skin irritation, altering skin function, initiating skin sensitization and miscible with skin secretion. Various approaches such as using mucoadhesive polymers, *in-situ* gelling system and drug delivery carriers such as the incorporation of different vesicles, nanoparticles, and nanocomposite into cosmetically improved creams and gels to provide the desired rate of drug release, be it local delivery or systemic delivery. For instance, drug-in-emulsion droplets of nanosize have successfully eliminated the requirement for the active ingredient's physicochemical properties to be responsible for the efficient drug permeation across the formidable barrier in the skin. Nanocomposite gels are another novel development in the field, which have the ability to control the drug release from the semisolid systems. Since the last few years, major efforts are being made to effectively characterize semisolid dosage forms including the rheological behavior and *in-vitro* drug release devices. These devices are able to produce reliable and reproducible results. Among the semisolid systems, much more attention is being given towards gel systems as compared to cream and ointments because of the gel's aesthetic appeal and better performance. The field of semisolid dosage forms have great future opportunities because of their unique characteristics, can be used for topical and TDD and both hydrophilic and lipophilic drugs with diverse classes can be incorporated into it.

KEYWORDS

- *in-situ* gelling systems
- *in-vitro* drug release
- permeation
- *Stratum corneum*
- transdermal drug delivery
- vesicular systems
- viscosity

REFERENCES

Abdel-Mottaleb, M. M. A., Mortada, N. D., Elshamy, A. A., & Awad, G. A. S., (2007). Preparation and evaluation of fluconazole gels, *Egypt. J. Biomed. Sci., 23*(1), 266–286.

Agrawal, A., Kulkarni, S., & Sharma, S., (2016). Recent advancements and applications of multiple emulsions. *Int. J. Adv. Pharm., 4*, 94–103.

Agrawal, V., Gupta, V., Ramteke, S., & Trivedi, P., (2010). Preparation and evaluation of tubular micelles of pluronic lecithin organogel for transdermal delivery of somatropin. *AAPS Pharm. Sci. Tech., 11*(4), 1718–1725.

Ahagon, A., & Gent, A., (1975). Effect of interfacial bonding on the strength of adhesion. *J. Polym. Sci. Polym. Phys. Ed., 13*(7), 1285–1300.

Ahmed, M. S., Ghoura, M. M., Shadeed, G. S., & Qushawy, M. K. E., (2014). Design, formulation, and evaluation of piroxicam niosomal gel. *Int. J. Pharm. Tech. Res., 6*(1), 185–195.

Ahmed, T. A., Ibrahim, H. M., Ibrahim, F., Samy, A. M., Kaseem, A., Nutan, M. T., & Hussain, M. D., (2012). Development of biodegradable *in situ* implant and microparticle injectable formulations for sustained delivery of haloperidol. *J. Pharm. Sci., 101*(10), 3753–3762.

Ahmed, T. A., Ibrahim, H. M., Samy, A. M., Kaseem, A., Nutan, M. T. H., & Hussain, M. D., (2014). Biodegradable injectable in situ implants and microparticles for sustained release of Montelukast: *In-vitro* release, pharmacokinetics, and stability. *AAPS Pharm. Sci. Tech., 15*(3), 772–780.

Albertini, B., Mezzena, M., Passerini, N., Rodriguez, L., & Scalia, S., (2009). Evaluation of spray congealing as technique for the preparation of highly loaded solid lipid microparticles containing the sunscreen agent, avobenzone. *J. Pharm. Sci., 98*(8), 2759–2769.

Alkilani, A. Z., McCrudden, M. T. C., & Donnelly, R. F., (2015). Transdermal drug delivery: Innovative pharmaceutical developments based on disruption of the barrier properties of the stratum corneum. *Pharm., 7*, 438–470.

Almeidaa, H., Amarala, M. H., Lobãoa, P., Silvaa, A. C., & Lobo, J. M. S., (2014). Applications of polymeric and lipid nanoparticles in ophthalmic pharmaceutical formulations: Present and future considerations. *J. Pharm. Pharm. Sci., 17*(3), 278–293.

Alsarra, I. A., Bosela, A. A., Ahmed, S. M., & Mahrous, G. M., (2005). Proniosomes as a drug carrier of ketorolac. *Eur. J. Pharm. Biopharm., 59*, 485–490.

Ammar, H. O., Ghorab, M., El-Nahhas, S. A., & Higazy, I. M., (2011). Proniosomes as a carrier system for transdermal delivery of tenoxicam. *Int. J. Pharm., 405*, 142–152.

Andrews, G. P., Laverty, T. P., & Jones, D. S., (2009). Mucoadhesive polymeric platforms for controlled drug delivery. *Eur. J. Pharm. Biopharm., 71*(3), 505–518.

Antunes, F. E., Gentile, L., Rossi, C. O., Tavano, L., & Ranieri, G. A., (2011). Gels of Pluronic F127 and nonionic surfactants from rheological characterization to controlled drug permeation. *Coll. Surf. B Biointerf., 87*, 42–48.

Azeem, A., Ahmad, F. J., Khar, R. K., & Talegaonkar, S., (2009). Nanocarrier for the transdermal delivery of an anti-parkinsonian drug. *AAPS Pharm. Sci. Tech., 10*(4), 1093–1103.

Bal, S. M., Ding, Z., Riet, E. V., Jiskoot, W., & Bouwstra, J., (2010). Advances in transcutaneous vaccine delivery: Do all ways lead to Rome? *J. Control. Release, 148*, 266–282.

Bansal, A., Saleem, M. A., Imam, S., & Singh, S., (2008). Preparation and evaluation of Valdecoxib Emulgel formulations. *Biomed. Pharmacol. J., 1*(1), 131–138.

Barot, B. S., Parejiya, P. B., Patel, H. K., Gohel, M. C., & Shelat, P. K., (2012). Microemulsion-based gel of terbinafine for the treatment of onychomycosis: Optimization of formulation using D-optimal design. *AAPS Pharm. Sci. Tech., 13*(1), 184–192.

Belgamwar, V. S., Pandey, M. S., Chauk, D. S., & Surana, S. J., (2008). Pluronic lecithin organogel. *Asian J of Pharm., 2*(3), 134–138.

Berger, J., Reist, M., Mayer, J. M., Felt, O., & Gurny, R., (2004). Structure and interactions in chitosan hydrogels formed by complexation or aggregation for biomedical applications. *Eur. J. Pharm. Biopharm., 57*(1), 35–52.

Berti, J. J., & Lipskys, J. J., (1995). Transcutaneous drug delivery: A practical review. *Mayo. Clin. Proc., 70*, 581–586.

Bhagurkar, A. M., Angamuthu, M., Patil, H., Tiwari, R. V., Maurya, A., Hashemnejad, S. M., Kundu, S., Murthy, S. N., & Repka, M. A., (2016). Development of an ointment formulation using hot-melt extrusion technology. *AAPS Pharm. Sci. Tech., 17*(1), 158–166.

Bharat, P., Paresh, M., Sharma, R. K., Tekade, B. W., Thakre, V. M., & Patil, V. R., (2011). A review: Novel advances in semisolid dosage forms & patented technology in semisolid dosage forms. *Int. J. Pharm. Tech. Res., 3*(1), 420–430.

Bhaskar, K., Anbu, J., Ravichandiran, V., Venkateswarlu, V., & Rao, Y. M., (2009). Lipid nanoparticles for transdermal delivery of flurbiprofen: Formulation, *in-vitro, ex vivo* and *in vivo* studies. *Lipids in Health Dis., 8*, 6.

Bhatia, A., Singh, B., Raza, K., Wadhwab, S., & Katare, O. P., (2013). Tamoxifen-loaded lecithin organogel (LO) for topical application: development, optimization and characterization. *Int. J. Pharm., 444*, 47–59.

Bhattarai, N., Gunn, J., & Zhang, M., (2010). Chitosan-based hydrogels for controlled, localized drug delivery. *Adv. Drug Deliv. Rev., 62*(1), 83–99.

Bhushan, B., (2003). Adhesion and stiction: Mechanisms, measurement techniques, and methods for reduction. *J. Vac. Sci. Technol., 21*(6), 2262–2296.

Bouchemal, K., Briançon, S., Perrier, E., & Fessi, H., (2004). Nano-emulsion formulation using spontaneous emulsification: Solvent, oil and surfactant optimization. *Int. J. Pharm., 280*, 241–251.

Burnham, R., Gregg, R., Healy, P., & Steadward, R., (1998). The effectiveness of topical diclofenac for lateral epicondylitis. *Clin. J. Sport Med., 8*, 78–81.

Camargo, P. H. C., Satyanarayana, K. G., & Wypych, F., (2009). Nanocomposites: Synthesis, structure, properties and new application opportunities. *Mater. Res., 12*, 1–39.

Carvalho, F. C., Bruschi, M. L., Evangelista, R. C., & Gremião, M. P. D., (2010). Mucoadhesive drug delivery systems. *Braz. J. Pharm. Sci., 46*(1), 1–17.

Center for Drug Evaluation and Research Website. http://www.fda.gov/cder/guidance/index.htm (Accessed on 19 November 2019).

Cevc, G., (1997). Drug delivery across the skin. *Expert Opinion on Investigational Drugs, 12*, 1887–1937.

Cevc, G., (2004). Lipid vesicles and other colloids as drug carriers on the skin. *Adv. Drug Deliv. Rev., 56*(5), 675–711.

Chandrababu, D., Rayudu, N. K., Kishorebabu, M., Surti, N., & Patel, D., (2013). Vesicular systems emerging as dermal and transdermal drug delivery systems. *Int. J. Pharm. Sci. Rev. Res., 18*(1), 176–182.

Chattaraj, S. C., & Kanfer, I., (1995). Release of acyclovir from semisolid dosage forms: A semiautomated procedure using a simple plexiglas flow-through cell. *Int. J. Pharm., 125*(2), 215–222.

Chattaraj, S. C., & Kanfer, I., (1996). "The insertion cell": A novel approach to monitor drug release from semi-solid dosage forms. *Int. J. Pharm., 133*(1), 59–63.

Chaudhary, H., Kohli, K., & Kumar, V., (2013). Nano-transfersomes as a novel carrier for transdermal delivery. *Int. J. Pharm., 454*(1), 367–380.

Chhatri, A., Bajpai, J., & Bajpai, A. K., (2011). Designing polysaccharide-based antibacterial biomaterials for wound healing applications, *Biomater., 1*, 189–197.

Ciribassi, J., Luescher, A., Pasloske, K. S., Plouch, C. R., Zimmerman, A., & Kaloostian-Whittymore, L., (2003). Comparative bioavailability of fluoxetine after transdermal and oral administration to healthy cats. *Am. J. Veter. Res., 64*, 994–998.

Dasari, S., Pereira, L., Reddy, A. P., Michaels, J. E., Lu, X., Jacob, T., Thomas, A., Rodland, M., Jr, Roberts, C. T., Gravett, M. G., & Nagalla, S. R., (2007). Comprehensive proteomic analysis of human cervical-vaginal fluid. *J. Proteome. Res., 6*(4), 1258–1268.

Date, A. A., Joshi, M. D., & Patravale, V. B., (2007). Parasitic diseases: Liposomes and polymeric nanoparticles versus lipid nanoparticles. *Adv. Drug Deliv. Rev., 59*(6), 505–521.

Davis, K. A., Burdick, J. A., & Ansetha, K. A., (2003). Photoinitiated crosslinked degradable copolymer networks for tissue engineering applications. *Biomater., 24*, 2485–2495.

Devi, D. R., Abhirami, M., Brindha, R., Gomathi, S., & Hari, B. N. V., (2013). In-situ gelling system-potential tool for improving therapeutic effects of drugs. *Int. J. Pharm. Pharm. Sci., 5*(3), 27–30.

Dodou, D., Breedveld, P., & Wieringa, P. A., (2005). Mucoadhesives in the gastrointestinal tract: Revisiting the literature for novel applications. *Eur. J. Pharm. Biopharm., 60*(1), 1–16.

Donnelly, R. F., & Wolfson, A. D., (2013). Polymeric biomaterial. In: Dumitriu, S., & Popa, V., (eds.), *Bioadhesive Drug Delivery Systems* (3rd edn., pp. 311–336). CRC Press, Boca Raton, NW.

Dubey, V., Mishra, D., Asthana, A., & Jain, N. K., (2006). Transdermal delivery of a pineal hormone: Melatonin via elastic liposomes. *Biomater., 27*, 3491–3496.

Dumortier, G., Grossiord, J. L., Agnely, F., & Chaumeil, J. C., (2006). A review of poloxamer 407 pharmaceutical and pharmacological characteristics. *Pharm. Res., 23*(12), 2709–2728.

Escobar-Chávez, J. J., López-Cervantes, M., Naik, A., Kalia, Y. N., Quintanar-Guerrero, D., & Quintanar, A. G., (2006). Applications of thermo-reversible Pluronic F-127 gels in pharmaceutical formulations. *J. Pharm. Pharm. Sci., 9*(3), 339–358.

Esposito, E., Ravani, L., Contado, C., Costenaro, A., Drechsler, M., Rossi, D., Menegatti, E., Grandini, A., & Cortesi, R., (2013). Clotrimazole nanoparticle gel for mucosal administration. *Mater. Sci. Eng. C. Mater. Biol. Appl., 33*(1), 411–418.

Fan, X., Chen, J., & Shen, Q., (2013). Docetaxel-nicotinamide complex-loaded nanostructured lipid carriers for transdermal delivery. *Int. J. Pharm., 458*, 296–304.

Farboud, E. S., Nasrollahi, S. A., & Tabbakhi, Z., (2011). Novel formulation and evaluation of a Q10-loaded solid lipid nanoparticles cream: *In-vitro* and *in vivo* studies. *Int. J. Nanomed., 6*, 611–617.

Fares, H. M., & Zatz, J. L., (1995). Measurement of drug release from topical gels using two types of apparatus. *Pharm. Tech., 19*, 52–58.

FDA, (1998). *Guidance for Industry, Nonsterile Semisolid Dosage Forms, Scale-Up and Post-Approval Changes, Chemistry, Manufacturing and Controls, In-Vitro Release Testing and In Vivo Bioequivalence.* "Documentation" (SUPAC-SS) and Manufacturing Equipment Addendum December.

Ferrari, F., Bertoni, M., Caramella, C., & Manna, A. L., (1994). Description and validation of an apparatus for gel strength measurements. *Int. J. Pharm., 109*(2), 115–124.

Flores, J. A., & Crowley, K. L., (1998). *Inventors, Process for the Preparation of Ketamine Ointment.* US patent, 5817699.

Flynn, G. L., Shah, V. P., Tenjarla, S. N., Corbo, M., De Magistris, D. M., Feldman, T. G., Franz, T. J., Miran, D. R., Pearce, D. M., Sequeira, J. A., Swarbrick, J., Wang, J. C. T., Yacobi, A., & Zatz, J. L., (1999). Assessment of value and applications of *in-vitro* testing of topical dermatological drug products. *Pharm. Res., 16*(9), 1325–1330.

Fouad, S. A., Basalious, E. B., El-Nabarawi, M. E., & Tayel, S. A., (2013). Microemulsion and poloxamer microemulsion-based gel for sustained transdermal delivery of diclofenac epolamine using in-skin drug depot: *In-vitro/in vivo* evaluation. *Int. J. Pharm., 453*, 569–578.

Franckum, J., Ramsay, D., Das, N. G., & Das, S. K., (2004). Pluronic lecithin organogel for local delivery of anti-inflammatory drugs. *Int. J. Pharm. Compound., 8*, 101–105.

Fung, P., Lim, C., Liu, X. Y., Kang, L., Chi, P., Ho, L., & Chan, S. Y., (2008). Physicochemical effects of terpenes on organogel for transdermal drug delivery. *Int. J. Pharm., 358*, 102–107.

Fung, P., Lim, C., Liu, X. Y., Kang, L., Chi, P., Ho, L., Chan, Y. W., & Chan, S. Y., (2006). Limonene GP1/PG organogel as a vehicle in transdermal delivery of haloperidol. *Int. J. Pharm., 311*, 157–164.

Gannu, R., Palem, C. R., Yamsani, V. V., & Yamsani, S. K., (2010). Enhanced bioavailability of lacidipine via microemulsion based transdermal gels: Formulation optimization, *ex vivo* and *in vivo* characterization. *Int. J. Pharm., 388*, 231–241.

Garg, V., Singh, H., Bhatia, A., Raza, K., Singh, S. A., Singh, B., & Beg, S., (2017). Systematic development of transethosomal gel system of piroxicam: Formulation optimization, *in-vitro* evaluation, and *ex vivo* assessment. *AAPS Pharm. Sci. Tech., 18*(1), 58–71.

Gide, P. S., Gidwani, S. K., & Kothule, K. U., (2013). Enhancement of transdermal penetration and bioavailability of poorly soluble acyclovir using solid lipid nanoparticles incorporated in gel cream. *Ind. J. Pharm. Sci., 75*(2), 138–142.

Gilani, S., Mir, S., Masood, M., Khan, A. K., Rashid, R., Azhar, S., Rasul, A., Ashraf, M. N., Waqas, M. K., & Murtaza, G., (2018). Triple-component nanocomposite films prepared using a casting method: Its potential in drug delivery. *J. Food Drug Anal., 26*(2), 887–902.

Giordano, J., Daleo, C., & Sacks, S. M., (1998). Topical ondansetron attenuates nociceptive and inflammatory effects of intradermal capsaicin in humans, *Eur. J. Pharmacol., 354*, R13–R14.

Giri, T., Bhowmick, M., Pal, S., & Bandyopadhyay, A., (2011). Polymer hydrogel from carboxymethyl guar gum and carbon nanotube for sustained transdermal release of diclofenac sodium. *Int. J. Biol. Macromol., 49*(5), 885–893.

Giri, T., Ghosh, A. B., Panda, P. S., & Bandyopdhyay, A., (2012). Tailoring carboxymethyl guar gum hydrogel with nanosilica for sustained transdermal release of diclofenac sodium, *Carbohydr. Polym., 87*, 1532–1538.

Gogna, D., Jain, S. K., Yadav, A. K., & Agrawal, G. P., (2007). Microsphere based improved sunscreen formulation of ethylhexyl methoxycinnamate. *Cur. Drug Deliv., 4*(2), 153–159.

Gönüllü, Ü., Üner, M., Yener, G., Karaman, E. F., & Aydoğmuş, Z., (2015). Formulation and characterization of solid lipid nanoparticles, nanostructured lipid carriers and nanoemulsion of lornoxicam for transdermal delivery. *Acta. Pharm., 65*, 1–13.

Goyal, P., Goyal, K., Gurusamy, S., Kumar, V., Singh, A., Katare, O. P., & Mishra, D. N., (2005). Liposomal drug delivery systems—clinical applications. *Acta. Pharm., 55*, 1–25.

Gu, J. M., Robinson, J. R., & Leung, S. H., (1988). Binding of acrylic polymers to mucin/epithelial surfaces: Structure-property relationships. *Crit. Rev. Ther. Drug Carrier Syst., 5*(1), 21–67.

Guidance for Industry., (1997). *Nonsterile Semisolid Dosage Forms: Scale-Up and Post-Approval Changes*. U.S. Food and Drug Administration, May, pp. 1–37.

Gulbake, A., Jain, A., Khare, P., & Jain, S. K., (2010). Solid lipid nanoparticles bearing oxybenzone: *In-vitro* and *in-vivo* evaluation. *J. Microencapsul., 27*(3), 226–233.

Gupta, A., Aggarwal, G., Singla, S., & Arora, R., (2012). Transfersomes: A novel vesicular carrier for enhanced transdermal delivery of sertraline: Development, characterization, and performance evaluation. *Sci. Pharm., 80*, 1061–1080.

Gupta, A., Mishra, A. K., Singh, A. K., Gupta, V., & Bansal, P., (2010). Formulation and evaluation of topical gel of diclofenac sodium using different polymers. *Drug Invent. Today, 2*, 250–253.

Gupta, P., & Garg, S., (2002). Recent advances in semisolid dosage forms for dermatological application. *Pharm. Technol.,* 144–162.

Haddadi, A., Aboofazeli, R., Erfan, M., & Farboud, E. S., (2008). Topical delivery of urea encapsulated in biodegradable PLGA microparticles: O/W and W/O creams. *J. Microencapsul., 25*(6), 379–386.

Hafeez, A., & Kazmi, I., (2017). Dacarbazine nanoparticle topical delivery system for the treatment of melanoma. *Scientific Reports, 7*, 16517.

Hajdukiewicz, K., Stachurska, A., Proczka, R., & Małecki, M., (2013). Study of angiogenic gene ointments designed for skin neovascularization. *Development Period Med., XVII*(1), 31–36.

Hathout, R. M., & Nasr, M., (2013). Transdermal delivery of betahistine hydrochloride using microemulsions: Physical characterization, biophysical assessment, confocal imaging and permeation studies. *Colloids and Surf. B: Biointerf., 110*, 254–260.

Hemelrijck, C. V., & Muller-Goymann, C. C., (2012). Rheological characterization and permeation behavior of poloxamer 407-based systems containing 5-aminolevulinic acid for potential application in photodynamic therapy. *Int. J. Pharm., 437*, 120–129.

Hoffman, A. S., (2013). Stimuli-responsive polymers: Biomedical applications and challenges for clinical translation, *Adv. Drug Deliv. Rev., 65*, 10–16.

Hussain, A. A., Hirai, S., & Bawarshi, R., (1983). *Nasal Dosage Forms of Propranol* (Vol. 394, p. 390). U.S. Patent 4.

Idson, B., & Lazarus, J., (1991). Semisolids. In: Lachman, L., Lieberman, H. A., & Kanig, J. L., (eds.), *The Theory and Practice of Industrial Pharmacy* (pp. 534–563). Varghese Publishing House: Bombay.

Jain, A., Gupta, Y., & Jain, S. K., (2007). Perspectives of biodegradable natural polysaccharides for site-specific drug delivery to the colon. *J. Pharm. Pharm. Sci., 10*, 86–128.

Jana, S., Manna, S., Nayak, A. K., Sen, K. K., & Basu, S. K., (2014). Carbopol gel containing chitosan-egg albumin nanoparticles for transdermal aceclofenac delivery. *Colloids and Surf. B: Biointerf., 114*, 36–44.

Jenning, V. J., Schäfer-Korting, M., & Gohla, S., (2000). Vitamin A-loaded solid lipid nanoparticles for topical use: Drug release properties. *J. Control. Release, 66*, 115–126.

Jenning, V., & Gohla, S. H., (2001). Encapsulation of retinoids in solid lipid nanoparticles (SLN). *J. Microencapsul., 18*, 149–158.

Jenning, V., Gysler, A., Schafer-Korting, M., & Gohla, S. H., (2000). Vitamin A loaded solid lipid nanoparticles for topical use: occlusive properties and drug targeting to the upper skin. *Eur. J. Pharm. Biopharm., 49*(3), 211–218.

Jeon, I. Y., & Baek, J. B., (2010). Nanocomposites derived from polymers and inorganic nanoparticles. *Mater., 3*, 3654–3674.

Jimenez-Castellanos, M. R., Zia, H., & Rhodes, C. T., (1993). Mucoadhesive drug delivery systems. *Drug Dev. Ind. Pharm., 19*, 143–194.

Joshi, B., Singh, G., Rana, A. C., & Saini, S., (2012). Development and characterization of clarithromycin emulgel for topical delivery. *Int. J. Drug Dev. Res., 4*(3), 310–323.

Jung, G., Yun, J., & Kim, H. I., (2012). Temperature and pH-responsive release behavior of PVAPAAc-PNIPAAm-MWCNTs nanocomposite hydrogels. *Carbon Lett., 13*, 173–177.

Kanfer, I., Rath, S., Purazi, P., & Mudyahoto, N. A., (2017). *In-vitro* release testing of semi-solid dosage forms. *Dissolution Technol.*, 52–59.

Kang, Y. O., Jung, J. Y., Cho, D., Kwon, O. H., Cheon, J. Y., & Park, W. H., (2016). Antimicrobial silver chloride nanoparticles stabilized with chitosan oligomer for the healing of burns. *Mater., 9*, 215.

Kanga, L., Liub, X. Y., Sawantb, P. D., Hoa, P. C., Chanc, Y. W., & Chan, S. Y., (2005). SMGA gels for the skin permeation of haloperidol. *J. Control. Release., 106*, 88–98.

Kapoor, D., Vyas, R. B., Lad, C., Patel, M., Lal, B., & Parmar, R., (2014). Formulation characterization of emulgel of NSAID. *Pharm. Chem. J., 1*, 9–16.

Khullar, R., Kumar, D., Seth, N., & Saini, S., (2012). Formulation and evaluation of mefenamic acid emulgel for topical delivery. *Saudi Pharm. J., 20*, 63–67.

Khurana, S., Bedi, P. M., & Jain, N. K., (2013). Preparation and evaluation of solid lipid nanoparticles based nanogel for dermal delivery of meloxicam. *Chem. Phys. Lipids., 175–176*, 65–72.

Khutoryanskiy, V. V., (2011). Advances in mucoadhesion and mucoadhesive polymers. *Macromol. Biosci., 11*(6), 748–764.

Kilfoyle, B. E., Sheihet, L., Zhang, Z., Laohoo, M., Kohn, J., & Michniak-Kohn, B. B., (2012). Development of paclitaxel-TyroSpheres for topical skin treatment. *J. Control. Release., 163*, 18–24.

Kim, Y. Y., Yun, J., Lee, Y. S., & Kim, H. I., (2010). Electro-responsive transdermal drug release of MWCNT/PVA nanocomposite hydrogels. *Carbon Lett., 11*, 211–215.

Kinloch, A., (1982). The science of adhesion. *J. Mater. Sci., 17*(3), 617–651.

Kogan, A., & Garti, N., (2006). Microemulsions as transdermal drug delivery vehicles. *Adv. in Colloid Interface Sci., 123–126*, 369–385.

Kossena, G. A., Charman, W. N., Boyd, B. J., & Porter, C. J., (2004). A novel cubic phase of medium chain lipid origin for the delivery of poorly water-soluble drugs. *J. Control. Release., 99*(2), 217–229.

Kouchak, M., (2014). *In Situ* gelling systems for drug delivery. *Jundishapur J. Nat. Pharm. Prod., 9*(3), e20126.

Krolow, M. Z., Hartwig, C. A., Link, G. C., Raubach, C. W., Pereira, J. S. F., Picoloto, R. S., Gonçalves, M. R. F., Carreño, N. L. V., & Mesko, M. F., (2013). Synthesis and characterization of carbon nanocomposites. In: Avellaneda, C., (ed.), *Carbon Nanostructures* (p. 3347), Springer-Verlag, Berlin Heidelberg, New York.

Kumar, L., & Verma, R., (2010). *In-vitro* evaluation of topical gel prepared using natural polymer. *Int. J. Drug Deliv., 2*(1), 58–63.

Kumar, R., & Katare, O. P., (2005). Lecithin organogels as a potential phospholipid-structured system for topical drug delivery: A review. *AAPS Pharm. Sci. Tech., 6*, E298–E310.

Kumbhar, A. B., Rakde, A. K., & Chaudhari, P. D., (2013). In situ gel-forming injectable drug delivery system. *Int. J. Pharm. Sci. Res., 4*(2), 597–609.

Kweon, J. H., Chi, S. C., & Park, E. S., (2004). Transdermal delivery of diclofenac using microemulsions. *Arch. Pharm. Res., 27*(3), 351–356.

Lakshmi, P. K., Kalpana, B., & Prasanthi, D., (2013). Invasomes-novel vesicular carriers for enhanced skin permeation. *Systemat. Rev. Pharm., 4*(1), 26–30.

Lane, M. E., (2013). Skin penetration enhancers. *Int. J. Pharm., 447*, 12–21.

Lang, J. C., Roehrs, R. E., Rodeheaver, D. P., Missel, P. J., Jani, R., & Chowhan, M. A., (2002). Design and evaluation of ophthalmic pharmaceutical products. In: Banker, G. S., & Rhodes, C. T., (eds.), *Modern Pharmaceutics*, Marcel Dekker, New York.

Li, Y., Dong, C., Cun, D., Liu, J., Xiang, R., & Fan, L., (2016). Lamellar liquid crystal improves the skin retention of 3-O-ethyl-ascorbic acid and potassium 4-methoxysalicylate *in-vitro* and *in vivo* for topical preparation. *AAPS Pharm. Sci. Tech., 17*(3), 767–777.

Liebenberg, W., Engelbrecht, E., Wessels, A., Devarakonda, B., Yang, W., & De Villiers, M. M., (2003). A comparative study of the release of active ingredients from semisolid cosmeceuticals measured with Franz, enhancer or flow-through cell diffusion apparatus. *J. Food and Drug Anal., 11*(4), 92–99.

Lieberman, H. A., Rieger, M. M., & Banker, G. S, (1989). *Pharmaceutical Dosage Forms: Disperse System* (Vol. 3, pp. 473–511). Marcel Dekker, Series 2, New York.

Limpongsa, E., & Umprayn, K., (2008). Preparation and evaluation of diltiazem hydrochloride diffusion-controlled transdermal delivery system. *AAPS Pharm. Sci. Tech., 9*, 464–470.

Lippacher, R. H., & Mader, M. K., (2001). Preparation of semisolid drug carriers for topical application based on solid lipid nanoparticles. *Int. J. Pharm., 214*, 9–12.

Lopez, R. F., Seto, J. E., Blankschtein, D., & Langer, R., (2011). Enhancing the transdermal delivery of rigid nanoparticles using the simultaneous application of ultrasound and sodium lauryl sulfate. *Biomater., 32*(3), 933–941.

Lu, M. F., Lee, D., & Rao, G. S., (1992). Percutaneous absorption enhancement of luprolide. *Pharm. Res., 9*(12), 1575–1579.

Madan, M., Bajaj, A., Lewis, S., Udupa, N., & Baig, J. A., (2009). *In Situ* forming polymeric drug delivery systems. *Indian J. Pharm. Sci., 71*(3), 242–251.

Mahalingam, R., Li, X., & Jasti, B. R., (2008). Semisolid dosages: Ointments, creams, and gels. In: Gad, S. C., (ed.), *Pharmaceutical Manufacturing Handbook* (pp. 267–312). John Wiley & Sons, Inc., New Jersey.

Małecki, M., Kolsut, P., & Proczka, R., (2005). Angiogenic and antiangiogenic gene therapy. *Gene !er., 12*, S159–S169.

Maqbool, Md. A., Mishra, M. K., Pathak, S., Kesharwani, A., & Kesharwani, A., (2017). Semisolid dosage forms manufacturing: tools, critical process parameters, strategies, optimization and recent advances. *Indo Ame. J. Pharm. Res., 7*(11), 882–893.

Marianecci, C., Marzio, L. D., Rinaldi, F., Celia, C., Paolino, D., Alhaique, F., Esposito, S., & Carafa, M., (2014). Niosomes from 80s to present: The state of the art. *Adv. Colloid and Interf. Sci., 205*, 187–206,

Mariano, M., El, K. N., & Dufresne, A., (2014). Cellulose nanocrystals and related nanocomposites: Review of some properties and challenges. *J. Polym. Sci. Part B: Polym. Phys., 52*, 791–806.

Markovich, R. J., (2001). Dissolution testing of semisolid dosage forms. *Am. Pharm. Rev., 4*(2), 100–105.

McGuinness, G. B., Vrana, N. E., & Liu, Y., (2015). Polyvinyl alcohol-based cryogels: Tissue engineering and regenerative medicine. In: Mishra, M., (ed.), *Encyclopedia of Biomedical Polymers and Polymeric Biomaterials* (pp. 6743–6753). CRC Press.

Meenakshi, & Ahuja, M., (2015). Metronidazole loaded carboxymethyl tamarind kernel polysaccharide polyvinyl alcohol cryogels: Preparation and characterization. *Int. J. Biol. Macromol., 72*, 931–938.

Mehnert, W., & Mader, K., (2001). Solid lipid nanoparticles production, characterization and applications. *Adv. Drug Deliv. Rev., 47*, 165–196.

Meno, G. K., (2002). New insights into skin structure: Scratching the surface. *Adv. Drug Deliv. Rev., 54*(1), S3–S17.

Menon, G., & Ghadially, R., (1997). Morphology of lipid alterations in the epidermis: A review, Microvas. *Res. Tech., 37*, 180–192.

Merino, S., Martin, C., Kostarelos, K., Prato, M., & Vazquez, E., (2015). Nanocomposite hydrogels: 3D polymer-nanoparticle synergies for on-demand drug delivery. *ACS Nano., 9*, 4686–4697.

Methods for Studying Percutaneous Absorption, (1983). In: Barry, B. W., (ed.), *Dermatological Formulations-Percutaneous Absorption* (pp. 234–295). Marcel Dekker, Inc., New York, NY.

Mills, P. C., & Cross, S. E., (2006). Transdermal drug delivery: Basic principles for the veterinarian. *Veter. J., 172*, 218–233.

Mishra, B., Patel, B. B., & Tiwari, S., (2010). Colloidal nanocarriers: A review on formulation technology, types and applications toward targeted drug delivery. *Nanomed.: Nanotechnol. Biol. Med., 6*, 9–24.

Moghassemi, S., & Hadjizadeh, A., (2014). Nano-niosomes as nanoscale drug delivery systems: An illustrated review. *J. Control. Release., 185*, 22–36.

Mohamed, M. I., (2004a). Optimization of chlorphenesin emulgel formulation. *AAPS J., 6*(3), 81–87.

Mohamed, M. I., (2004b). Topical emulsion gel composition comprising diclofenac sodium. *Am. Assn. Pharm. Sci., 6*(3), 1–7.

Mokhtar, M., Sammour, O. A., Hammad, M. A., & Megrab, N. A., (2008). Effect of some formulation parameters on flurbiprofen encapsulation and release rates of niosomes prepared from proniosomes. *Int. J. Pharm., 361*(1&2), 104–111.

Montenegro, L., (2017). Lipid-based nanoparticles as carriers for dermal delivery of antioxidants. *Curr. Drug Metab., 18*, 469–480.

Montenegro, L., Pasquinucci, L., Zappalà, A., Chiechio, S., Turnaturi, R., & Parenti, C., (2017). Rosemary essential oil-loaded lipid nanoparticles: *In vivo* topical activity from gel vehicles. *Pharm., 9*, 48.

Mudshinge, S. R., Deore, A. B., Patil, S., & Bhalgat, C. M., (2011). Nanoparticles: Emerging carriers for drug delivery. *Saudi Pharm. J., 19*, 129–141.

Murdan, S., (2003). Electro-responsive drug delivery from hydrogels. *J. Control. Release., 92*, 1–17.

Murdan, S., (2005). A review of pluronic lecithin organogels as a topical and transdermal drug delivery system. *Hospital Pharmacist, 12*(7), 267–270.

Nagai, N., & Ito, Y., (2014). Therapeutic effects of gel ointments containing tranilast nanoparticles on paw edema in adjuvant-induced arthritis rats. *Biol. Pharm. Bull., 37*(1), 96–104.

Nagai, N., Iwamae, A., Tanimoto, S., Yoshioka, C., & Ito, Y., (2015). Pharmacokinetics and Antiinflammatory effect of a novel gel system containing ketoprofen solid nanoparticles. *Biol. Pharm. Bull., 38*, 1918–1924.

Nair, R., Kumar, K. S. A., Priya, K. V., & Sevukarajan, M., (2011). Recent advances in solid lipid nanoparticles based drug delivery systems. *J. Biomed. Sci. Res., 3*, 368–384.

Neha, M. V., Namita, M. T., Srendran, C. S., & Viral, H. S., (2013). Formulation optimization and evaluation of liposomal gel of prednisolone by applying statistical design. *Ind. J. Res. Pharm. Biotechnol., 1*(2), 180–187.

Niemiec, S. M., Ramachandran, C., & Weiner, N., (1995). Influence of nonionic liposomal composition on topical delivery of peptide drugs into pilosebaceous units: An *in vivo* study using the hamster ear model. *Pharm. Res., 8*, 1184–1188.

Nirmal, H. B., Bakliwal, S. R., & Pawar, S. P., (2010). *In situ* gel: New trends in controlled and sustained drug delivery system. *Int. J. Pharm., 2*, 1398–1408.

Paduraru, O. M., Ciolacu, D., Darie, R. N., & Vasile, C., (2012). Synthesis and characterization of polyvinyl alcohol/cellulose cryogels and their testing as carriers for a bioactive component. *Mater. Sci. Eng. C., 32*(8), 2508–2515.

Pakhare, V., Deshmane, S. V., Deshmane, S. S., & Biyani, K. R., (2017). Design and development of emulgel preparation containing diclofenac potassium. *Asian J. Pharm., 11*(4), S712.

Pandey, M. S., Belgamwar, V. S., & Surana, S. J., (2009). Topical delivery of flurbiprofen from pluronic lecithin organogel. *Ind. J. Pharm. Sci., 71*(1), 87–90.

Pandit, R. S., Gaikwad, S. C., Agarkar, G. A., Gade, A. K., & Rai, M., (2015). Curcumin nanoparticles: Physico-chemical fabrication and its *in-vitro* efficacy against human pathogens. *3 Biotech., 5*, 991–997.

Parhi, R., & Swain, S., (2018). Transdermal evaporation drug delivery system: Concept to commercial products. *Adv. Pharm. Bull., 8*(4), 535–550.

Parhi, R., (2016a). Development and optimization of pluronic® F127 and HPMC based thermosensitive gel for the skin delivery of metoprolol succinate. *J. Drug Deliv. Sci. Technol., 36*, 23–33.

Parhi, R., (2017). Cross-linked hydrogel for pharmaceutical applications: A review. *Adv. Pharm. Bull., 7*(4), 515–530.

Parhi, R., (2018). Nanocomposite for transdermal drug delivery. In: Inamuddin, A. A. M., & Ali, M., (eds.), *Applications of Nanocomposite Materials in Drug Delivery* (Vol. 2, p. 353–390). Woodhead Publishing, Elsevier, Oxford, U.K.

Parhi, R., Suresh, P., & Pattnaik, S., (2016b). Pluronic lecithin organogel (PLO) of diltiazem hydrochloride: Effect of solvents/penetration enhancers on *ex vivo* permeation. *Drug Deliv. Transl. Res., 6*, 243–253.

Park, K., & Robinson, J. R., (1984). Bioadhesive polymers as platforms for oral-controlled drug delivery: Method to study bioadhesion. *Int. J. Pharm., 19*(2), 107–127.

Patel, H. K., Barot, B. S., Parejiya, P. B., Shelat, P. K., & Shukla, A., (2013). Topical delivery of clobetasol propionate loaded microemulsion based gel for effective treatment of vitiligo: *Ex vivo* permeation and skin irritation studies. *Colloids and Surf. B: Biointerf., 102*, 86–94.

Patel, N. R., Patel, D. A., Bharadia, P. D., Pandya, V., & Modi, D., (2011). Microsphere as a novel drug delivery. *Int. J. Pharm. Life Sci., 2*(8), 992–997.

Patel, P., Tyagi, S., Patel, C. J., Patel, J., Chaudhari, B., & Kumar, U., (2013). Recent advances in novel semisolid dosage forms: An overview. *J. Biomed. Pharm. Res., 2*(1), 9–14.

Pazos, V., Mongrain, R., & Tardif, J. C., (2009). Polyvinyl alcohol cryogel: Optimizing the parameters of cryogenic treatment using hyperelastic models. *J. Mech. Behav. Biomed. Mater., 2*(5), 542–549.

Perez-Martınez, C. J., Chavez, S. D. M., Del Castillo-Castro, T., Ceniceros, T. E. L., Castillo-Ortega, M. M., Rodrıguez-Felix, D. E., Carlos, J., & Ruize, G., (2016).

Electroconductive nanocomposite hydrogel for pulsatile drug release. *React. Funct. Polym., 100*, 12–17.

Pharmaceutical Machinery. *Ointment Manufacturing Plant, Planetary Mixer, Tube Filling Machine.* http://www.pharmaceuticalmachinery.in/ointment_section.htm (Accessed on 19 November 2019).

Pina, S., Oliveira, J. M., & Reis, R. L., (2015). Natural-based nanocomposites for bone tissue engineering and regenerative medicine: a review. *Adv. Mater., 27*, 1143–1169.

Ponnaian, P. K., Oommen, R., Kannaiyan, S. K. C., Jayachandran, S., Natarajan, M., & Santhanam, A., (2015). Synthesis and characterization of silver nanoparticles for biological applications. *J. Environ. Nanotechnol., 4*(1), 23–26.

Preeti, M., & Kumar, S., (2014). Development of celecoxib transfersomal gel for the treatment of rheumatoid arthritis. *Ind. J. Pharm. Biol. Res., 2*(2), 7–13.

Qiu, Y., & Park, K., (2012). Environment-sensitive hydrogels for drug delivery. *Adv. Drug Deliv. Rev., 64*, 49–60.

Rajalakshmi, R., Mahesh, K., & Kumar, C. K. A., (2011). A critical review on nanoemulsions. *Int. J. Innov. Drug Discov., 1*, 1–8.

Ramachandran, S., Chen, S., & Etzler, F., (1999). Rheological characterization of hydroxypropyl cellulose gels. *Drug Dev. Ind. Pharm., 25*(2), 153–161.

Rao, J. P., & Geckeler, K. E., (2011). Polymer nanoparticles: Preparation techniques and size-control parameters. *Prog. Polym. Sci., 36*, 887–913.

Rao, M., Sukre, G., Aghav, S., & Kumar, M., (2013). Optimization of metronidazole emulgel. *J. Pharm.*, 1–9.

Rege, P. R., Vilivalam, V. D., & Collins, C. C., (1998). Development in release testing of topical dosage forms: Use of the Enhancer Cell TM with automated sampling. *J. Pharm. Biomed. Anal., 17*(8), 1225–1233.

Rheological Studies, (2016). *Kulkarni-Shaw Essential Chemistry for Formulators of Semisolid and Liquid Dosages* (pp. 145–182). Academic Press: USA.

Schäfer-Korting, M., Mehnert, W., & Korting, H. C., (2007). Lipid nanoparticles for improved topical application of drugs for skin diseases. *Adv. Drug Deliv. Rev., 59*, 427–443.

Selzer, D., Abdel-Mottaleb, M. M. A., Hahn, T., Schaefer, U. F., & Neumann, D., (2013). Finite and infinite dosing: Difficulties in measurements, evaluations and predictions. *Adv. Drug Deliv. Rev., 65*, 278–294.

Semisolid Drug Products-Performance Tests. In: *The United States Pharmacopoeia and National Formulary USP 37–NF 32* (pp. 1273–1284). The United States Pharmacopoeial Convention, Inc.: Rockville, MD, 2014.

Shaikh, R., Singh, T. R. R., Garland, M. J., Woolfson, A. D., & Donnelly, R. F., (2011). Mucoadhesive drug delivery systems. *J. Pharm. Bioallied Sci., 3*(1), 89–100.

Shetty, P. K., Venuvanka, V., Jagani, H. V., Chethan, G. H., Ligade, V. S., Musmade, P. B., Nayak, U. Y., Reddy, M. S., Kalthur, G., Udupa, N., Rao, C. M., & Mutalik, S., (2015). Development and evaluation of sunscreen creams containing morin-encapsulated nanoparticles for enhanced UV radiation protection and antioxidant activity. *Int. J. Nanomed., 10*, 6477–6491.

Shrotriya, S. N., Ranpise, N. S., & Vidhate, B. V., (2017). Skin targeting of resveratrol utilizing solid lipid nanoparticle-engrossed gel for chemically induced irritant contact dermatitis *Drug Deliv. Transl. Res., 7*, 37–52.

Shuwaili, A. H. A. L., Abdul, B. K., Rasool, A. B. K., & Abdulrasool, A. A., (2016). Optimization of elastic transfersomes formulations for transdermal delivery of pentoxifylline. *Eur. J. Pharm. Biopharm., 102*, 101–114.

Siddique, M. I., Katas, H., Jamil, A., Iqbal, M. C., Amin, M., Ng, S. F., Zulfakar, M. H., & Nadeem, S. M., (2017). Potential treatment of atopic dermatitis: Tolerability and safety of cream containing nanoparticles loaded with hydrocortisone and hydroxytyrosol in human subjects. *Drug Deliv. Transl. Res.,* (Epub ahead of print).

Smart, J. D., (2005). The basics and underlying mechanisms of mucoadhesion. *Adv. Drug Deliv. Rev., 57*(11), 1556–1568.

So, J. W., Kim, S., Park, J. S., Kim, B. H., Jung, S. H., Shin, S. C., & Cho, C. W., (2010). Preparation and evaluation of solid lipid nanoparticles with JSH18 for skin-whitening efficacy. *Pharm. Dev. Technol., 15*(4), 415–420.

Souto, E. B., & Müller, R. H., (2010). Lipid nanoparticles: Effect on bioavailability and pharmacokinetic changes. *Handb. Exp. Pharmacol., 197*, 115–141.

Tavano, L., Gentile, L., Rossi, C. O., & Muzzalupo, R., (2013). Novel gel-niosomes formulations as multicomponent systems for transdermal drug delivery. *Colloids and Surf. B: Biointerf., 110*, 281–288.

Ueda, C. T., Shah, V. P., Derdzinski, K., Ewing, G., Flynn, G., Maibach, H., Marques, M., Rytting, H., Shaw, S., Thakker, K., & Yacobi, A., (2009). Topical and transdermal drug products: The topical/transdermal ad hoc advisory panel for the USP performance tests of topical and transdermal dosage forms. *United States Pharmacopoeia Convention Inc., 35*, 750–764.

Umalkar, D. G., & Rajesh, K. S., (2013). Formulation and evaluation of liposomal gel for treatment of psoriasis. *Int. J. Pharm. Bio. Sci., 4*(4), 22–32.

Valenzuela, P., & Simon, J. A., (2012). Nanoparticle delivery for transdermal HRT. *Nanomed., Suppl. 1*, S83–89.

Varde, N. M., Thakor, N. M., Srendran, C. S., & Shah, V. H., (2013). Formulation optimization and evaluation of liposomal gel of prednisolone by applying statistical design. *Ind. J. Res. Pharm. Biotechnol., 2*(1), 180–187.

Varma, V. N. S. K., Maheshwari, P. V., Navya, M., Reddy, S. C., Shivakumar, H. G., & Gowda, D. V., (2014). Calcipotriol delivery into the skin as emulgel for effective permeation. *Saudi Pharm. J., 22*, 591–599.

Varshosaz, J., Sadrai, H., & Heidari, A., (2006). Nasal delivery of insulin using bioadhesive chitosan gels. *Drug Deliv., 13*, 31–36.

Vasir, J. K., Tambwekar, K., & Garg, S., (2003). Bioadhesive microspheres as a controlled drug delivery system. *Int. J. Pharm., 255*(1&2), 13–32.

Venkataharsha, P., Maheshwara, E., Raju, Y. P., Reddy, V. A., Rayadu, B. S., & Karisetty, B., (2015). Liposomal Aloe vera trans-emulgel drug delivery of naproxen and nimesulide: A study. *Int. J. Pharm. Investig., 5*(1), 28–34.

Vintiloiu, A., & Leroux, J. C., (2008). Organogels and their use in drug delivery—A review. *J. Control. Release, 125(3)*, 179–192.

Wang, L., Hu, X., Shen, B., Xie, Y., Shen, C., Lu, Y., Qi, J., Yuan, H., & Wu, W., (2015). Enhanced stability of liposomes against solidification stress during freeze-drying and spray-drying by coating with calcium alginate. *J. Drug Deliv. Sci. Technol., 30*, 163–170.

Werys, K., Pieniak, K., Lesniak-Plewinska, B., Zmigrodzki, J., & Cygan, S., (2015). Validation of the polyvinyl alcohol cryogel with glycerol as a material for phantoms in magnetic resonance imaging. *The 8*[th] *IEEE International Conference on Intelligent Data Acquisition and Advanced Computing Systems: Technology and Applications* (pp. 656–659). Warsaw, Poland.

Yapar, E. A., & Inal, O., (2014). Transdermal spray in hormone delivery. *Trop. J. Pharm. Res., 13*(3), 469–474.

Yapar, E. A., (2017). Herbal cosmetics and novel drug delivery systems. *Ind. J. Pharm. Edu. Res., 51*(3s), s152–s158.

Yu, T., Andrews, G., & Jones, D., (2014). Mucoadhesion and characterization of mucoadhesive properties. In: Das Neves, J., & Sarmento, B., (eds.), *Mucosal Delivery of Biopharmaceuticals* (pp. 35–58). Springer, Boston, MA.

Zahedi, P., Souza, R. D., Miller, P. M., & Allen, C., (2011). Docetaxel distribution following intraperitoneal administration in mice. *J. Pharm. Pharm. Sci., 14*, 90–99.

Zhang, J., & Michniak-Kohn, B., (2011). Investigation of microemulsion microstructures and their relationship to transdermal permeation of model drugs: Ketoprofen, lidocaine, and caffeine. *Int. J. Pharm., 421*, 34–44.

Zheng, W., Xia, F., Wang, L., & Zhang, Y., (2012). Preparation and quality assessment of itraconazole transfersomes. *Int. J. Pharm., 436*(1&2), 291–298.

CHAPTER 7

Recent Advancements in Transdermal Drug Delivery System

MOHAMMED ASADULLAH JAHANGIR,[1] ABDUL MUHEEM,[2] CHETTUPALLI ANAND[3] and SYED SARIM IMAM*[4]

[1]Department of Pharmaceutics, Nibha Institute of Pharmaceutical Sciences, Rajgir–803116, Nalanda, Bihar, India

[2]School of Pharmaceutical Education and Research, Jamia Hamdard, New Delhi–110062, India

[3]Department of Pharmaceutics, Anurag Group of Institutions, School of Pharmacy, Venkatapur, Ghatkesar, Telangana–500088, India

[4]Department of Pharmaceutics, College of Pharmacy, King Saud University, Riyadh–11451, Saudi Arabia

*Corresponding author. E-mail: sarimimam@gmail.com

ABSTRACT

Sir Ronald Fisher introduced the concept of applying statistical analysis in the beginning of the twentieth century. Recently, regulatory guidelines issued by the key federal agencies to implement the practice of 'quality by design (QbD)' approach to the researchers in the industrial milieu, in particular, to use experimental designs during drug product development. The aim to introduce the design approach is to build quality into the product. The implementation of the QbD approach in the transdermal/topical formulation is the key enabler of assuring quality in the final product. The optimization processes are required for accurate research in these fields and therefore, the right implementation is carried out for different design approaches at an industrial scale. This chapter illustrates the principles of QbD design and their contributions to the background of the design of experiments in different transdermal/topical nanoformulations.

7.1   INTRODUCTION

Transdermal drug delivery has made an impressive contribution to medical practice but has yet to achieve its potential as a go-to alternative to oral delivery and hypodermic injection. Its non-invasive mode of administration and ease of self-administered represents an attractive alternative to oral delivery of drugs. Since human civilization, humans have placed substances on the skin for therapeutic effects and, in the modern era, a variety of topical formulations have been developed to treat local indications. It can protect the drug from a significant first-pass effect of the liver that can prematurely metabolize drugs (Prausnitz and Langer, 2008; Imam and Aqil, 2016). It is capable of providing extended release of drugs and also able to improve patient compliance and are comparatively inexpensive. The potential meritorious features associated with transdermal drug delivery are well documented in numerous researches and review scientific contents. These include by-passing first-pass effect, administration of lower doses, potentially decreased side effects, constant plasma levels, and improved patient compliance. In the development of a transdermal drug delivery system (TDDS), the skin penetration enhancement of the drug plays a key factor in its application because of the barrier properties of the stratum corneum to drug permeation.

To identify, analyze and control all causes that could alter quality and safety of a new drug, the United States Food and Drug Administration (USFDA) proposed in 2000 a risk-based approach of drug engineering, which was finally came to be known as Quality-by-Design (QbD) in the year 2008 by the International Council for Harmonization of technical requirements for pharmaceuticals for human use (ICH) (Hafner et al., 2014; Bastogne, 2017). Conversely to the traditional approaches that only test the quality of the product, the Design of Experiment (DoE) (Singh et al., 2004) and QbD (Bhoop, 2014) fundamentally aims at building quality and safety from the very first design steps. It is often regarded as a new drug development paradigm in the pharmaceutical industry. It is, in reality, the inheritance of the experience gained from the manufacturing industry over the years. In the 1970s, J.M. Juran created the QbD concept and popularized it in the late 1990s (Juran, 1992). All those contributions generally use common graphical, scoring and similar statistical tools such as the Ishikawa and Pareto diagrams, Failure Mode Effect Analysis, Design of Experiments, and Statistical Process Control. However, in his book, Juran did not consider drugs or medical devices.

7.2 DOE-BASED TRANSDERMAL/TOPICAL NANOCARRIERS

The pharmaceutical sector is a process-based and quality-oriented industry, thus it was expected that the aforementioned paradigms will be adapted soon after their introduction (Politis et al., 2008). However, Quality by Design was actually suggested by the regulatory authorities (FDA, EMA) at the beginning of the new millennium, recognizing that quality cannot be tested into products, but the quality should be built in by design (Prausnitz and Langer 2008). It should be noted that there are different mathematical modeling techniques available for addressing pharmaceutical development and more specifically within the QbD (Figure 7.1). It gives an understanding of the different formulation components interaction(s) at the different levels and helps in selecting "the best" formulation with minimal time, effort (Singh et al., 2005; Singh et al., 2014 and 2015; Beg et al., 2017a,b and 2019)

There are wide ranges of different transdermal and topical formulations have been formulated and statistically optimized using the different optimization process. The different formulations have been widely published in the literature using the different QbD approaches [Plackett-Burman design (PBD); central composite design (CCD); Box-Behnken design (BBD), Taguchi design (TD)] for optimization. The formulation was optimized using the different independent variables and their effects were observed on the dependent variables. This optimization approach was particularly selected because it requires lesser runs and may take different variables at a different level for optimization. The collected data for each response in each run were statistically analyzed and fitted into the different regression models.

There are many nanotransdermal/topical formulations (vesicles, colloidal particle, nanoparticles) have been widely optimized and reported in the literature using different formulation design approach (Table 7.1). These delivery systems reported for their better applicability for the local and systemic absorption of drugs across the skin. In this chapter, an attempt was made to provide an overall overview of information about QbD-based transdermal delivery systems and to summarize the different major QbD approaches used in transdermal/topical drug delivery systems (Table 7.1).

7.2.1 LIPID-BASED VESICULAR CARRIER

The application of neovascular carriers has shown a promising response in drug permeation and bioavailability enhancement. These vesicular

TABLE 7.1　QbD Used Different Transdermal/Topical Nano-Formulation with Their Used Variables

S.No	Formulation	Drug	QbD Design	Independent variables	Dependent variables	Reference
1	NLCs	Lappacontine, Ranaconitine	Uniform design	Lipid (%); Surfactant (%); Solid/Liquid (w/w); Drug/Lipid (w/w).	Size (nm), Encapsulation efficiency (%), Drug loading (%)	Guo et al., 2015
2	Transfersomes	Raloxifene HcL	Box-Behnken design	Phospholipon® 90G; Sodium deoxycholate; Sonication time.	Entrapment efficiency; Vesicle size; Transdermal flux.	Mahmood et al., 2014
3	Glycerosomes	Paeoniflorin	Uniform design	Phospholipid; cholesterol; glycerol in water.	Particle size; Polydispersity index; Zeta potential; Encapsulation efficiency	Zhang et al., 2017.
4	Polymeric mixed micelles	Terconazole	2^3 full factorial design	Weight ratio of total Pluronics to drug; Weight ratio of Pluronic P123 to Pluronic F127; Percent of Cremophor EL in an aqueous medium.	MIE (%); micellar size (nm); PDI; Zeta potential (mV)	Abd-Elsalam et al., 2018
5	Nanoethosomes	Vardenafil	Box–Behnken design	Lipid composition, Sonication time, Ethanol	Particle size; Encapsulation efficiency	Fahmy, 2015
6	Nanoemulsion	Ceramide IIIB	Central composite design	Water content (30%–70%, w/w), Mixing rate (400–720 rpm), Temperature (20°C–60°C), Addition rate (0.3–1.8 mL/min).	Droplet size; Polydispersity index.	Su et al., 2017

TABLE 7.1 *(Continued)*

S.No	Formulation	Drug	QbD Design	Independent variables	Dependent variables	Reference
7	Nanoemulsion	Chalcone	Full factorial	Type of surfactant; Type of co-surfactants	Physicochemical characteristics; Skin permeation/retention	de Mattos et al., 2015
9	Pronioomes	Pioglitazone	Box–Behnken design	Tween80 (A), phospholipid (B), and cholesterol (C)	Particle size, percentage entrapment and transdermal flux	Prasad et al., 2015
10	NlCs	Nimesulide	Box–Behnken design	Ratio of stearic acid: oleic acid; Poloxamer 188 concentration; Lecithin concentration.	Particle size; Entrapment Efficiency.	Moghaddam et al., 2016
11	Nanoethosome	Tramadol	Box–Behnken design	Phospholipid; Ethanol; Sonication time.	Vesicle size; Entrapment efficiency; Transflux	Ahmed et al., 2016
12	Niosomes	Lacidipine	Box–Behnken design	Span 60 concentration; Cholesterol concentration; Hydration time; Sonication time.	Vesicle size; Entrapment efficiency Flux.	Qumbar et al., 2016
13	Ethosomes	Tropisetron HCl	Full factorial design	Concentrations of both phosphatidylcholine; Ethanol; Phosphatidylcholine type.	Entrapment efficiency; Vesicle size; Polydispersity index; Zeta potential	Abdel Messih et al., 2017
14	Liposomes	Alprazolam	Central composite design	Solvent/nonsolvent volume ratio; Phospholipid concentration; Alprazolam concentration; Cholesterol content.	Vesicle size; Encapsulation efficiency.	Hashemi et al., 2018

TABLE 7.1 *(Continued)*

S.No	Formulation	Drug	QbD Design	Independent variables	Dependent variables	Reference
15	Niosomes	Sumatriptan Succinate	Taguchi design	Time lapsed to hydrate the lipid film	Vesicle size; Zeta potential; Drug entrapment.	González-Rodríguez et al., 2012
16	Microemulasion	Agomelatine	Mixture design	Percentages of capryol 90 as an oily phase (X_1); Cremophor RH40 and Transcutol HP in a ratio of (1:2) as surfactant/cosurfactant mixture 'S_{mix}' (X_2); Water (X_3).	Globule size; Optical clarity; Cumulative amount permeated after 1 and 24h.	Said et al., 2017
17	Nanolipid vesicular	Phosphatidylcholine	Two-level factorial design	Concentration of PC; Concentration of edge activator; Edge activator type.	—	ElAfify et al., 2018
18	Transfersomes	Buspirone hydrochloride	Full factorial design	Oleic acid; Ethanol.	Particle size; Poly dispersity index; Zeta potential; Encapsulation efficiency.	Shamma et al., 2013
19	NLCs	Aceclofenac	Box–Behnken design	Lipids; Oil: lipid ratio; Concentration of surfactants.	Entrapment efficiency; Particle size.	Garg et al., 2017
20	NLCs	Silymarin	Full factorial design	HHPH pressure; Number of cycles; Stirring speed.	Particle size; Polydispersity index; Zeta potential.	Singh et al., 2016

carriers have shown several advantages such as the ability to entrap drugs with different solubility profile, the possibility of being produced using natural ingredients, can accommodate both hydrophilic and lipophilic drugs (Khan et al., 2018). Many vesicular carriers have been reported in the literature which includes liposomes, niosomes, Transfersomes® (Idea AG, Germany), and invasomes (Imam and Aqil, 2016). The success of the first generation of vesicular systems (liposome carriers) are widely used systems in recent days as a delivery system (Bsieso et al., 2015).

7.2.1.1 NIOSOMES

Niosomes are unilamellar or multilamellar vesicles made up of phospholipids and nonionic surfactants with or without incorporation of cholesterol or other lipids. It has gained much attention as vesicular drug delivery systems in the last three decades due to their unique characteristics for providing the enhanced solubility and bioavailability for poorly soluble drugs (Abidin et al., 2016; Sayeed et al., 2017). It has a high potential to act as carriers for poorly soluble drugs (Jamal et al., 2015).

The application of formulation design was applied by Aziz et al. (2018a) to formulate and optimize diacerein niosomes using film hydration technique. They applied central composite design for the optimization by taking three-level three-factor to get an optimal niosomes formulation with the desired characteristics. The three formulations used were the amount of salt in hydration medium (X_1), lipid amount (X_2) and number of surfactant parts (X_3) and their effects were assessed on entrapment efficiency percent (Y_1), particle size (Y_2), polydispersity index (Y_3), and zeta potential (Y_4). The design-based optimize formulation showed high entrapment efficiency (95.63%), low particle size (436.65 nm) and polydispersity index (0.47) with zeta potential (–38.80 mV). The results revealed that the CCD based niosomal system was successfully optimized which will result in delivering diacerein efficiently (Aziz et al., 2018a). The topical niosomes delivery system was developed and reported by the research group using methotrexate (MTX) as a drug for the treatment of psoriasis. They used Box-Behnken's design to optimize MTX proniosome gels using span 40, cholesterol, (Chol-X_1) and tween 20 (X_2) and short-chain alcohols (X_3) [namely ethanol (Et), propylene glycol (Pg), and glycerol (G)]. The responses showed a significant effect on vesicles size (Y_1), entrapment efficiency (EE%-Y_2) and zeta potential (Y_3). MTX

loaded niosomes were formed immediately upon hydration of the proniosome gels with the employed solvents. The optimized formula of MTX
loaded niosomes showed vesicle size of 480 nm, high EE% (55%) and zeta
potential of −25.5 mV, at Chol and T20 concentrations of 30% and 23.6%,
respectively (Zidan et al., 2017).

Another research group formulates and optimize diacerein loaded
cholesterol-rich niosomes by employing a 3-factor, 3-level Box-Behnken
design (Moghaddam et al., 2016). The results of the study indicated that
Span 60 (90 mg) and cholesterol (10 mg), and hydration time (45 min) were
found to be optimum for niosomes preparation. The optimized formulation
F2 entrapped the drug with 83.02% efficiency, size 477.8 nm, and flux of
2.820 µg/cm²/h, and followed the Higuchi model and non-Fickian transport
mechanism. Concisely, the results showed that BBD optimized diacerein
delivery might be used for enhanced treatment of psoriasis. Imam et al.
(2016) fabricated and optimized 4-factor 3-level QbD-based proniosome
for transdermal delivery of risperidone. The independent factors used for
the optimization study were span 60, cholesterol, phospholipon 90 G,
and risperidone concentration and their responses were assessed on the
vesicle size (nm), encapsulation efficiency (%) and transdermal flux (µg/
cm²/h). The selection of optimized risperidone niosome formulation was
done on the criteria of attaining the minimum vesicles size and maximum
% encapsulation efficiency and transdermal flux, by applying the point
prediction method. The results showed the optimized niosomes formulation exhibited the vesicles size of 498.43 ± 1.27 nm, entrapment efficiency
of 90.43 ± 1.21%, and the transdermal flux across rat skin was 117.42 ±
8.61 mg/cm²/h. Similarly, another research group Soliman et al. (2016)
prepared lacidipine encapsulated proniosomes and optimized using 2^3 full
factorial design for improved transdermal delivery. They used cholesterol,
soya lecithin, and cremophor RH 40 as independent variables and their
effects were observed on the vesicle size (nm), entrapment efficiency
(%), and release efficiency (%). The results indicated that the optimized
niosomal formulation composition developed using cholesterol (10 mg),
soya lecithin (80 mg) and cremophore RH 40 (270 mg) exhibited the low
vesicles size (162.43±0.77 nm), high entrapment efficiency (98.01±0.68%)
and release efficiency (88.33±2.43%). Moreover, the optimized formulation exhibited significantly improved $AUC_{0 \to a}$ was evaluated for its
bioavailability compared with the commercial product. In another study
Kumar and Goindi (2014), statistically, Taguchi design and D-optimal

design optimized itraconazole hydrogel using nonionic surfactant vesicles (NSVs). They used different factors surfactant type, content and molar ratio of cholesterol: surfactant for the screening of optimized niosomes. The ex vivo studies in rat skin depicted that optimized formulation augmented drug skin retention and permeation in 6h than conventional cream and oily solution. Abdelbary et al. (2015), used Design-Expert(®) software to apply BBD design for the optimization of MTX niosomes using different formulation variables for the management of psoriasis. The formulation was prepared using thin-film hydration technique using three independent variables as MTX concentration in hydration medium (X_1), total weight of niosomal components (X_2) and surfactant: cholesterol ratio (X_3) and their effects were observed on the encapsulation efficiency (Y_1) and particle size (Y_2) as dependent variables. The optimal formulation (F12) displayed spherical morphology under transmission electron microscopy (TEM), the optimum particle size of 1375.00 nm and high EE% of 78.66%. In-vivo skin deposition study showed that the highest value of percentage drug deposited (22.45%) and AUC_{0-10} (1.15 mgh/cm²) of MTX from niosomes were significantly greater than that of drug solution (13.87% and 0.49 mg.h/cm², respectively). In another study by Aboelwafa et al. (2010) used different non-ionic surfactants like polyoxyethylene alkyl ethers, namely Brij 78, Brij 92, and Brij 72; and sorbitan fatty acid esters (Span 60) to evaluate the possible factors of CAR proniosomal gels. A $2^{(3)}$ full factorial design was employed to evaluate individual and combined effects of formulation variables. The proniosomes prepared with Brij 72 and Span 60 showed better noisome forming ability and higher EE% than those prepared with Brij 78 and Brij 92. The skin permeation study result revealed that higher permeation was mainly affected by the weight of proniosomes. The proniosomes gel prepared with Span 60 showed higher permeation enhancing effect than Brij 72.

7.2.1.2 TRANSFEROSOMES

Transfersomesare also called elastic or deformable vesicles containing an edge activator in the lipid bilayer structure. In the year 1992, Cevc and Blume introduced a new class of ultra-flexible vesicles termed Transfersomes™ (Idea AG, Germany). They are prepared with phospholipids, such as phosphatidylcholine and surfactants (Cevc 1996).

Recently, Moolakkadath et al., (2018) implemented Box–Behnken design to evaluate the optimization of fisetin based transethosomes formulation for dermal delivery. The optimization of the formulation was carried out using Lipoid S 100, ethanol and sodium cholate and the prepared transethosomes were characterized for vesicle size, entrapment efficiency and in vitro skin penetration study. The findings of the present study demonstrated that the optimized formulation shown the size of 74.21 ± 2.65 nm, entrapment efficiency of $68.31 \pm 1.48\%$ and flux of 4.13 ± 0.17 mg/cm^2/h. the study results data revealed that the developed statistically optimized transethosomes vesicles formulation was found to be a potentially useful drug carrier for fisetin dermal delivery. In another study, the topical drug delivery against cutaneous leishmaniasis (CL) was developed by preparing sodium stibogluconate (SSG) nano-deformable liposomes (NDLs) (Dar et al., 2018). The formulations were prepared by a modified thin-film hydration method and optimized *via* Box–Behnken statistical design. The results of the developed formulation showed physicochemical properties of SSG-NDLs were established in terms of vesicle size (195.1 nm), polydispersity index (0.158), zeta potential (-32.8 mV), and entrapment efficiency (35.26%). The *ex vivo* skin permeation study revealed that SSG-NDLs gel provided 10-fold higher skin retention towards the deeper skin layers, attained without the use of classical permeation enhancers. The *in vivo* results displayed higher anti-leishmanial activity by efficiently healing lesion and successfully reducing parasite burden.

Sildenafil citrate (SLD) loaded optimized nano-transfersomal transdermal films with enhanced and controlled permeation were prepared using modified lipid hydration technique (Badr-Eldin et al., 2016). Central composite design was applied for the optimization of transfersomes using the independent variables as drug-to-phospholipid molar ratio, surfactant hydrophilic-lipophilic balance, and hydration medium pH. The optimized transfersomes showed the nanometric size and exhibited enhanced ex vivo permeation parameters in compare to SLD control films. Further, the SLD transfersomes film depicted enhanced bioavailability and extended absorption as shown by their higher maximum plasma concentration (C_{max}) and area under the curve (AUC) and longer time to maximum plasma concentration (T_{max}) compared to control films.

The optimized ethosomal formulation of glimepiride was formulated and evaluated for the transdermal films (Ahmed et al., 2016). The four formulation factors were optimized for their effects on vesicle size (Y_1), entrapment efficiency (Y_2), and vesicle flexibility (Y_3). The percent of alcohol was significantly affecting all the studied responses while the other factors and their interaction effects were varied on their effects on each response. The ex-vivo permeation of films loaded with optimized ethosomal formulation was superior to that of the corresponding pure drug transdermal films. So, the ethosomal formulation could be considered a suitable drug delivery system especially when loaded into transdermal vehicle with possible reduction in side effects and controlling the drug release.

Timolol maleate (TiM), designed to formulate and optimize trans-fersomal TiM gel for transdermal delivery using 2^3 full factorial designs (Morsi et al., 2016). TiM transfersomal gel was optimized using the variables effects of egg phosphatidylcholine (PC): surfactant (SAA) molar ratio, solvent volumetric ratio, and the drug amount were assessed on particle size, entrapment efficiency (%EE), and release rate. The opti-mized transfersomal gel was prepared with PC:SAA molar ratio (4.65:1), solvent volumetric ratio (3:1), and drug amount (13 mg) with particle size of 2.72 μm, EE of 39.96%, and a release rate of 134.49 μg/cm²/h. The study revealed that factorial design optimized transfersomal transdermal system was successfully developed.

In one of the studies, Ahmed (2015) utilizes Plackett–Burman design to evaluate the effect of different processing and formulation parameters on the preparation of sildenafil (SD) transferosomes. The formulation with optimum desirability showed entrapment efficiency and vesicle size in the range of 97.21% and 610 nm respectively. In vitro permeation of the drug-loaded transferosome showed more than 5-fold higher permeation rate compared with a standard drug suspension. The significant variables were further optimized using point prediction optimization method to produce smaller vesicle size that could increase the permeation of sildenafil from optimized transferosomes formulation.

Another research group prepared and evaluated raloxifene hydrochlo-ride-loaded transferosomes (Mahmood et al., 2014). The transfersomes were evaluated using response surface methodology (Box-Behnken design) using phospholipon® 90G, sodium deoxycholate, and sonication time as independent variables at three levels. The developed formulation was evaluated for entrapment efficiency, vesicle size, and transdermal flux as the dependent variables. The size was found to be in the range of 134±9 nm with an entrapment efficiency of 91.00%±4.90% and transdermal flux of 6.5 ± 1.1 µg/cm^2/hour. The research group concluded that prepared raloxifene hydrochloride transferosomes were found significantly superior in terms of the amount of drug permeated and skin deposition.

González-Rodríguez et al. (2012) applied Taguchi orthogonal experimental design using the amount of cholesterol (F1), the amount of edge-activator (F2), the distribution of the drug into the vesicle (F3), the addition of stearylamine (F4) and the type of edge-activator (F5) as causal factors. Their effect was assessed on deformability index, phosphorus recovery, vesicle size, polydispersity index, zeta potential and percentage of drug entrapped as dependent variables. From the study, it was concluded that the lipid to surfactant ratio and type of surfactant are the main key factors for determining the flexibility of the bilayer of transferosomes.

7.2.1.3   ETHOSOMES

Ethosomes are soft malleable lipid vesicles composed of phospholipids, a high concentration of ethanol and water. It is widely used vesicles to delivers the enable drugs to reach the deep skin layers and/or systemic circulation. It differs from liposome vesicles because it contains a large amount of ethanol, which gives enhanced transdermal property for both hydrophilic as well as hydrophobic drugs.

The transdermal delivery of colchicine loaded transethosomal gels as potential carriers were prepared by the cold method and statistically optimized using three sets of 2^4 factorial design experiments (Abdulbaqi et al., 2018). The optimized colchicine-loaded transethosomal gels were further characterized for rheological behavior and ex vivo skin permeation through Sprague Dawley rats' back skin. The results of the study showed that the colchicine-loaded TEs shown nanometric size and high entrapment efficiency. The developed colchicine's transethosomal gels were able to enhance the skin permeation in comparison to the non-ethosomal gel.

In another study, Aziz et al., (2018b) assessed diacerein (DCN) elastosomes (edge activator (EA)-based vesicular nanocarriers) as a novel transdermal system were prepared according to $4^1.2^1$ full factorial design using different EAs in varying amounts. The prepared formulae were characterized for different parameters and the desirability function was employed using Design-Expert® software to select the optimal elastosomes (E1) which showed EE% of $96.25\pm2.19\%$, PS of 506.35 ± 44.61 nm, PDI of

0.46 ± 0.09, ZP of -38.65 ± 0.91 mV, and DI of 12.74 ± 2.63 g. In addition, E1 was compared to DCN-loaded bilosomes and both vesicles exhibited superior skin permeation potential and retention capacity compared to drug suspension. *The o*verall, results of the study confirmed the admirable potential of E1 to be utilized as novel carrier for transdermal delivery of DCN using the full factorial design.

In another study, Mishra et al. (2013) developed and optimized ethosomes using different concentrations of phospholipids (2–5 % w/v), ethanol (20–50 % w/v), ropinirole HCl (5 % w/v) and water. The ethosomes were optimized using $3^{(2)}$ full factorial designs to study the effect of independent variables on dependent variables as entrapment efficiency and in-vitro drug release (24 h). The regression analysis of the study concluded that the used independent variables shown significant effect on response variables. The contour plot and response surface plot showed that the optimized formulation was containing 30 % w/v ethanol and 4% w/v lecithin.

7.2.1.4 INVASOMES

Invasomes are lipid-based vesicles with very high membrane fluidity, containing single or blend of terpenes, which act as penetration enhancement. The presence of terpenes (1–5%) and ethanol provided them with this unique feature.

The transdermal risperidone invasomes were prepared by Imam et al. (2017), using phospholipid, safranal, and ethanol. The study was performed with 3-factor 3-level Box-Behnken design to optimize the soft lipid vesicles and their effects were observed on the dependent variables vesicle size (81.28–153.87 nm), entrapment efficiency (70.43–89.74%) and flux (97.43–182.65 $\mu g/cm^2/h$). The optimized risperidone soft lipid vesicles were prepared with safranal (0.85% w/v), ethanol (5.78% w/v) and phospholipid (8.65 mg). The extent of absorption from the optimized formulation was found to be superior when compared to oral risperidone suspension with a relative bioavailability of 177%.

The same research group formulated isradipine invasomes by using phospholipon 90G, b-citronellene (terpene) and ethanol utilizing Box-Behnken design (Qadri et al., 2017). The results of the study revealed that prepared isradipine-loaded invasomes deliver ameliorated flux (22.80

± 2.10 mg/cm²/h through rat skin), reasonable entrapment efficiency (88.46%), and more effectiveness for transdermal delivery. In their study, the researchers concluded that with better flux and permeation through the skin the developed isradipine invasomes can be potentially used for the management of hypertension. Further in another research reported by Kamran et al. (2016), formulated, optimized and evaluated Olmesartan nano-invasomes for transdermal delivery by applying Box-Behnken design. The optimized formulation showed promising results with vesicles size of 83.35±3.25nm, entrapment efficiency of 65.21±2.25% and flux of 32.78±0.703 μg/cm²/h. The values of all parameters were found in agreement with the predicted value generated by Box-Behnken design. The researchers concluded that the response surfaces estimated by the Design Expert confirmed the relationship between formulation factors and response variables and the developed olmesartan invasomes were found to be a better transdermal carrier.

7.2.1.5 LIPOSOMES

Liposomes are microscopic vesicles (size ranges from 50 nm to several hundred nm) enclosed aqueous spaces containing phospholipid bilayers. They are mainly composed of phospholipids along with or without other additives, like cholesterol. There are different types of liposomes classified as unilamellar lipid vesicles (ULV) and multilamellar lipid vesicles (MLV) (Imam and Aqil, 2016).

A four-factor five-level CCD design was used to optimize alprazolam-loaded nanoliposomes by taking the different variables used for the study were the solvent/nonsolvent volume ratio (0.2–0.5), phospholipid concentration (mg/mL), alprazolam concentration (mg/mL), and cholesterol content (2.5%–10%, w/w) (Hashemi et al. 2018). The formulations alprazolam nanoliposomes were evaluated by taking variables for the used responses were vesicle size (nm) and entrapment efficiency. The results of the study showed the optimized composition of nanoliposomes were solvent/nonsolvent volume ratio (0.425), phospholipid (15.87 mg/mL), alprazolam (0.875 mg), and cholesterol (7.5%) showed the vesicle size and entrapment efficiency of 121.63 nm and 93.08%, respectively.

In another study reported by Li et al. (2016), about the application of response surface methodology in the optimization of madecassoside (MA) liposomes. The optimized liposomes formulation showed the optimal formulation conditions of double-emulsion based liposomes with a mean size of 151 nm and encapsulation efficiency of 70.14%.

The optimization of Naringenin-loaded elastic liposomes was done by two-factor three-level factorial design containing different amounts of Tween 80 and cholesterol (Tsai et al., 2015). The effects of used variables were assessed on the physicochemical properties including vesicle size, surface charge, encapsulation efficiency, and permeability capacity. The result showed that the skin deposition amounts of naringenin were significantly increased about 7.3~11.8-fold and 1.2~1.9-fold respectively in comparison to the saturated aqueous solution and Tween 80 solution-treated groups.

The application of response surface method incorporating multivariate spline interpolation (RSM-S) has been applied by another researcher (Duangjit et al., 2014). They have used penetration enhancer (PE) factors as formulation factors (Zn), with the type of PE (Z_1) and content of PE (Z_2) and their effects were assessed on vesicle size (X_1), size distribution (X_2), zeta potential (X_3), elasticity (X_4), drug content (X_5), entrapment efficiency (X_6), and release rate (X_7) as causal factors. From the optimization data, the simultaneous optimal solutions were estimated using RSM-S indicated that X_4, X_5, and Z_2 were the prime factors affecting Y_1 and Y_2.

Shi et al. (2012) designed and optimized paeonol-loaded transdermal liposomes gel formulation using 3-factor and 3-level Box-Behnken design. The design showed a second-order polynomial equation to construct three-dimensional (3D) contour plots for the prediction of responses. During the study, the independent variables were the DC-Chol concentration, the molar ratio of lipid/drug, the polymer concentration and the levels of each factor were taken as low, medium, and high. The BBD design based formulation demonstrated the role of the derived polynomial equation and 3-D contour plots in predicting the values of dependent variables for the preparation and optimization of the optimized formulation.

Vitamin E acetate encapsulated liposome was successfully optimized by a factorial design approach for improving its topical delivery. The liposomes were optimized by taking the amount of phospholipid (PL) and cholesterol (CH) was taken at three different levels. The liposomes were prepared using the ethanol injection method and characterized for encapsulation efficiency, vesicle size, zeta potential, and drug deposition in the rat skin. The results of regression analysis revealed that vesicle size and drug deposition in the rat skin were dependent on the lipid concentration and lipid:drug ratio. The factorial design was found to be well suited to identify the key variables affecting drug deposition. Improved drug deposition from liposomal preparations demonstrates its potential for dermal delivery (Padamwar and Pokharkar., 2006).

7.2.2 LIPID NANOPARTICLES

Nowadays, the uses of lipid-based nanoparticles (SLN, NLCs, LDC) are the most common areas of research because these delivery systems have shown higher drug load, encapsulation, and better release. Lipid nanoparticles have shown the capability to enhancement in the solubility and bioavailability of poorly water-soluble and/or lipophilic drugs. It can easily encapsulate more drug load, minimize drug expulsion, and modify the drug release profile by varying the lipid matrix (Mishra et al., 2016; Hasnain et al., 2018). Solid lipid nanoparticles (SLN) comprises of a solid lipid and nanolipid carriers (NLC) are composed of a blend of oil with a solid lipid.

Kaur et al. (2017) formulated DIF-phospholipid complex (DIF-PL complex) by using the solvent-evaporation method and supramolecular nano-engineered lipidic carriers (SNLCs). The developed formulation was optimized using face centered cubic design (FCCD) after the screening of variables by L8 Taguchi orthogonal array design. The results of the optimized SNLC formulation depicted average particle size (188.1 nm), degree of entrapment (86.77±3.33%), permeation flux (5.47±0.48 µg/cm^2/h) and skin retention (17.72±0.68 µg/cm^2). The results of the study concluded that FCCD optimized dual formulation strategy-based SNLCs showed a promising future in the treatment of pain and inflammation associated with rheumatoid arthritis.

In another study by Garg et al., (2017) prepared and characterized aceclofenac nanostructured lipid carriers (NLCs) exploiting Quality by Design (QbD)-oriented technique. The different lipids and surfactants were chosen to prepare NLCs using the microemulsion method. A 3^3 factorial design was used for optimization and evaluation of NLCs for different critical quality attributes (CQAs) using CMAs such as lipids, oil: lipid ratio and concentration of surfactants on CQAs like drug entrapment efficiency and particle size. The result of the study concluded that the optimized ACE-NLCs shown spherical structure, nanosize with higher drug loading and entrapment efficiency. The *in-vitro* drug release study showed that the developed formulation followed the Korsmeyer-Peppas model showing Fickian diffusion. The optimized NLCs-based gel formulation showed superior texture, rheological profile and better cell uptake efficiency on hyperkeratinocytic cells (HaCaT cell lines) in comparison to the marketed formulation.

Pioglitazone loaded nanostructured lipid carriers (PZNLCs) were successfully developed to investigate the application of BBD design for the improvement of bioavailability by transdermal delivery (Alam et al., 2016). The research group used high-pressure homogenization followed by ultrasonication method for formulation development. The statistically optimized (BBD) NLCs were evaluated for particle size, drug loading, *ex-vivo* skin transport studies and in vivo bioactivity study. The optimized formulation showed a mean size of 166.05 nm and drug loading of 10.41% with flux value of 47.36 $\mu g/cm^2/h$. The in vivo pharmacokinetic and pharmacodynamic study showed 2.17 times enhancement in bioavailability and lowers blood sugar level in a sustained pattern for a prolonged period of time.

The double emulsion solvent evaporation (DESE) method was employed to formulate and optimize sildenafil-loaded poly (lactic-co-glycolic acid) (PLGA) nanoparticles (NPs) (Ghasemian et al., 2013). The relationship between design factors and experimental data was evaluated using response surface methodology (BBD). The design was made considering the mass ratio of drug to polymer (D/P), the volumetric proportion of the water to oil phase (W/O) and the concentration of polyvinyl alcohol (PVA) as the independent agents and evaluated for size (nm), entrapment efficiency (EE), drug loading (DL) and cumulative release of drug from NPs post 1 and 8 hrs as the responses. The optimized formulation with a desirability factor of 0.9 was selected, characterized and the shown particle size of 270 nm, EE of 55%, DL of 3.9% and cumulative drug release of 79% after 12 hrs. Sildenafil citrate NPs prepared with optimum formulae provided by an evaluation of experimental data, showed no significant difference between calculated and measured data.

The Box–Behnken design optimized capsaicin-loaded nanolipoidal carriers (NLCs) were designed to increase permeation and achieve the enhanced analgesic and anti-inflammatory effect (Wang et al., 2017). The developed formulations exhibited sustained release and significantly enhance the penetration amount, permeation flux, and skin retention amounts. *In vivo* therapeutic experiments demonstrated that capsaicin-loaded NLCs and capsaicin-loaded NLCs gel could improve the pain threshold in a dose-dependent manner and inhibit inflammation. The overall conclusion of the study stated that BBD optimized NLCs may be a potential carrier for topical delivery of capsaicin.

In another research, the hot-melt extrusion (HME) method was used for the production of Fenofibrate (FBT), and solid lipid nanoparticles (SLN) (Patil et al., 2015). The Quality by Design (QbD) principles were used to achieve continuous production of SLN by combining two processes: HME technology for melt-emulsification and high-pressure homogenization (HPH) for size reduction. The varying process parameters enabled the production of SLN below 200 nm. The pharmacokinetic study results demonstrated a statistical increase in C_{max}, T_{max}, and AUC_{0-24} h in the rate of drug absorption from SLN formulations as compared to the crude drug and marketed micronized formulation. In summary, the present QbD based optimized study demonstrated the potential use of hot-melt extrusion technology for continuous and large-scale production of SLN.

Keshri and Pathak (2013), successfully optimized central composite design based topical econazole nitrate nanostructured lipid carriers by solvent injection technique. The design suggested the selection of five NLC formulations which were converted to hydrogels (G1–G5) using Carbopol 934. The permeation studies of gels demonstrated G3 with a flux rate of 3.21 ± 0.03 µg/cm^2/min as the best formulation that exhibited zero order permeation.

7.2.3   NANOEMULSION/MICROEMULSION

Nanoemulsion is a transparent, thermodynamically stable isotropically clear dispersion of two immiscible liquids, such as oil and water, stabilized by an interfacial film of surfactant molecules (Shakeel et al., 2014). The dispersed phase is composed of small particles or droplets, with a size range of 5–200 nm, and has a very low oil/water interfacial tension (Aqil et al., 2016).

In another study by Tripathi et al. (2018) to develop doxorubicin (Dox) loaded folate functionalized nanoemulsion (NE) for profound therapeutic activity against mammary gland cancer. Box-Behnken design was employed to systematically develop the NE and the optimized NE (f-Dox-NE) was evaluated for in vitro and in vivo activity. F-Dox-NE, with globule size 55.2 ± 3.3 nm, zeta potential -31 ± 2 mV, entrapment $92.51 \pm 3.62\%$, drug loading $0.42 \pm 0.08\%$ and percent drug release $94.86 \pm 1.87\%$ in 72 h, was found to be capable of reducing cell viability in MCF-7 cell lines in comparison to pure and marketed drug. In another study, dexiprofen loaded microemulsion comprising ethyl oleate, Tween 80:PG (2:1), and water were prepared and optimized by simplex lattice design and characterized (Ali et al., 2017). The impact of drug loading, surface area, membrane thickness, adhesive, and agitation speed on drug release and permeation was studied. The result suggests that a membrane-based patch with zero-order release rate, Q_{24} of $79.13 \pm 3.08\%$, and maximum flux of $331.17 \mu g/$ cm^{2}h can be obtained exhibiting suitable anti-inflammatory activity with no visible skin sensitivity reaction.

Olmesartan transdermal nanoemulsion formulation was optimized using the independent variables were clove oil (X_1), Smix (X_2) and water (X_3) while particle size (Y_1), polydispersity index (Y_2), and olmesartan transdermal flux (Y_3) were the dependent variables. The results indicate that the developed olmesartan nanoemulsion provides reasonable particle size, polydispersity index, and transdermal flux. The in vivo pharmacokinetic study of optimized formulation showed a significant increase in bioavailability (1.23 times) compared with the oral formulation of olmesartan by virtue of better permeation through rat skin (Aqil et al., 2016). Another research reported by Negi et al. (2015) endeavors for systematic optimization and evaluation of NEs of local anesthetic drugs namely lidocaine and prilocaine, employing the systematic approach of Quality by Design. A 3(3) Box-Behnken design was employed for systematic optimization of the factors obtained from screening studies exploiting Plackett-Burman design and risk assessment studies. Better permeation rates, and higher concentrations of the drugs in skin layers from the optimized NE carriers, were achieved in permeation and dermatokinetic studies in comparison to the marketed cream.

The application of response surface methodology used by the research group in the year 2014 by Ngan et al. (2014) to assess the process parameters for the optimization of fullerene nanoemulsions. The optimization of independent variables was investigated by using a combined statistical design approach of Box-Behnken design and central composite rotatable design. The parameters used to investigate the effect of the homogenization

Aboelwafa, A., El-Setouhy, D. A., & Elmeshad, AN., (2010). Comparative study on the effects of some polyoxyethylene alkyl ether and sorbitan fatty acid ester surfactants on the performance of transdermal carvedilol proniosomal gel using experimental design. *AAPS Pharm. Sci. Tech., 11*, 1591–1602.

Ahmed, S., Imam, S. S., Ameeduzzafar, Ali, A., Aqil, M., & Gull, A., (2016). *In vitro* and preclinical assessment of factorial design based nanoethosomestransgel formulation of an opioid analgesic. *Art. Cells. Nanomed. and Biotech., 44*(8), 1793–1802.

Ahmed, T. A., (2015). Preparation of transfersomes encapsulating sildenafil aimed for transdermal drug delivery: Plackett-Burman design and characterization. *J. Liposome Res., 25*(1), 1–10.

Ahmed, T. A., El-Say, K. M., Aljaeid, B. M., Fahmy, U. A., & Abd-Allah, F. I., (2016). Transdermal glimepiride delivery system based on optimized ethosomal nano-vesicles: Preparation, characterization, *in vitro*, *ex vivo* and clinical evaluation. *Int. J. Pharm., 500*(1&2), 245–254.

Alam, S., Aslam, M., Khan, A., et al., (2016). Nanostructured lipid carriers of pioglitazone for transdermal application: From experimental design to bioactivity detail. *Drug Deliv., 23*(2), 601–609.

Ali, F. R., Shoaib, M. H., Yousuf, R. I., Ali, S. A., Imtiaz, M. S., Bashir, L., & Naz, S., (2017). Design, development, and optimization of dexibuprofen microemulsion based transdermal reservoir patches for controlled drug delivery. *Biomed Res. Int.,* 4654958.

Aqil, M., Ahmed, K., Imam, S. S., & Ahad, A., (2016). Development of clove oil based nanoemulsion of olmesartan for transdermal delivery: Box-Behnken design optimization and pharmacokinetic evaluation. *J. of Molecular Liq., 214*, 238–248.

Aziz, D. E., Abdelbary, A. A., & Elassasy, A. I., (2018 a). Fabrication of novel elastosomes for boosting the transdermal delivery of diacerein: Statistical optimization, *ex-vivo* permeation, *in-vivo* skin deposition and pharmacokinetic assessment compared to oral formulation. *Drug Deliv., 25*(1), 815–826.

Aziz, D. E., Abdelbary, A. A., & Elassasy, A. I. (2018b). Implementing Central Composite Design for Developing Transdermal Diacerein-Loaded Niosomes: Ex vivo Permeation and In vivo Deposition. *Curr Drug Deliv. 15*(9),1330–1342.

Badr-Eldin, S. M., & Ahmed, O. A. A., (2016). Optimized nano-transfersomal films for enhanced sildenafil citrate transdermal delivery: *Ex vivo* and *in vivo* evaluation. *Drug Des. Devel. Ther., 10*, 1323–1333.

Bastogne, T., (2017). Quality-by-design of nanopharmaceuticals—a state of the art. *Nanomed. Nanotech. Biol. and Med., 13*, 2151–2157.

Beg, S., Rahman, M., Kohli, K., (2019). Quality-by-design approach as a systematic tool for the development of nanopharmaceutical products. *Drug Discovery Today.* 24(3), 717–725.

Beg, S., Akhter, S., Rahman, M., Rahman, Z., (2017a). Perspectives of Quality by Design approach in nanomedicines development. *Current Nanomedicine,* 7, 1–7.

Beg, S., Rahman, M., Panda, S.S., (2017b). Pharmaceutical QbD: Omnipresence in the product development lifecycle. *European Pharmaceutical Review.* 22(1), 2–8.

Bhoop, S. B., (2014). Quality by design (QbD) for holistic pharma excellence and regulatory compliance. *Pharma Times, 46*(8), 26–33.

Bsieso, E. A., Nasr, M., Moftah, N. H., Sammour, O. A., & Abd El Gawad, N. A., (2015). Could nanovesicles containing a penetration enhancer clinically improve the therapeutic outcome in skin fungal diseases? *Nanomed., 10*, 2017–2031.

Cevc, G., (1996). Transfersomes, liposomes and other lipid suspensions on the skin: Permeation enhancement, vesicle penetration, and transdermal drug delivery. *Crit. Rev. Ther. Drug Carrier Syst., 13*(3&4), 257–388.

Dar, M. J., Fakhar, U. D., & Khan, G. M., (2018). Sodium stibogluconate loaded nanodeformable liposomes for topical treatment of leishmaniasis: Macrophage as a target cell. *Drug Deliv., 25*(1), 1595–1606.

De Mattos, C. S., Argenta, D. F., Melchiades, G. L., et al., (2015). Nanoemulsions containing a synthetic chalcone as an alternative for treating cutaneous leishmaniasis: Optimization using a full factorial design. *Int. J. Nanomedicine, 10*, 5529–5542.

Duangjit, S., Opanasopit, P., & Rojanarata, T., (2014). Bootstrap resampling technique to evaluate the reliability of the optimal liposome formulation: Skin permeability and stability response variables. *Biol. Pharm. Bull., 37*(9), 1543–1549.

ElAfify, M. S., ZeinEl, D. E. A., et al., (2018). Development and optimization of novel drug free nanolipid vesicular system for treatment of osteoarthritis. *Drug Dev. Ind. Pharm., 44*(5), 767–777.

Fahmy, U. A., (2015). Nanoethosomal transdermal delivery of vardenafil for treatment of erectile dysfunction: Optimization, characterization, and *in vivo* evaluation. *Drug Des. Devel. Ther., 9*, 6129–6137.

Garg, N. K., Sharma, G., Singh, B., et al., (2017). Quality by design (QbD)-enabled development of aceclofenac loaded-nano structured lipid carriers (NLCs): An improved dermatokinetic profile for inflammatory disorder(s). *Int. J. Pharm., 517*(1&2), 413–431.

Ghasemian, E., Vatanara, A., Najafabadi, A. R., Rouini, M. R., Gilani, K., & Darabi, M., (2013). Preparation, characterization and optimization of sildenafil citrate loaded PLGA nanoparticles by statistical factorial design. *Daru., 21*(1), 68.

Gonzalez-Rodriguez, M. L., Mouram, I., Cozar-Bernal, M. J., et al., (2012). Applying the Taguchi method to optimize sumatriptan succinate niosomes as drug carriers for skin delivery. *J. Pharm. Sci., 101*(10), 3845–3863.

Guo, T., Zhang, Y., Zhao, J., Zhu, C., & Feng, N., (2015). Nanostructured lipid carriers for percutaneous administration of alkaloids isolated from *Aconitum sinomontanum. J. Nanobiotechnology, 13*, 47.

Hafner, A., Lovric, J., Lakos, G. P., & Pepic, I., (2014). Nanotherapeutics in the EU: An overview on current state and future directions. *Int. J. Nanomedicine, 9*, 1005–1023.

Hashemi, S. H., Montazer, M., Naghdi, N., et al., (2018). Formulation and characterization of alprazolam-loaded nanoliposomes: Screening of process variables and optimizing characteristics using RSM. *Drug Dev. Ind. Pharm., 44*(2), 296–305.

Hasnain, M., Imam, S. S., Aqil, M., et al., (2018). Application of lipid blend-based nanoparticulate scaffold for oral delivery of antihypertensive drug: Implication on process variables and *in vivo* absorption assessment. *J. Pharm. Innov.* https://doi.org/10.1007/s12247-018-9329-x (Accessed on 19 November 2019).

Huang, C. T., Tsai, M. J., Lin, Y. H., Fu, Y. S., Huang, Y. B., Tsai, Y. H., & Wu, P. C., (2013). Effect of microemulsions on transdermal delivery of citalopram: Optimization studies using mixture design and response surface methodology. *Int. J. Nanomedicine., 8*, 2295–2304.

Imam, S. S., & Aqil, M. (2017). Penetration enhancement strategies for dermal and transdermal drug delivery: An overview of recent research studies and patents. Dragicevic & Maibach, (eds.), *"Drug Penetration Into/Through the Skin: Methodology and General Considerations"* (pp. 337–350). Springer Publisher. doi: 10.1007/978-3-662-53273-7_20.

Imam, S. S., Aqil, M., Ahad, A., et al., (2017). Formulation by design based risperidone nano soft lipid vesicle as a new strategy for enhanced transdermal drug delivery: *In-vitro* characterization, and *in-vivo* appraisal. *Material. Sci. and Eng. C., 75,* 1198–1205.

Imam, S. S., Aqil, M., Akhtar, M., et al., (2016). Formulation by design based proniosome for accentuated transdermal delivery of risperidone: *In vitro* characterization and *in vivo* pharmacokinetic study. *Drug Delivery, Early Online,* 1–12. doi: 10.3109/10717544.2013.870260.

Jamal, M., Imam, S. S., Aqil, M., et al., (2015). Transdermal potential and anti-arthritic efficacy of ursolic acid from niosomalgel systems. *Int. Immunopharm., 29,* 361–369.

Juran, J. M., (1992). *On Quality by Design the New Steps for Planning Quality Into Goods and Services* (pp. 1, 2). New York Free Press.

Kamran, M., Ahad, A., Aqil, M., et al., (2016). Design, formulation and optimization of novel soft nano-carriers for transdermal olmesartan medoxomil delivery: *In vitro* characterization and *in vivo* pharmacokinetic assessment. *Int. J. Pharm., 505*(1&2), 147–158.

Kaur, A., Bhoop, B. S., Chhibber, S., et al., (2017). Supramolecular nano-engineered lipidic carriers based on diflunisal-phospholipid complex for transdermal delivery: QbD based optimization, characterization and preclinical investigations for management of rheumatoid arthritis. *Int. J. Pharm., 533*(1), 206–224.

Keshri, L., & Pathak, K., (2013). Development of thermodynamically stable nanostructured lipid carrier system using central composite design for zero order permeation of econazole nitrate through epidermis. *Pharm. Dev. Technol., 18*(3), 634–644.

Khan, K., Aqil, M., Imam, S. S., Ahad, A., & Moolakkadath, T., (2018). Ursolic acid loaded intranasal nano lipid vesicles for brain tumor: Formulation, optimization, *in-vivo* brain/plasma distribution study and histopathological assessment. *Biomed. and Pharm., 106,* 1578–1585.

Kumar, N., & Goindi, S., (2014). Statistically designed nonionic surfactant vesicles for dermal delivery of itraconazole: Characterization and *in vivo* evaluation using a standardized *Tinea pedis* infection model. *Int. J. Pharm., 472*(1&2), 224–240.

Li, Z., Liu, M., Wang, H., et al., (2016). Increased cutaneous wound healing effect of biodegradable liposomes containing madecassoside: preparation optimization, *in vitro* dermal permeation, and *in vivo* bioevaluation. *Int. J. Nanomed., 11,* 2995–3007.

Mahmood, S., Taher, M., & Mandal, U. K., (2014). Experimental design and optimization of raloxifene hydrochloride loaded nanotransfersomes for transdermal application. *Int. J. Nanomedicine, 9,* 4331–4346.

Mishra, A. D., Patel, C. N., & Shah, D. R., (2013). Formulation and optimization of ethosomes for transdermal delivery of ropinirole hydrochloride. *Curr. Drug Deliv., 10*(5), 500–516.

Mishra, A., Imam, S. S., Aqil, M., et al., (2016). Carvedilol nano lipid carriers: Formulation, characterization and *in-vivo* evaluation, *Drug Deliv., 23*(4), 1486–1494.

Moghddam, S. M. M., Ahad, A., Aqil, M., Imam, S. S., & Sultana, Y., (2017). Optimization of nanostructured lipid carriers for topical delivery of nimesulide using Box-Behnken design approach. *Art. Cells. Nanomed. and Biotech., 45*(3), 617–624.

Moghddam, S. R. M., Aqil, M., Imam, S. S., & Sultana, Y., (2016). Formulation and optimization of niosomes for topical diacerein delivery using 3-factor, 3-level Box-Behnken design for the management of psoriasis. *Material Sci. and Eng. C., 69,* 789–797.

Moolakkadath, T., Aqil, M., Ahad, A., Imam, S. S., & Iqbal, Z., (2018). Development of transethosomes formulation for dermal fisetin delivery: Box-Behnken design, optimization, *in vitro* skin penetration, vesicles-skin interaction and dermatokinetic studies, *Artif. Cells, Nanomed. and Biotech.*, doi: 10.1080/21691401.2018.1469025.

Morsi, N. M., Aboelwafa, A. A., & Dawoud, M. H. S., (2016). Improved bioavailability of timolol maleate via transdermal transfersomal gel: Statistical optimization, characterization, and pharmacokinetic assessment. *J. Adv. Res., 7*(5), 691–701.

Negi, P., Singh, B., Sharma, G., et al., (2015). Biocompatible lidocaine and prilocaine loaded-nanoemulsion system for enhanced percutaneous absorption: QbD-based optimization, dermatokinetics and *in vivo* evaluation. *J. Microencapsul., 32*(5), 419–431.

Ngan, C. L., Basri, M., Lye, F. F., Masoumi, H. R. F., Tripathy, M., Roghayeh, A. K. R. A., & Malek, E. A., (2014). Comparison of process parameter optimization using different designs in nanoemulsion-based formulation for transdermal delivery of fullerene. *Int. J. Nanomedicine., 9,* 4375–4386.

Padamwar, M. N., & Pokharkar, V. B., (2006). Development of vitamin loaded topical liposomal formulation using factorial design approach: Drug deposition and stability. *Int. J. Pharm., 320*(1&2), 37–44.

Patil, H., Feng, X., Ye, X., Majumdar, S., & Repka, M. A., (2015). Continuous production of fenofibrate solid lipid nanoparticles by hot-melt extrusion technology: A systematic study based on a quality by design approach. *AAPS J., 17*(1), 194–205.

Politis, S. N., Colombo, P., Colombo, G., & Rekkas, D. M., (2017). Design of experiments (DoE) in pharmaceutical development. *Drug Dev and Ind. Pharm., 43*(6), 889–901.

Prasad, P. S., Imam, S. S., Aqil, M., Sultana, Y., & Ali, A., (2016). QbD-based carbopoltransgel formulation: Characterization, pharmacokinetic assessment and therapeutic efficacy in diabetes. *Drug Del., 23*(3), 1047–1056.

Qadri, G. R., Ahad, A., Aqil, M., et al., (2017). Invasomes of isradipine for enhanced transdermal delivery against hypertension: Formulation, characterization, and *in vivo* pharmacodynamic study. *Artif. Cells Nanomed. Biotech., 45*(1), 139–145.

Qumbar, M., Ameeduzzafar., Imam, S. S., Ali, J., Ahmad, J., & Ali, A., (2017). Formulation and optimization of lacidipine loaded niosomal gel for transdermal delivery: *In-vitro* characterization and *in-vivo* activity. *Biomed & Pharmacoth., 93,* 255–266.

Said, M., Elsayed, I., Aboelwafa, A. A., & Elshafeey, A. H., (2017). Transdermal agomelatine microemulsion gel: Pyramidal screening, statistical optimization and *in vivo* bioavailability. *Drug Deliv., 24*(1), 1159–1169.

Sayeed, S., Imam, S. S., Najmi, A. K., et al., (2017). Nonionic surfactant based thymoquinone loaded nanoproniosomal formulation: *In vitro* physicochemical evaluation and *in vivo* hepatoprotective efficacy. *Drug Dev. Ind. Pharm., 43*(9), 1413–1420.

Shakeel, F., Haq, N., Al-Dhfyan, A., Alanazi, F. K., & Alsarra, I. A., (2014). Double w/o/w nanoemulsion of 5-fluorouracil for self-nanoemulsifying drug delivery system. *J. Mol. Liq., 200*, 183–190.

Shamma, R. N., & Elsayed, I., (2013). Transfersomal lyophilized gel of buspirone HCl: Formulation, evaluation and statistical optimization. *J. Liposome Res., 23*(3), 244–254.

Shi, J., Ma, F., Wang, X., et al., (2012). Formulation of liposomes gels of paeonol for transdermal drug delivery by Box-Behnken statistical design. *J. Liposome Res., 22*(4), 270–278.

Singh, B., & Beg, S., (2015). Attaining product development excellence and federal compliance employing Quality by Design (QbD) paradigms. *The Pharma Review.* 13(9), 35–44.

Singh, B., & Beg, S., (2014). Product development excellence and federal compliance via QbD. *Chronicle PharmaBiz.* 15(10), 30–35.

Singh, B., Dahiya, M., Saharan, V., et al., (2005). Optimizing drug delivery systems using systematic "design of experiments." Part II: Retrospect and prospects, *Crit. Rev. Ther. Drug Carrier Syst., 22*(3), 215–293.

Singh, B., Kumar, R., & Ahuja, N., (2004). Optimizing drug delivery systems using systematic "design of experiments." Part I: Fundamental aspects critical reviews™. *In Therapeutic Drug Carrier Systems, 22*(1), 27–105.

Soliman, S. M., Abdelmalak, N. S., El-Gazayerly, O. N., et al., (2016). Novel non-ionic surfactant proniosomes for transdermal delivery of lacidipine: Optimization using 2^3 factorial design and *in vivo* evaluation in rabbits. *Drug Deliv., 23*(5), 1608–1622.

Su, R., Yang, L., Wang, Y., Yu, S., Guo, Y., Deng, J., Zhao, Q., & Jin, X., (2017). Formulation, development, and optimization of a novel octyldodecanol-based nanoemulsion for transdermal delivery of ceramide IIIB. *Int. J. Nanomedicine., 12*, 5203–5221.

Tripathi, C. B., Parashar, P., Arya, M., Singh, M., Kanoujia, J., Kaithwas, G., & Saraf, S. A., (2018). QbD-based development of α-linolenic acid potentiated nanoemulsion for targeted delivery of doxorubicin in DMBA-induced mammary gland carcinoma: *In vitro* and *in vivo* evaluation. *Drug Del. and Transl. Res., 10*, 1–22.

Tsai, M. J., Huang, Y. B., Fang, J. W., Fu, Y. S., & Wu, P. C., (2015). Preparation and characterization of naringenin-loaded elastic liposomes for topical application. *PLoS One., 10*(7), e0131026.

Wang, X. R., Gao, S. Q., Niu, X. Q., Li, L. J., Ying, X. Y., Hu, Z. H., & Gao, J. Q., (2017). Capsaicin-loaded nanolipoidal carriers for topical application: Design, characterization, and *in vitro/in vivo* evaluation. *Int. J. Nanomed., 12*, 3881–3898.

Zhang, K., Zhang, Y., Li, Z., Li, N., & Feng, N., (2017). Essential oil-mediated glycerosomes increase transdermal paeoniflorin delivery: Optimization, characterization, and evaluation *in vitro* and *in vivo*. *Int. J. Nanomedicine, 12*, 3521–3532.

Zidan, A. S., Mokhtar, I. M., & Megrab, N. A. E., (2017). Optimization of methotrexate loaded niosomes by Box-Behnken design: An understanding of solvent effect and formulation variability. *Drug Dev. Ind. Pharm., 43*(9), 1450–1459.

CHAPTER 8

Recent Advances in the Formulation Development of Inhalational Dosage Forms

A. A. SALLAM

Al-Taqaddom Pharmaceutical Industries, Amman, Jordan

Corresponding author. E-mail: a.sallam@tqpharma.com

8.1 INTRODUCTION

8.1.1 HISTORY OF INHALATION DRUG DELIVERY SYSTEMS (IDDS)

A historical perspective of IDDS was reviewed and revealed that inhalation therapy as smokes and mist aerosols for the treatment of disease was known in many old cultures like ancient Egypt. In India, about 2000 BC, Indians used to smoke through pipe leaves of *Datura stramonium* preparations containing along with datura, ginger, and pepper as a remedy for chest conditions (Hickey, 2018a; Preedy and Prokopovich, 2013). In ancient China 2600 BC, Chinese medicine as inhalation therapy in the forms of smoke, steam vapor, medicated pillows, and aromatic sachets were reported for the treatment of respiratory disease (Miao et al., 2015). Fire fumigation of herbs and direct inhalation through a funnel was reported in Europe in the 12th century. The first pressurized inhaler was presented in Paris in 1858 while the first dry powder inhaler was used in London in 1864 using dry finely pulverized medicated powders. Combustion of herbal powder and cigarettes containing herbal components were common to treat asthma and other lung ailments (Sanders, 2007).

The formulation of aerosols started early with the progress of discoveries in pharmacology in the 18th century. The mass commercialization of inhaled drugs was not achieved until 1948 when Abbot Laboratories developed the Aerohaler for inhaled penicillin-G powder (Young et al., 2008). Development of pressurized metered-dose inhaler (pMDI) started in 1956 and followed by different forms of dry powder inhalers (DPI) in the 1960s and 1970s. Nebulizer therapies were known since the 19th century, while the progress in the device design and the use of a combination of drugs were reported in the second half of the 20th century (Hickey, 2018a). Chlorofluorocarbon (CFCs) the well-known propellants were replaced in 1989 with hydrofluoroalkane (HFA) propellants due to their contribution to the depletion of the ozone layer. Consequently, the phase-out of CFC propellants gave rise to the progress and advances in DPI devices (de Boer et al., 2017; Preedy and Prokopovich, 2013; Sanders, 2007).

8.1.2   CLINICAL USES AND PERSPECTIVES OF IDDS

The lung has a high surface area, circa 100 m^2, offering the possibility of high absorption and non-hepatic drug delivery, which results in pharmacological advantages. IDDS therapy has been used mainly for a pulmonary disease like asthma, and chronic obstructive pulmonary disease (COPD) delivering bronchodilators and corticosteroids (Lavorini et al., 2014). However, IDDS has been also used in the treatment of diabetes to deliver insulin; and cystic fibrosis to deliver antibiotics, recombinant human deoxyribonuclease I (RH DNase) and other drugs (Wang et al., 2014; Hickey, 2018a; Agent and Parrott, 2015). The particle size of aerosols is expressed as mass aerodynamic particle size distribution (APSD). The effective respiratory dose of any drug is achieved if it has an APSD of less than 5 μm. Although the deposition, adsorption, diffusion, clearance, and residence of particles in the lung are still not fully understood, it is generally accepted that APSD of 0.5–5 μm is regarded as respirable whereas, particles of lower size get exhaled and larger particles get accumulated in the upper airways (Young et al., 2008; Rangaraj et al., 2019; Beck-Broichsitter et al., 2012). Inhaled particles of less than 2.5 μm are deposited mainly in the alveoli where they may exert no pharmacodynamic effect and are rapidly absorbed, increasing the risk of systemic side effects (Pritchard, 2001).

A recent review (Wang et al., 2014) has shown that lung pathophysiology factors may have an impact on the fate of inhaled drugs which may affect aerosol deposition, dissolution, absorption, and clearance. Such parameters shall affect the biopharmaceutical and pharmacodynamical behavior of inhaled drugs. The fate of inhaled drugs after deposition of inhaled particles primarily depends on the site of their deposition. The review has concluded that on developing IDDS for the treatment of lung diseases, the dosing regimen, safety, and pharmacokinetic studies should be conducted on patients with lung diseases, in addition to healthy subjects. Furthermore, it is worth to mention that the lack of desired clinical outcome along with the problem regarding efficacy or any adverse drug effect may arise due to improper training and education in use of the device to control the actuation and aerosol inhalation (Chandel, 2019; Klijn, 2017). Consequently, it is very important to train patients on how to use and manipulate inhalation devices and procedures.

8.1.3 INHALATION DRUG DELIVERY SYSTEMS (IDDS)

There are different types of IDDS; the major three types of IDDS are pMDI, DPIs, and nebulizers in addition to soft mist inhalers. This chapter reviews recent advances in the development of inhalation dosage forms with special emphasis on product formulations.

Formulation of pMDI is very complex because of the presence of high vapor pressure and low dielectric constant propellants (Rangaraj et al., 2019). The challenge for IDDS formulators and device engineers has been how to produce a product, which meets the specifications required by the pharmaceutical regulatory authorities and, importantly, patient acceptability and compliance. Furthermore, there are challenges in IDDS development in terms of material and formulation characterization and scale-up (Young et al., 2008). The development of IDDS product must take into consideration the following factors (Hou et al., 2015, Sallam, 2019): (1) type of drugs, either local or systemic action, chemical or biological macromolecule, and dose and frequency of administration; (2) physico-chemical characteristics of the drug substance, such as solubility profile, pKa, Log P, particle size, polymorphic transformation and tendency of crystal growth, cohesiveness and agglomeration tendency, morphology and density, as these determine the formulation development; (3) type of formulation (e.g., DPI, pMDI, or aqueous inhalation formulation) being selected to deliver the drug; (4) device design for compatibility with the formulation to be suitable for the targeted patient with regard to age; (5) propellant nature, and vapor pressure.

Recently in 2018, the US Food and Drug Administration (FDA) has revised its draft guidance for developing pMDIs and DPIs, updated to reflect current standards and requirements to enhance understanding of appropriate development approaches for these products consistent with the quality by design (QbD) paradigm (FDA, 2018). QbD is defined as a systematic approach to pharmaceutical development for drug products that begins with predefined objectives and emphasizes product and process understanding and process control, based on sound science and Quality Risk Management (ICH Q8(R2)). Furthermore, QbD is achieved by identifying the Critical Material Attributes (CMAs), which together with the Critical Process Parameters (CPPs), both defined as inputs, will deliver through their proper selection and interaction the output (Singh et al., 2014 and 2015; Beg et al., 2017a,b and 2019). This is the drug product with the desired quality obtained by the continuous optimization of its critical quality attributes (CQAs) in order to meet the predefined Quality Target Product Profile (QTPP) and the patient's needs during the entire lifecycle of the product (Buttini et al., 2018). Under the quality by design (QbD) paradigm, systematic investigations are necessary to understand how changes in critical quality attributes (CQAs) of formulation, device, and manufacturing process influence key product performance parameters, such as delivered dose uniformity (DDU) and fine particle dose (FPD) (Sheth and Sandell et al., 2017). Recent reviews have discussed the application of the QbD approach in the development of IDDS (Thorat and Meshram, 2015; Cooper, 2016; Buttini et al., 2018; Sallam, 2019).

8.2   FORMULATION OF PMDIS

The drug in pMDIs is normally formulated in propellants, which are liquefied compressed gas that gives rise to high pressures within the canister. Hence, propellants function as a driving force for the atomization of the formulation upon actuation. The propellant also serves as the medium in which to disperse drugs in either solution or suspension. When the canister's valve is actuated the propellant flash evaporates at atmospheric pressure, and the ability to control and make use of this property is the basis for pMDI performance. The payload of the propellant evaporates rapidly, leaving it suspended as very fine particles or droplets. As a result of passing extensive toxicology studies in 1990s, the most used propellants are HFA 134a (1,1,1,2-tetrafluoroethane) and 227 (1,1,1,2,3,3,3-hepta-fluoroethane). In pMDIs formulations, the propellants are combined with the drug, in addition to volatile and nonvolatile cosolvents, surfactants, polymers, suspension stabilizers, and bulking agents (Hickey, 2018b; Myrdal et al., 2014). The device consists of the vial (either aluminum can or plasticized glass vial), metering valve, actuator, and recently a dose counter. Thus, it is important to note that, the formulations and the device are functioning together to determine the eventual performance characteristics of the pMDIs. Critical quality attributes of pMDIs include the delivered dose content uniformity, APSD of the delivered aerosol, the fine particle fraction (FPF) which represents the amount of drug that is considered respirable, mass median aerodynamic diameter (MMAD; aerodynamic diameter at which 50% of the aerosolized mass lies below the stated value), chemical and physical shelf-life stability of the drug, and extent of leachable materials from device components (Myrdal et al., 2014).

8.2.1 PROPELLANTS

The most common used propellants are hydrochlorofluorocarbons (CFC), while hydrofluorocarbons (HFA) are alternative propellants. The use of CFC is not allowed due to the presence of chlorine in their structure, which may cause ozone depletion. The Montreal Protocol provided motivation to the pharmaceutical industry to develop non-CFC containing inhaler products. They are to be phased out during 2015–2030 and the pMDIs developed with these propellants may require replacement with other propellants such as HFA. Thus, HFAs may be called 'bridging agents' rather than alternatives of CFCs (Rangaraj et al., 2019, Ibiapina et al., 2004).

The propellants HFA 134a and HAF 227 characteristics are shown in Table 8.1. They have an excellent safety profile, a high degree of purity, and are chemically stable under normal storage conditions. Both propellants have relatively low boiling points, which afford sufficient vapor pressure, even at reduced temperatures, to enable efficient propellant performance. These propellants are capable of maintaining constant pressure throughout the device life because of their high expansion ratio; vaporization 1 ml of propellant would occupy 240 ml (Rangaraj et al., 2019). Furthermore, they are completely miscible in one another and vapor pressure upon mixing behaves ideally, thus they may be blended in different proportions to obtain a specific vapor pressure or density (Myrdal et al., 2014). The difference between the density of 1.23 and 1.41 does not look that much. However, many drugs may have crystal densities in this range so the choice of a HFA can determine whether a particular drug crystal floats, or quickly sinks to the bottom. If the drug crystal settles rapidly then it is difficult to get a reliable dose, a problem, which is further, complicated by a tendency for crystals either to stick together or result in crystal growth particularly in the presence of moisture. The use of blends of HFA may help to match the density of the formulation to the density of the suspended drug particles.

TABLE 8.1 Physicochemical Properties of HFA 134a and HFA 227

Propellant	HFA 134a	HFA 227
Molecular weight	102	170
Liquid density at 20°C (g/mL)	1.23	1.41
Dipole moment (debye)	2.06	0.93
Vapor pressure at 20°C (psi)	83	56.6
Water solubility in liquid phase (g/kg) at 25°C	2.22	0.61
Log P (octanol/water)	1.1	2.1
Purity	> 99.9	> 99.9
Solubility parameter (calculated value)	6.8	5.4
Safety profile	Safe	Safe
Miscibility in one another	Miscible	Miscible

(Modified from Myrdal et al., 2014; Solvay Special Chemicals).

Furthermore, partition coefficient, polarity and solubility parameter differences of HFAs as shown in Table 8.1 may be significant for formulating a certain drug in the formulation. Water has nearly 4-fold increased solubility in HFA 134a versus 227 (2.2 and 0.610 g/kg, respectively). In such cases, the polarity of HFA 134a can make the recrystallization problem worse due to the higher level of moisture affinity. This also has a very deleterious impact on chemical stability, as the uptake of moisture is one of the most common reasons for the degradation of drugs on storage in pMDIs. Generally, problems of this nature with HFA 134a are few and not common, in some cases HFA 227 has proven the better choice in the formulation of such drugs. The migration rate of water will depend not only on the propellant and additional excipients (e.g., ethanol) but also on the valve components and storage conditions. It was shown that the emitted particle size and FPF can change depending on the drug and extent of moisture ingress (Myrdal et al., 2014; Ivey, et al., 2017).

Other propellants have been reported such as 1,1-difluoroethane (HFA 152a), propane, n-butane, isobutane, n-pentane, isopentane, neopentane, dimethyl ether, and hydro-fluoro olefins (HFOs). Many of these propellants are flammable materials and the safety and toxicology studies of them are not yet fully known, and thus cause an inherent safety risk (Myrdal et al., 2014).

8.2.2 SOLUTION FORMULATIONS

Solution formulations are homogeneous molecular dispersion of the drug completely dissolved in the propellant alone or by the addition of solubilizing excipients. The solution formulation of pMDIs has an advantage over suspension pMDIs, because being the homogeneous solution the patients do not need to shake the vial immediately prior to use, a finer residual aerosol and a higher percentage of fine particle mass per actuation. Furthermore, any issues with flocculation, sedimentation, Oswald ripening, particle-device/component adhesion, and metering consistency are overcome (Young et al., 2008). Examples of solubilizing excipients are water, ethanol, glycerol, propylene glycol, polyethylene glycols, lecithin (Soya), Spans and Tweens, and complexing agents. Cosolvents are often added as solubilizing agents because of their high miscibility with the propellants. These excipients may also alter the dissolution of residual particles from the aerosol spray in the lungs, which results in modulating the pharmacological effect (Myrdal et al., 2014; Grainger et al., 2012; Riley et al., 2012).

The spray pattern, final APSD and FPF of a solution pMDI are affected by the vapor pressure of the propellant, the percentage and volatility of cosolvent (Shethand Grimes et al., 2017), the concentration of the dissolved drug and the dimensions of the actuator orifice (Newman, 2005; Myrdal et al., 2014). The main function of using volatile cosolvents such as ethanol in solution formulation of pMDI, is to increase drug or excipient solubility in the propellant HFA or to enhance valve function. It has been reported that changes in the surface tension or viscosity of the formulation as the ethanol concentration changes may have influenced the atomization process (Dalby and Byron 1988; Stein and Myrdal, 2006). The delivery efficiency of pMDI was experimentally shown to decrease with increasing ethanol concentration because of the following changes: (1) by changing the formulation density and thus changing the total mass of formulation atomized during actuation of the device, (2) by changing atomization of the formulation and the size of the atomized droplets, and (3) by changing the evaporation rate of these droplets towards their residual particle sizes. The results showed that the formulation was atomized into coarser droplets as the ethanol concentrations increased with the mass median aerodynamic diameter (MMAD) of more than 11 µm, which might lead to a decrease in FPF and fine particle mass, thereby decreasing the overall dosing efficiency (Stein and Myrdal, 2006). This could be due to the fact that ethanol concentration affects both the ability of the formulation to be atomized into fine droplets (due to a decrease in vapor pressure) and the time required for the droplets to evaporate into the smaller residual particles (slower rate of evaporation).

It is essential to optimize the percentage of the volatile cosolvent, in order to obtain the proper ASPD or MMAD of pMDI. It may result in particles with APSD in the range of 0.8–1.2 µm. Although this size range is clearly suitable for respiratory delivery, it will generally result in a product targeted largely to the alveoli as described above, which for generic pMDI formulations, may not be comparable to existing deposition patterns, pharmacokinetic and clinical efficacy of the originator pMDI (Young et al., 2008). Additionally, as in the case of a high proportion of ethanol coarser ASPD might be produced which will influence drug delivery efficiency with oropharyngeal deposition being more likely to be observed. Such deposition also affects the pharmacokinetics and clinical efficacy of pMDI (Stein and Gabrio, 2000).

The presence of a non-volatile additive in a solubilized HFA volatile cosolvent system will result in an increase in the final droplet size (Brambilla et al., 1999; Ganderton et al., 2002). The final aerosol droplets will be containing both drug and non-volatile additive. After evaporation of the volatile components, the resultant particulate size will be dependent on the concentration of the non-volatile component which will dominate the particle size. Meanwhile, this approach has been employed by the addition of the nonvolatile concentration of glycerol or polyethylene glycol, which resulted in the ability to modify the aerodynamic diameter of the resultant aerosol, the MMAD increased from 1 µm to 3 um by adding 2% w/w of glycerol and to 4 μm by adding 6.5% w/w of glycerol (Ganderton, et al., 2002). Furthermore, the addition of nonvolatile excipients such as nonionic surfactant is expected to increase the residual MMAD of the formulation and consequently decrease the FPF. A published data showed that, with the addition of 1.22% (w/w) Pluronic L81 to a formulation with 0.04% (w/w) dissolved drug in HFA 227 with ethanol, the residual MMAD increased from 1.56 ± 0.05 μm to 3.70 ± 0.08 μm while the % FPF did not change significantly (49.63 ± 2.00 and 50.72 ± 0.69, respectively). However, further increase in Pluronic L81 concentration (up to 5.45%), resulting in a significant increase in the MMAD (5.93 ± 0.49 μm) and decrease in the FPF (33.2 ± 3.37) compared to formulations with 0% and 1.22% Pluronic L81 (Saleem and Smith, 2013).

Furthermore, the type of propellant has an influence on the APSD of solution-based pMDI formulations. A published data (Leach et al., 1998) describes HFA solution pMDI formulation of dissolved beclomethasone dipropionate (BDP) of 80 μg/actuation, which has been formulated to produce a residual MMAD of 1.1 μm (Product I). With a small MMAD, it is expected that a greater extent of the drug deposits in the peripheral airways (airway diameters, ≤2 mm), compared with another formulation of BDP in CFC with a MMAD of approximately 3 μm (Product II), which primarily deposited in the central airways. The extra-fine solution of pMDI (Product I) permits the product to have a lower product drug concentration, increased inhalation process tolerance and increased ratio of therapeutic efficacy to adverse side effects because of the deposition of the drug in the peripheral airways compared to the Product II (Price et al., 2013; Robinson and Tsourounis, 2013). Commercially, there are many HFA solution pMDIs products which produce extra fine MMAD and available in the market such as ciclesonide (Alvesco® HFA), flunisolide hemihydrate (Aerospan® HFA), formoterol fumarate (Atimos®), and combination product with BDP and formoterol (Fostair®). Furthermore, salmeterol xinafoate HFA solution pMDI utilizes a cosolvent, a mineral acid to adjust pH and up to 2% (w/w) water to dissolve the drug and produce extra fine MMAD (Church et al., 2012).

8.2.3 SUSPENSION FORMULATIONS

Generally, HFA propellants have poor drug solubilization power, hence suspension formulations become more common in the preparation of their pMDIs (Young et al., 2008). Suspension formulations are heterogeneous systems where drug particles are suspended in HFA solution formulations. Subsequently, pharmaceutical suspensions may suffer phase separation, flocculation, agglomeration, caking, crystal growth, Ostwald ripening, drug particle interaction with other drug particles or device material, or moisture ingress (O'Donnell and Williams III, 2013). Thus, HFA suspension formulations of pMDI require the use of other additives to stabilize the micronized drug and support uniform dose and aerodynamic particle size characteristics. As with IDDS, the drug particles used in suspension pMDI should ideally have a diameter of less than 5 μm to achieve a therapeutic effect upon administration. Such drug powders are micronized powders, characterized by having a high surface area to mass ratio and therefore they are cohesive in nature and have a tendency to form agglomerates. Moreover, broad particle size distribution of the micronized drug particles, the presence of solvation, van der Waals, and electrical double layer forces, as well as density difference effects, may lead to physical instability, and uncontrolled agglomeration and/or caking of the suspensions (Young et al., 2008; Myrdal et al., 2014).

Drug particle engineering and formulation optimization of inhalation suspension provide suspended drug particles with a proper particulate size distribution, density, and dispersibility. Many reviews and published articles have dealt with this subject (Williams III et al., 1999; Shoyele and Cawthorne, 2006; Chow et al., 2007; Young et al., 2008; Vehring, 2008; Jones, 2011; O'Donnell and Williams III, 2013; Weers and Tarara, 2014; Myrdal et al., 2014; Chan, et al., 2014; Hickey and Holt, 2014; Yang et al., 2015; Stein et al., 2015; Thorat and Meshram, 2015; Hickey 2016; Sheth and Sandell et al., 2017; Lia and Xu, 2017; Ivey, et al., 2017; Biddiscombe and Usmani, 2018; Ferguson et al., 2018; Taylora et al., 2018, Chandel, 2019). The drug particles can be engineered to match the density of the formulation, which is the approach utilized by the PulmoSpheres®, and similarly, the excipients can be utilized to ensure decreased agglomeration of suspended drug particles (Rougeda, 2005; Weers and Tarara, 2014). PulmoSpheres® are small porous sponge-like particles, which are made up of two materials endogenous to the lungs: di-stearoyl phosphatidylcholine and calcium chloride, in a 2:1 molar ratio. The drug is incorporated within PulmoSpheres® particles which have a mass median diameter (geometric size) between 1 and 5 μm, and a tapped density between 0.01 and 0.5 g/cm^3 (Dellamary, at al., 2011; Weers and Tarara, 2014). The final composition of the drug product is dependent on the dose of the drug. In case of highly potent drugs, the PulmoSpheres® excipients may comprise more than 99% w/w of the particles, while for high doses of drugs, the PulmoSpheres® excipients may be incorporated in small quantities as small as 5% w/w of the drug product (Weers and Tarara, 2014). The porous structure of the particles allows the propellant to penetrate into the particles creating particles with an effective density that is almost similar to the propellant, and hence reducing the tendency of either sedimentation or creaming regardless of the formulation temperature (Dellamary, at al., 2000; O'Donnell and Williams III, 2013). PulmoSpheres® have particles with relatively large geometric size which results in lower surface area available for contact and thereby reducing the tendency of particulate agglomeration. The penetration of the propellant into the particles generates particles with similar polarizability as the propellant, which reduces the van der Waals potential between particles, and hence reduce the tendency of particulate agglomeration (Myrdal et al., 2014). However, PulmoSphere® technology has limitations because it cannot be used in case of drugs having low glass transition temperatures (e.g., glycopyrrolate), high propellant solubility (e.g., mometasone furoate), or known physical instability and chemical lability (i.e., proteins and peptides).

Spray drying techniques were used to prepare large highly porous nanoparticle particles with advantageous aerodynamic properties and low cohesive forces (Tsapis et al., 2002; Ivey, et al., 2017). Similar techniques were also used to prepare spray-drying of micronized budesonide microcrystals in the presence of phospholipid-coated emulsion droplets which resulted in the production of low-density lipid-coated microcrystals with low surface energy and excellent colloidal stability in the suspension of HFA formulations (Tarara et al., 2004). Meanwhile, matching the density of the propellants to the density of the drug can be achieved by adding cosolvents like ethanol (0.789 g/cm^3 at 20°C) or propylene glycol (1.036 g/cm^3 at 20°C) or blending propellants to increase or decrease the overall density of the HFA pMDI suspension formulations. The limitation of this approach is related to the fact that the density of propellant formulations varies significantly with temperature changes (Lechuga-Ballesteros et al., 2011). Nanosized particles with unimodal size distribution were prepared by combination techniques of spray-drying and W/O microemulsion for either salbutamol sulfate or insulin. Subsequently, these nanoparticles were used to prepare stable suspension in the propellant HFA 134a, and have an efficient deposition in the lower respiratory tract represented by achieving very fine particle (<5.8 um) with high FPF (70% w/w) (Lia and Xu, 2017).

Co-milling with a pharmaceutical stabilizer such as hydrophilic polymers and nonionic surfactants was used to improve the stability of pMID. For example, co milled product of triamcinolone acetonide (TAA) with nonionic surfactant Pluronic F when formulated with HFA suspension pMDI exhibited reduced propellant solubility, increased formulation stability and improved aerosol dispersion (resulting in increased FPF) (Williams III et al., 1999).

An example of the influence of formulation variables is the surface modifications of drug particles by the use of HFA soluble surfactants, cosolvents and/or stabilizing agents. The association of the cosolvent, stabilizing polymer or the surfactant at the surface of the drug particles suspended in HFA, may either reduce interfacial tension, produce steric hindrance between particles, or form colloid bridges to increase flocculation which in turn reduce the tendency for the particles to aggregate and thereby allows them to remain suspended in the low polarity propellant. In the case of controlled flocculation, the suspension upon standing can be readily deflocculated by shaking, allowing redispersion of drug particles and hence can deliver drug particles in an acceptable APSD. It was found that an increase in chain length, of low molecular weight polyethylene glycol, added to salbutamol sulfate (SS) suspensions of HFA, showed a decrease in inter-particulate cohesion and hence sterically stabilized pMDI suspensions. Similarly, when polyvinyl pyrrolidone (PVP) was added to HFA, a large reduction of up to 70% in force of cohesion was observed when compared to HFA only. However, any further addition of different concentrations of PEG 400 to the HFA–PVP/drug suspension did not result in a significant reduction of the force of cohesion. The large planar rigid molecules of PVP spread over and covered most of the surface of SS particles in the suspension, hindering any interaction of PEG with SS particles and hence preventing any further stabilizing effect due to the added concentration of PEG (Traini et al., 2006).

A simulation model predicted the residual APSDs of dissolved and suspended drug dually present as a combination in HFA-134a pMDIs. Simulated and experimental data showed that APSDs of the dissolved and suspended components of the pMDI were significantly affected by concentrations of the nonvolatile dissolved and micronized suspended drugs, in addition to suspended drug particle size. The particle size distribution (PSD) of the residual APSD produced from the dissolved drug was shown both theoretically and experimentally to consist of a bimodal lognormal distribution. This bimodal distribution consists of a smaller PSD that is made up of residual particles containing only the dissolved drug and a larger PSD that is made up of residual particles containing both the dissolved and suspended drugs. Furthermore, it was shown that a formulation that contained only dissolved drugs at a low concentration produced a relatively small residual APSD and a narrow distribution, compared to that of the solution component of combination formulations (Stein et al., 2015). A physically stable micro-suspension of budesonide was formulated by an in situ-precipitation process using a hydrophilic stabilizer such as hydroxypropyl beta-cyclodextrin (HPBCD) with PEG 300 and ethanol as cosolvents in relatively hydrophobic HFA 227 propellant pMDI. Moreover, it was observed that in the absence of HPBCD, a supersaturated solution formed which re-crystallized at the container inner surfaces and led to crystal growth upon storage (Steckel and Wehle, 2004).

A recent review article has described co-suspension delivery technology for the formulation of pMDIs. The technology uses micronized drug crystals strongly associated with porous, low-density phospholipid particles which are engineered in HFA propellant to deliver the combination of drugs to the airways with accurate and consistent dosing, independent of medication types and combinations. This sort of pMDI technology has the advantage of formulating multiple therapies in one IDDS and consequently improving patient compliance (Ferguson et al., 2018). While suspension formulations of HFA pMDI are briefly discussed above, articles of an extensive review of the topic should be considered for further readings (Newman, 2005; Shoyele and Cawthorne, 2006; Chow et al., 2007; Young et al., 2008; Myrdal et al., 2014; Ferguson et al., 2018).

8.3 FORMULATIONS OF DPIS

8.3.1 LOW DOSE DPIS

DPIs are powder blends of micronized drug particles with coarse lactose which are known formulations since the 1970s (Hickey, 2018b). The main objective of DPI formulation is to achieve a balance of the forces of interaction between micronized drug particles and coarse lactose particles that will stabilize the DPI through filling and storage but allow ease of aerosolization and hence dispersion when inhaled by the patient (Hickey et al., 2007). The performance of DPIs is dependent on the design of the DPI device and aerodynamic properties of the powder formulation. The scope of this review chapter deals with the recent development in the formulation of DPIs rather than their devices. Generally, powder formulations are either composed of micronized drug powder mixed with carrier excipients in case of potent drugs or only micronized drug powder in case of high dose drugs (de Boer et al., 2017).

The drug powder in DPIs is micronized and normally has a particle size in the range of 1–5 μm to allow aerodynamic deposition in the tracheobronchial airways of the lungs. Micronized drug particles have a high surface area to mass ratio, rendering these particles highly cohesive/ adhesive in nature. Cohesive and adhesive forces play the major roles in the interaction between drug and carrier particles in the powder blends which will be influencing aerodynamic properties and hence the percentage of FPF that aerosolized from the DPIs. Surface characteristics, particle size, shape, density, surface roughness or rugosity, and morphology of either drug or carrier particles may influence their inter-particulate forces and aerodynamic properties (Rudén et al., 2019). The particles are bound by van der Waals forces, electrostatic forces, capillary forces, and mechanical interlocking. Formulation of the DPIs should be able to deliver the aerosolized drug powder, where coordination between the patient breathing and actuation of the device subjected it to larger dispersion forces in order to deagglomerate and/or detach into individual particles. Thus, recent powder formulation developments aim at a reduction of the adhesive and cohesive forces between the particles, and/or modification of surface characteristics of powders in order to generate and increase the percentage of FPF delivered to the lungs (Young et al., 2007; Yang et al., 2014; Grasmeijer et al., 2015; Carvalho et al., 2015).

A range of carrier-based dry powder formulations consisting of micronized drug, and carrier lactose with or without fine lactose were prepared and tested for dispersibility, i.e., generating fine particle fraction (FPF). A model based on the total amount of fines (drug, carrier fines and the fines inherent to the carrier) and the cohesive energy (derived from regular solutions theory), which allows calculation of interparticle interaction parameters of the formulation was proposed. Beclomethasone dipropionate and budesonide the model drugs were found to be 5.3 times and 1.8 times more cohesive than lactose fines respectively, and the macroscopic behavior of the dry powder formulation was dependent on the inter particulate interaction between the different components of the powder blends. Furthermore, the model showed that a decrease in FPF was associated with the increase in the proportion of the cohesive drug powder at a constant total fine (drug and carrier) (Thalberg et al., 2012).

A drug powder detachment model was developed and used in the simulation of airflow and carrier particle motion through the inhaler, which could be applied for optimization of DPI device geometry and formulation. The simulation was dependent on the Lattice Boltzmann method as a class of computational fluid dynamics and Reynolds-averaged Navier–Stokes equations which primarily used to describe turbulent flows (Cui et al., 2014; Mahmoudi et al., 2019). For the detachment of the drug particles from the carrier through the aerodynamic flow, the adhesion force (van der Waals) and the friction force have to be overcome. It was shown that drug particle detachment was governed by a balance of the moments of aerodynamic drag and rough-surface pull-off forces which were based on three detachment mechanisms namely lift-off, sliding or rolling (Cui et al., 2014; Ibrahim et al., 2003; Cui and Sommerfeld, 2015; Cui and Sommerfeld, 2019).

It was previously reported that the prior saturation of high adhesive-energy surface sites of coarse lactose particles (CL) with fine lactose particles (FL), the drug can be detached easily during aerosolization (Thalberg et al., 2012; Grasmeijer et al., 2015). This was due to the fact that FL particles would compete with the drug on the active sites of the CL particles. A study proposed a mathematical approach to evaluate aerosolization behavior of micronized drug particles alone and in the formulation with FL and CL (Parisini et al., 2015). This study investigated the deagglomeration behavior of micronized drug particles having different polarities (salmeterol xinafoate (SX) as a model hydrophobic drug and salbutamol sulfate (SS) as a model hydrophilic drug). SX and SS have a different deagglomeration mechanism, while SX had cohesively balanced mechanism when added to the lactose, due to its tendency to form agglomerates on the lactose surface (Kendall and Stainton, 2001; Adi et al., 2006), SS had adhesively balanced mechanism when added to lactose as previously reported (Adi et al., 2006). FL, SX, and SS showed different deagglomeration processes to each other indicating variability in agglomerate size and strength between agglomerates. Consequently, greater energy was required for the deagglomeration process to occur for SS compared to SX and FL. Furthermore, SX and FL reached the maximum deagglomeration earlier than SS. When FL was mixed with either SS or SX, increased deagglomeration was observed when the pressure was increased more than 0.5 Bar. However, at low pressure (0.5 Bar) SS– FL deagglomeration did not occur completely as indicated by the bimodal distribution of particle size. However, when mixed with CL and FL the deagglomeration process was modified and resulted in the identification of two different types of fractions of dispersed particles upon increasing dispersing airflow. It was also found that SS:FL:CL powder blends produced a greater number of free agglomerates than SX:FL:CL, resulting in a higher dispersion of the micronized material. Therefore, adding the fine lactose would modify the adhesive strength between particles and enhance the detachment of the drug particles.

The drug-carrier cohesive-adhesive balance (CAB) ratio in DPI formulations containing different drugs and carriers was studied using colloidal probe atomic force microscopy (Jones et al., 2008). It was shown in this study that fluticasone propionate was strongly adhesive and SX was strongly cohesive with respect to lactose, while formoterol fumarate was only slightly cohesive with respect to lactose. A high cohesive drug-carrier CAB ratio indicates a stronger drug-drug cohesion, and relatively weaker drug-carrier adhesion. Subsequently, the study concluded that carrier-based DPI formulation performance would be optimized when the drug-carrier CAB ratio is slightly cohesive.

Supercritical fluid technology (SCFT) was applied to modify the surface physicochemical properties of the drug substance (Ober, et al., 2013; Miyazaki et al., 2016; Sun, 2016; Miyazaki et al., 2017; Wu, et al., 2018). The particles produced by SCFT had reduced interparticulate forces because of their low density, the irregular surface structure and/or reduced surface free energy. It was shown that reduced surface energy of SCFT produced particles, related to their low adhesion, plays an important role in the good performance of these particles in the DPI formulation. A carrier-free DPI containing budesonide (BUD) was prepared using supercritical fluid technology. In contrary to the milled powder, the obtained BDS powder exhibited large specific surface area, homogenous and lower work of cohesion, better flowability, and lower surface energy, hence showed better aerodynamic performances (Sun, 2016). The APSD was less than

5 um with FPF of approximately 33% comparable to the commercially available BUD/DPI, which showed FPF of 28.4%. In another study, the SCFT along with the freeze-drying technique (SCFT/FD) was used for the preparation of budesonide (BDS) powder. The SCFT/FD/BDS powder showed in stage 2 of twin impinge, a deposition 4-fold higher than that obtained with unprocessed raw BDS. The improved inhalation properties were related to an increase in surface roughness and a decrease in surface energy (Miyazaki et al., 2017). However, the residual amount of SCFT/FD/BDS in the capsule was increased due to the increase in the adhesion to the capsule shell. This drawback was overcome by the use of various additives such as monoglyceride stearate (MGS), which improved both the release from the capsule and the inhalation properties. The improved inhalation properties found with MGS was attributed to MGS adsorbed to the drug particle surface and reduced interparticulate cohesion, although the particles had a smooth surface (Miyazaki et al., 2017). The quantity of drug powder retention in the capsule shell of DPIs depends on the interaction between the surface physicochemical properties of the capsule shell, the characteristics of the interactive powder mixture (composed of micronized drug particles and coarse and /or fine carrier particles), and the functioning of the DPI device. With a given formulation and device, powder mixture retention can be modified by changing the surface characteristics of the capsule shell (Lavorini et al., 2017, Saim and Horhota, 2002) or changing the surface characteristics of the interactive powder mixture (Miyazaki et al., 2017) in order to achieve the optimal performance target. Different shapes and sizes of water-soluble mannitol (MN) particles were prepared using a supercritical assisted atomization technique. In vitro aerosolization tests using an Andersen cascade impactor showed that the spheroidal particles of MN exhibited a faster rate of deagglomeration arising from the lower contact area between the spheroidal particles. Furthermore, the percentage of FPF was increased due to the excellent powder flowability of the larger MN microparticles (Wu, et al., 2018).

The use of dual excipients as a platform for DPI formulations such as lactose monohydrate and magnesium stearate was discussed. The commercialization of DPI products having dual excipients in a form of either capsule, blister or reservoir has been achieved (Shur et al., 2016). An investigation of the effect of co- milling 1% w/w beclomethasone dipropionate (BDP)/lactose with 5%w/w magnesium stearate (MgSt) on the physicochemical properties and aerosol performance of powder blends was done (Lau, 2017). The results showed that a significant reduction in agglomerate size and strength, and improvement of aerosolization performance was observed for co- milled formulations with MgSt compared to the co-milled formulation without MgSt. Furthermore, another advantage of adding MgSt was increasing stability because deterioration in samples performance after storage at 25°C and 75% relative humidity for 2 weeks was greater for the co-milled formulation without MgSt, compared with co-milled formulation with MgSt. Magnesium stearate is a hydrophobic substance that would provide a barrier and hinder the adsorption of water on the surface of micronized lactose particles. Moreover, surface coverage by Mgst would reduce the extent of cohesive/adhesive interactions between micronized particles. It may also act by coating the amorphous sites on lactose particles, preventing recrystallization after storage at high humidity, and decreasing the formation of new amorphous regions during the co-milling process. These functions of Mgst led to a reduction in the degree of agglomerate formation and strength (Lau, 2017).

PulmoSphere® technology (Weers and Tarara, 2014) is spray-dried formulations comprise of phospholipid-based small, hollow, porous particles and can be used in both MDI and DPI delivery systems, as discussed in Section 8.3.3. These particles have reduced contact area and lower density which results in improved powder aerosolization efficiency and reduced aerodynamic diameter. A dry powder budesonide PulmoSpheres were prepared using an emulsion-based spray-drying process reported to exhibit improved in vivo respiratory deposition when compared to a conventional micronized formulation (Duddu, et al., 2002). For carrier-based PulmoSphere® formulations, small porous PulmoSphere® particles were used as carrier particles, forming adhesive mixtures with micronized drug particles and delivered as respirable agglomerates (Weers and Tarara, 2014). Carrier-based PulmoSphere® formulations of formoterol fumarate and glycopyrronium bromide and a fixed-dose combination of the two drugs were developed for the treatment of COPD. A triple combination by adding a corticosteroid such as mometasone was also developed. PulmoSphere® formulations were also used to develop large dose IDDS such as tobramycin and ciprofloxacin for treatment of cystic fibrosis, and Amphotericin B for prophylaxis against invasive pulmonary aspergillosis. Furthermore, PulmoSphere® technology could be employed for formulation of most drugs legible for IDDS independent of its physical form, physicochemical properties; molecular weight (small molecule and macromolecule including proteins, RNAs and viruses, and stability (Dellamary, at al., 2011; Weers and Tarara, 2014).

A spray-dried porous particle for sodium cromoglycate DPI was developed using ammonium bicarbonate(1.25%w/w) as a pore-forming agent (Gallo et al., 2019). After spray drying at 170°C, the dried particles were amorphous powder free of ammonium carbonate. The porous spherical shape powder exhibited good aerosolization performance (FPF of 56%) with MMAD < 5 um, and good stability (for 12 months) under dry condition (silica gel), however, further studies are required to evaluate the in-vivo deposition pattern of sodium cromoglycate porous particles.

The in-vitro aerosol performance of two commercially available combination DPI products was investigated using single-particle aerosol mass spectrometry (SPAMS) (Jetzer et al., 2018). This instrument is capable of generating APSD and chemical composition for single particles for real-time analysis, along with a very high data acquisition rate and chemometric analysis, allows the determination of the chemical composition for the particles. The first product contains fluticasone propionate (FP), salmeterol xinafoate (SX) and lactose monohydrate (LMH) in a blister DPI, while the second product contains beclomethasone dipropionate (BDP), formoterol fumarate (FF), LMH and magnesium stearate (MgSt) in a reservoir DPI. The SPAMS technique had been used to characterize the particulate interactions whether drug-drug or drug-excipient in the APSD of DPI products (single component or more), by the determination of the chemical structure for each component in the agglomerate (Jetzer et al., 2017). The results showed that DPI of BDP/FF produced a higher fraction of FPF (< 5 um) for either BDP or FF and also produced a significantly higher fraction of extra-fine particle (EFPF < 2um). Thus, a much higher number of particles with a small MMAD were detected from DPI of BDP/FF compared to DPI of FP/SX with prominent different particulate characteristics. Moreover, the DPI of FP/SX showed APSD composed of a high number of agglomerated drug particles of FP and SX, while the DPI of BDP/FF showed a negligible number of agglomerated drug particles of BDP and FF. Consequently, it was concluded that the interactions between the drug particles and excipient particles in both DPIs were significantly different. It was observed that MgSt was detected in the mass spectra of BDP in DPI of BDP/FF, which indicated that MgSt particles were co-associated with BDP particles rather than with FF particles. An explanation was related to either co milling of BDP with MgSt before mixing with FF and LMH or the BDP or the LMH were coated with MgSt. Such treatment would hinder the co-association or agglomeration of the drug-drug or drug-excipient particles and facilitate detachment from the carrier (Jetzer et al., 2018). This explanation for the role of MgSt was in agreement with a previous study, which used SPAMS and described it as being a force control agent in DPIs capable of influencing the inter particulate forces in DPI formulations (Jetzer et al., 2016).

A published study (Singh et al., 2015) described the preparation of surface-modified lactose (SML) particles by light coating with force control agents (FCA) such as Pluronic F-68, Cremophor RH 40, glyceryl monostearate, polyethylene glycol 6000, magnesium stearate, and soya lecithin. Such surface treatment would reduce the high surface free energy, decrease surface roughness or rugosity and consequently would increase the flowability of SML particles. Fluticasone propionate (1% w/w) as a model drug was blended with SML formulations and used with two different DPI devices, Rotahaler and Diskhaler. The results of both devices showed that the FPF value of all Fluticasone propionate/SML formulations were higher than the FPF value of the same formulations containing untreated lactose. This means that particle engineering technique applying a surface modification of the carrier by using FCAs is a successful process in the inhalational properties of DPI. A recent study has shown the use of leucine as spray-dried mannitol–leucine as a single carrier to enhance the aerosolization performance of SS. Formulation containing 10%w/w leucine has produced almost 53% FPF of SS (Molina et al., 2019). Force control agent particles may be coated onto drug particles by applying a process known as "mechanofusion" or mechanical dry coating (Begat et al., 2009; Qu et al., 2015; Mehta, 2018).

The effects of surface enrichment by hydrophobic drugs or excipients on aerosolization performance of DPIs particularly hygroscopic ones were reported (Cuvelier et al., 2015; Chan et al., 2017; Wang et al., 2015; Zhou et al., 2016; Momin et al., 2, 2018.). The adsorption of water on the surface of particles changes in the interparticulate forces by changing the surface energy of the particles, and hence increasing interaction via capillary forces (Zhu et al., 2008; Brunaugh et al., 2018). An example is the hygroscopic disodium cromoglycate powder when the surface of the drug particles was enriched by spray dry coating with the hydrophobic amino acid L-leucine, protected from moisture, improved dispersibility and hence increased aerosolization (Chan et al., 2017).

8.3.2 HIGH DOSE DPIS

There are different IDDS for delivering the high dose drugs to the lungs, including pMDIs, nebulizers, and DPIs, however, DPIs are considered the most suitable IDDS for high drug doses (Momin et al., 2018). A recent publication has shown that three major barriers to achieving the desired pharmacokinetics and hence pharmacodynamic effect with these compounds: aerosol delivery, lung deposition, and clearance (Hatipoglu et al., 2018). Drug plasma concentration remains much higher and for a longer time after pulmonary administration of high dose relative to oral administration. Furthermore, concentrations in the lung tissue dosed as DPI can be many folds higher than in plasma after oral administration.

Moreover, the increasing presence of poorly water-soluble drugs in the lung may raise a health concern or even hazards because it is associated with adverse lung changes leading to, allergic inflammatory responses, lung damage and fibrosis (Momin et al., 2018; Brunaugh et al., 2018). Thus, all these parameters should be carefully investigated in order to reduce the likelihood of adverse effects as a result of high blood concentrations of the drugs and residues of insoluble particles (Hatipoglu et al., 2018, Brunaugh et al., 2018).

DPIs of potent drugs have been used for many years for the treatment of asthma and COPD, which requires 'low' drug doses of 5–500 μg (Smith and Parry-Billings, 2003; Brunaugh et al., 2018). High dose inhaled antibiotics or antivirals like colistin (55 mg or 125/dose) and tobramycin (28 mg/dose), zanamivir (5 mg /dose), and laninamivir octanoate (20-40mg/dose) DPIs are already on the market, and further development is going on amikacin, kanamycin, gentamycin and isoniazid, loxapine, levodopa, voriconazole, amikacin, kanamycin, gentamycin, amphotericin, tacrolimus (as liposomes), cyclosporin A (as cyclodextrin complexes), low molecular weight heparin, ciprofloxacin amongst others. Generally, DPIs containing drugs of 5 mg or greater and even more than 100 mg, referred to as high dose DPIs (Sibum et al., 2018). In order to achieve deep lung delivery for formulations of high dose DPIs, the APSD should be lower than 5 μm with a narrow size distribution. Furthermore, the particles should have a spherical shape with low tapped density, low surface energy and consequently low particle interactions. Crystalline materials with a low level of surface roughness and hydrophobic surface characteristics shall result in lower particle interactions and lower sensitivity to moisture.

Uptake of water leads to increase particle interactions by changing the surface energy, particularly for hygroscopic drugs, which are very sensitive to water, hinder de-agglomeration and decrease aerosolization of the powders.

The carrier-based formulation in small dose DPIs is not considered applicable for the development of high drug dose DPIs. In carrier-free formulations, powders are formulated as agglomerates containing either drug powder only, drug powder blended with fine lactose or suitable additives such as FCAs. Hence the agglomerates should be de-agglomerated during aerosolization in order to reach deeply into the lungs. De-agglomeration efficiency in the formulation of high drug dose DPIs has been achieved using several particle-engineering techniques and different formulation approaches. Examples of used particle-engineering techniques are micronization (well established and most used technique), crystallization (preparation of crystalline particles with predetermined size distribution shape and polymorphic form), spray-drying (well established technique, and applicable for solution, suspension and emulsion-based formulations) supercritical fluid technology (suitable for compounds sensitive to micronization and soluble in the supercritical fluids), spray freeze-drying (suitable for thermosensitive drugs), freeze-drying (suitable for thermosensitive drugs) amongst others. Furthermore, Pulmo Sphere technology also has been shown applicable for the delivery of high dose antibiotics (up to doses >100 mg) along with the spray drying technique (Geller et al., 2011). Therefore, particle engineering is considered a proper approach for the production of carrier-free (or with a minimum amount of carriers or additives) DPIs of high drug doses with good flowability and superior aerosolization properties.

Different formulation approaches for high dose DPIs have been extensively reviewed (Momin et al., 2018; Sibum et al., 2018; Brunaugh et al., 2018; Zhou et al., 2015; Lau, 2017). Many of these approaches have already mentioned in Section 8.4.1which may be applied in the formulation of high dose DPIs. Other approaches are as follows:

1. Preparation of low-density porous particles (LPP) which have large geometric size. LPPs exhibit better lung deposition, bioavailability and prolongs drug release, particularly when using biodegradable polymers such as poly(lactic-co-glycolic acid) copolymer (Edward et al., 1997).

2. Particle surface modification by applying hydrophobic barriers such as Leucine. In case of high dose hygroscopic drug the degree of moisture protection is dependent on the amount of leucine enriched onto the particle surface (Li et al., 2016); however, this must be considered as an additional bulk material and its potential inhalation burden (Brunaugh et al., 2018).

3. To target deep lung delivery of drugs and minimize oropharyngeal deposition excipient-enhanced growth is another formulation approach, where submicrometer aerosol particles combining a drug and hygroscopic excipient are delivered through inhalation. The size of the aerosol increases after entering the highly moist airways and the large size improves retention in the lung (Momin et al., 2018). However, this approach may not be suitable for high dose delivery of drugs because a high percentage (50% w/w) of hygroscopic excipient is required.

4. Controlled crystallization of drugs over micronization in the manufacturing of inhalable dry powder particles as it may produce highly crystalline particles with a predetermined size, size distribution shape, and polymorphic form. In comparison with micronization, the crystals of drug particles have better aerosolization efficiency and physical stability (Rasenack et al., 2003). The use of a crystalline form of inhalable rifapentine powder improved FPF compared to the amorphous form, which was hypothesized to be due to the elongated morphology (Brunaugh et al., 2018).

5. Co-formulation of hydrophobic and hygroscopic drugs has been utilized in order to improve the aerosol performance of hygroscopic drug particles (Zhou et al., 2014; Zhou et al., 2016; Momin et al., 2018). Zhou et al., (Zhou et al., 2014, 2016) reported that improved aerosol performance and protection against moisture-induced performance deterioration of hygroscopic colistin particles when cospray dried with hydrophobic drugs (rifampin or azithromycin) was achieved. The improved aerosolization was related to the hydrophobic surface enrichment of the co-spray dried powder particles by optimizing of spray drying conditions (Momin and Tucker et al., 2018). Momin et al., highlighted that in the co-formulation approach, the drugs are generally selected based on their known synergistic effect. However, the number of synergistic combinations is very limited (Momin et al., 2018).

Recent DPIs formulation approaches include the use of drug nanoparticles for enhancing drug delivery, the use of microspheres of drugs with polymeric carriers for prolonging drug activity and the use of DPIs for delivery of proteins, peptides and vaccines as an alternative route to injectable. These recent approaches along with others have been discussed in many review articles (Rangaraj et al., 2019; Chan, et al., 2014; Yurdasiper et al., 2018; Weers et al., 2010; Mehta 2016; Javadzadeh and Yaqoubi, 2017). However, de Boer et al reported that DPIs may not be suitable for large biopharmaceuticals, but suitable for smaller molecules (having molecular weights < $1KD_a$), such as levodopa, loxapine, iloprost, or sildenafil (de Boer et al., 2017).

8.4 NEBULIZERS AND SOFT MISTS

Nebulizers are IDDS used for asthma therapy to deliver fine droplets of drugs to the lungs. All nebulizer formulations are aqueous solutions. Generally they are solutions of drugs, however, some are aqueous suspensions (Young et al., 2008; Hickey, 2018a). Formulation parameters such as viscosity, surface tension, and electrolyte concentration are influencing droplet aerosol properties such as droplet size distribution and FPF (Chan, et al., 2014). The viscosity is only important in case cosolvents such as glycerol, propylene glycol, or polyethylene glycol are added in quantities significantly change the water properties. However, the major considerations for the preparation and stability of solutions for nebulization are pH and ionic strength. An increase in viscosity and conductivity reduced the aerodynamic size, while increased electrolyte concentrations enhanced aerosol output (Beck-Broichsitter et al., 2013; Chan et al., 2012). Furthermore, the droplet size of nebulized aerosols was significantly reduced by adding micromolar concentrations of nonionic surfactant Pluronic polymers to the nebulizer solutions (Haddrell et al., 2013). Suspension nebulizers are usually formulated with drug particles alone or lipid-based systems representing drug encapsulation such as liposomal amphotericin B formulation and sustained-release (liposomal) ciprofloxacin among other new formulations (Young et al., 2008; Alexander et al., 2011). The types of devices for nebulization are numerous such as jet, ultrasonic, and vibrating mesh, however other models are commercially available (Misik et al., 2018; A310). A recent study using budesonide suspension and albuterol inhalation solution has shown that the flow pattern, device, and formulation are the main parameters affecting the APSD of nebulizers (Misik et al., 2018). In 2003 Boehringer Ingelheim produced a new nebulizer, the Respimat Soft Mist™ Inhaler which was considered as combining form of nebulizer and pMDI and characterized by being a propellant-free, multi-dose system with aerosol-cloud fall into the fine particle fraction of droplets (high proportion of the droplets < 5.8 μm) (Young et al., 2008, Dalby et al., 2004). The aerosol-cloud is generated by mechanical power from a spring rather than a liquid-gas propellant as used by pMDI (Misik et al., 2018). Furthermore, because of the high amount of drug deposited in the lungs by the aerosol clouds, it is expected that inhaled drugs would maintain their efficacy even when smaller doses were administered (Dalby et al., 2004).

8.5 CONCLUDING REMARK

Inhaled drug delivery systems (IDDS) include three major dosage forms; pressurized metered-dose inhalers (pMDIs), dry powder inhalers (DPIs), and nebulizers. This review has discussed IDDS in terms of the development of their formulations. Particle engineering technologies for the formulation of suspension or powdered IDDS have been investigated which demonstrated a major role in the development of a new generation of inhaler formulations. This review also discusses the development of high dose dry powder formulations, their challenges and the potential for pulmonary delivery.

KEYWORDS

- **advanced formulations of DPIs**
- **advanced formulations of pMDIs**
- **formulations of DPIs**
- **formulations of pMDIs**
- **inhalation delivery systems**

REFERENCES

Adi, H., et al., (2005). Influence of cohesive properties of micronized lactose powders on particle size analysis by laser diffraction. *CHEMECA, Australasian Chemical Engineering*. Brisbane, Australia.

Adi, H., et al., (2006). Agglomerate strength and dispersion of salmeterol xinafoate from powder mixtures for inhalation. *Pharm Res., 23*(11), 2556–2565. doi: 10.1007/s11095-006-9082-6.

Agent, P., & Parrott, H., (2015). Inhaled therapy in cystic fibrosis: Agents, devices and regimens. *Breathe, 11*(2), 111–118. doi: 10.1183/20734735.021014.

Alexander, B. D., (2011). *In vitro* characterization of nebulizer delivery of liposomal amphotericin B aerosols. *Pharm Dev Technol., 16*(6), 577–582. doi: 10.3109/10837450.2011.591803.

Beck-Broichsitter, M., et al., (2012). Controlled pulmonary drug and gene delivery using polymeric nano-carriers. *J. Control. Release., 161*, 214–224.10.1016/j.jconrel.2011.12.004.

Beck-Broichsitter, M., et al., (2013). On the correlation of output rate and aerodynamic characteristics in vibrating-mesh-based aqueous aerosol delivery. *Int. J. Pharm., 461*(1&2), 34–37. doi: 10.1016/j.ijpharm.2013.11.036.

Beg, S., Rahman, M., Kohli, K., (2019). Quality-by-design approach as a systematic tool for the development of nanopharmaceutical products. *Drug Discovery Today.* 24(3), 717–725.

Beg, S., Akhter, S., Rahman, M., Rahman, Z., (2017a). Perspectives of Quality by Design approach in nanomedicines development. *Current Nanomedicine, 7*, 1–7.

Beg, S., Rahman, M., Panda, S.S., (2017b). Pharmaceutical QbD: Omnipresence in the product development lifecycle. *European Pharmaceutical Review.* 22(1), 2–8.

Begat, P., et al., (2009). The role of force control agents in high-dose dry powder inhaler formulations. *J. Pharm. Sci., 98*, 2770–2783. doi: 10.1002/jps.21629.

Biddiscombe, M. F., & Usmani, O. S., (2018). Is there room for further innovation in inhaled therapy for airways disease? *Breathe, 14*(3), 216–224. doi: 10.1183/20734735.020318.

Brambilla, G., et al., (1999). Modulation of aerosol clouds produced by pressurized inhalation aerosols. *Int. J Pharm., 186*, 53–61.

Brunaugh, A. D., et al., (2018). Formulation techniques for high dose dry powders. *Int. J. Pharm., 547*, 489–498. doi: 10.1016/j.ijpharm.2018.05.036.

Buttini, F., et al., (2018). The application of quality by design framework in the pharmaceutical development of dry powder inhalers. *Eur. J. Pharm. Sci., 113*, 64–76. doi: 10.1016/j.ejps.2017.10.042.

Carvalho, S. R., et al., (2015). Dry powder inhalation for pulmonary delivery: Recent advances and continuing challenges. In: Nokhodchi, A., & Martin, G., (eds.), *Pulmonary Drug Delivery: Advances and Challenges* (pp. 35–62). Wiley & Sons, Ltd, Chichester, West Sussex.

Chan, J. G. Y., et al., (2014). Advances in device and formulation technologies for pulmonary drug delivery. *AAPS Pharm. Sci. Tech., 15*(4), pp. 1–16. doi: 10.1208/s12249-014-0114-y.

Chan, J. G., et al., (2012). Delivery of high solubility polyols by vibrating mesh nebulizer to enhance mucociliary clearance. *J. Aerosol. Med. Pulm. Drug Deliv.*, *25*(5), 297–305. doi: 10.1089/jamp.2011.0961.

Chan, K. H., et al., (2017). Protection of hydrophobic amino acids against moisture-induced deterioration in the aerosolization performance of highly hygroscopic spray-dried powders. *Eur. J. Pharm. Biopharm.*, *119*, 224–234. doi: 10.1016/j.ejpb.2017.06.023.

Chandel, A., et al., (2019). Recent advances in aerosolized drug delivery. *Biomed Pharmacother.*, *112*(4), 108601, 1–11. DOI: 10.1016/j.biopha.2019.108601.

Chow, A. H. L., et al., (2007). Particle engineering for pulmonary drug delivery. *Pharm Res.*, *24*(3), 411–437. doi: 10.1007/s11095-006-9174-3.

Church, T. K., et al., (2012). *Salmeterol Superfine Formulation*. US Patents 8, 088, 362 B2.

Cooper, A., (2016). A QbD method development approach for a generic pMDI. *Pharm. Tech.*, *40*(5), 30–36, 63.

Cui, Y., & Sommerfeld, M., (2015). Forces on micron-sized particles randomly distributed on the surface of larger particles and possibility of detachment. *Int. J. Multiphase Flow*, *72*, 39–52. doi: 10.1016/j.ijmultiphaseflow.2015.01.006.

Cui, Y., & Sommerfeld, M., (2019). The modeling of carrier-wall collision with drug particle detachment for dry powder inhaler applications. *Powder Technol.*, *344*, 741–755. doi: 10.1016/j.powtec.2018.12.067.

Cui, Y., et al., (2014). Towards the optimisation and adaptation of dry powder inhalers. *Int. J. Pharm.*, *470*, 120–132. doi: 10.1016/j.ijpharm.2014.04.065.

Cuvelier, B., et al., (2015). Minimal amounts of dipalmitoylphosphatidylcholine improve aerosol performance of spray-dried temocillin powders for inhalation. *Int. J. Pharm.*, *495*, 981–990. doi: 10.1016/j.ijpharm.2015.10.019.

Dalby, R. N., & Byron, P. R., (1988). Comparison of output particle size distributions from pressurized aerosols formulated as solutions or suspensions. *Pharm. Res.*, *5*(1), 36–39.

Dalby, R., et al., (2004). A review of the development of Respimat® Soft MistTM Inhaler. *Int. J. Pharm.*, *283*, 1–9. 10.1016/j.ijpharm.2004.06.018.

De Boer, H. A., et al., (2017). Dry powder inhalation: Past, present and future. *Expert Opin. Drug Deliv.*, *14*(4), 499–512. doi: 10.1080/17425247.2016.1224846.

Dellamary, L. A., et al., (2000). Hollow porous particles in metered dose inhalers. *Pharm Res.*, *17*(20), 168–174. doi: 10.1023/A:1007513213292.

Dellamary, L. A., et al., (2011). Stable metal ion-lipid powdered pharmaceutical compositions for drug delivery and methods of use. *US Patent 7, 871*, 598 B1, 1–27.

Duddu, S. P., et al., (2002). Improved lung delivery from a passive dry powder inhaler using an Engineered PulmoSphere powder. *Pharm. Res.*, *19*(5), 689–695. doi: 10.1023/A:1015322616613.

Edwards, D. A., et al., (1997). Large porous particles for pulmonary drug delivery. *Science*, *276*(5320), 1868–1871.

FDA, (2018). *USA, Metered Dose Inhaler (MDI) and Dry Powder Inhaler (DPI) Products—Quality Considerations Guidance for Industry*, 1–50.

Federico Lavorini, F., et al., (2014). New inhaler devices—the good, the bad and the ugly. *Respiration*, *88*, 3–15. doi: 10.1159/000363390.

Ferguson, G. T., et al., (2018). Co-suspension delivery technology in pressurized metered-dose inhalers for multi-drug dosing in the treatment of respiratory diseases. *Respir. Med.*, *134*, 16–23. doi: 10.1016/j.rmed.2017.09.012.

Gallo, L., et al., (2019). Development of porous spray-dried inhalable particles using an organic solvent-free technique. *Powder Technol.*, *342*, 642–652. doi: 10.1016/j. powtec.2018.10.041.

Ganderton, D., et al., (2002). Modulite (R): A means of designing the aerosols generated by pressurized metered dose inhalers. *Respir. Med.*, *96*, S3–S8.

Geller, D. E., et al., (2011). Development of an inhaled dry-powder formulation of tobramycin using pulmosphere™ technology. *J. Aerosol Med. Pulm. Drug Deliv.*, *24*(4), 175–182. doi: 10.1089/jamp.2010.0855.

Grainger, C., et al., (2012). Critical characteristics for corticosteroid solution metered dose inhaler bioequivalence. *Mol. Pharmaceutics.*, *9*(3), 563–569. doi: 10.1021/mp200415g.

Grasmeijer, F., et al., (2015). Recent advances in the fundamental understanding of adhesive mixtures for inhalation. *Curr. Pharm. Des.*, *21*, 5900–5914. doi: 10.2174/1381 612821666151008124622.

Haddrell, A. E., et al., (2013). Control over hygroscopic growth of saline aqueous aerosol using pluronic polymer additives. *Int. J. Pharm.*, *443*(1&2), 183–192. doi: 10.1016/j. ijpharm.2012.12.039.

Hartwig, S. H., & Wehle, S., (2004). A novel formulation technique for metered dose inhaler (MDI) suspensions. *Int. J. Pharm.*, *284*, 75–82. doi: 10.1016/j.ijpharm.2004.07.005.

Hatipoglu, K., et al., (2018). Pharmacokinetics and pharmacodynamics of high doses of inhaled dry powder drugs. *Int. J. Pharm.*, *549*(1&2), 306–316. doi: 10.1016/j. ijpharm.2018.07.050.

Hickey, A. J., & Holt, J., (2014). Surface interactions in propellant driven metered dose inhaler product design. In: *Colloid and Interface Science in Pharmaceutical Research and Development* (pp. 79–102). Elsevier B. V., NY.

Hickey, A. J., (2016). Pulmonary drug delivery: Pharmaceutical chemistry and aero sol technology. In: Wang, B., et al., (eds.), *Drug Delivery: Principles and Applications* (2nd edn., pp. 186–205). John Wiley & Sons, Inc, NY.

Hickey, A. J., (2018a). Chapter 2: Dosage forms. In: *Inhaled Pharmaceutical Product Development Perspectives: Challenges and Opportunities* (pp. 15–33). Elsevier Inc. RTI International, Research Triangle Park, North Carolina.

Hickey, A. J., (2018b). Introduction: historical perspective. In: *Inhaled Pharmaceutical Product Development Perspectives: Challenges and Opportunities* (pp. 1–13). Elsevier Inc. RTI International, Research Triangle Park, North Carolina.

Hickey, A. J., et al., (2007). Physical characterization of component particles included in dry powder inhalers. I. Strategy review and static characteristics. *J. Pharm. Sci.*, *96*(5), 1282–1301. doi: 10.1002/jps.20916.

Hou, S., et al., (2015). Practical, regulatory and clinical considerations for development of inhalation drug products. *Asian J. Pharm. Sci.*, *10*, 490–500. doi: 10.1016/j. ajps.2015.08.008.

Ibiapina, C. C., et al., (2004). Hydrofluoroalkane as a propellant for pressurized metered-dose inhalers: History, pulmonary deposition, pharmacokinetics, efficacy and safety. *J. Pediatr. (Rio J).*, *80*, 441–446. doi: 10.1590/S0021–75572004000800004.

Ibrahim, A. H., et al., (2003). Microparticle detachment from surfaces exposed to turbulent airflow: Controlled experiments and modeling. *J Aerosol Sci.*, *34*, 765–782. doi: 10.1016/ S0021–8502(03)00031–4.

Imran, Y., Saleem, I. Y., & Smyth, H. D. C., (2013). Tuning aerosol particle size distribution of metered dose inhalers using cosolvents and surfactants. *Bio. Med. Research International*, Article ID, 574310, 1–7. doi: 10.1155/2013/574310.

Ivey, J. W., et al., (2017). Humidity affects the morphology of particles emitted from beclomethasone dipropionate pressurized metered dose inhalers. *Int. J. Pharm.*, *520*, 207–215. doi: 10.1016/j.ijpharm.2017.01.062.

Javadzadeh, Y., & Yaqoubi, S., (2017). Therapeutic nanostructures for pulmonary drug delivery. In: *Nanostructures for Drug* (pp. 619–638). Elsevier, Inc.

Jetzer, M. W., et al., (2016). Investigating the effect of the force control agent magnesium stearate in fluticasone propionate dry powder inhaled formulations with single particle aerosol mass spectrometry (SPAMS). *Drug Delivery to the Lungs*, *27*, 1–4.

Jetzer, M. W., et al., (2017). Particle interactions of fluticasone propionate and salmeterol xinafoate detected with single particle aerosol mass spectrometry (SPAMS). *Int. J. Pharm.*, *30*, *532*(1), 218–228. doi: 10.1016/j.ijpharm.2017.08.113.

Jetzer, M. W., et al., (2018). Probing the particulate microstructure of the aerodynamic particle size distribution of dry powder inhaler combination products. *Int. J. Pharm.*, *538*(1&2), 30–39. doi: 10.1016/j.ijpharm.2017.12.046.

Jones, M. D., et al., (2008). An investigation into the relationship between carrier-based dry powder inhalation performance and formulation cohesive-adhesive force balances. *Eur. J. Pharm. Biopharm.*, *69*, 496–507. doi: 10.1016/j.ejpb.2007.11.019.

Jones, S. A., (2011). Suspension versus solution metered dose inhalers: Different products, different particles? *J. Drug Del. Sci. Tech.*, *21*(4), 319–322. doi: 10.1016/S1773–2247(11)50049–8.

Kendall, K., & Stainton, C., (2001). Adhesion and aggregation of fine particles. *Powder Technol.*, *121*, 223–229. doi: 10.1016/S0032–5910(01)00386–2.

Klijn, S. L., et al., (2017). Effectiveness and success factors of educational inhaler technique interventions in asthma & COPD patients: A systematic review. *NPJ Prim Care Respir. Med.*, *27*(24), 1–10. doi: 10.1038/s41533–017–0022–1.

Lau, M., et al., (2017). Co-milled API-Lactose systems for inhalation therapy: Impact of magnesium stearate on physicochemical stability and aerosolization performance. *Drug Dev. Ind. Pharm.*, *43*(6), 980–988. doi: 10.1080/03639045.2017.1287719.

Lavorini, F., et al., (2017). Recent advances in capsule-based dry powder inhaler technology. *Multidiscip. Respir. Med.*, *12*(11), 1–7. doi: 10.1186/s40248–017–0092–5.

Leach, C., et al., (1998). Improved airway targeting with the CFC-free HFA-beclomethasone metered-dose inhaler compared with CFC-beclomethasone. *Eur. Respir. J.*, *12*(6), 1346–1353.

Lechuga-Ballesteros, D., et al., (2011). Novel cosuspension metered-dose inhalers for the combination therapy of chronic obstructive pulmonary disease and asthma. *Future Med. Chem.*, *3*(13), 1703–1718. doi: 10.4155/fmc.11.133.

Li, L., et al., (2016). l- Leucine as an excipient against moisture on *in vitro* aerosolization performances of highly hygroscopic spray-dried powders. *Eur. J. Pharm. Biopharm.*, *102*, 132–141. doi: 10.1016/j.ejpb.2016.02.010.

Lia, H. Y., & Xu, E. Y., (2017). Innovative pMDI formulations of spray-dried nanoparticles for efficient pulmonary drug delivery. *Int. J. Pharm.*, *530*(1&2), 12–20. doi: 10.1016/j.ijpharm.2017.07.040.

Mahmoudi, S., et al., (2019). Fluidisation characteristics of lactose powders in simple turbulent channel flows. *Exp. Therm. Fluid Sci.*, *103*, 201–213. doi: 10.1016/j. expthermflusci.2019.01.012.

Mehta, P., (2016). Dry powder inhalers: A focus on advancements in novel drug delivery systems. *J. Drug Deliv.*, Article ID, 8290963, 1–17. doi: 10.1155/2016/8290963.

Mehta, P., (2018). Imagine the superiority of dry powder inhalers from carrier engineering. *J. Drug Deliv.*, Article ID, 5635010, 1–19. doi: 10.1155/2018/5635010.

Miao, X., et al., (2015). Chinese medicine in inhalation therapy: A review of clinical application and formulation development. *Curr. Pharm. Des.*, *21*(27), 3917–3931. doi: 10.2174/1381612821666150820110550.

Misik, O., et al., (2018). Inhalers and nebulizers: Basic principles and preliminary measurements. *EPJ Web of Conferences, 180*, 02068, 1–6.

Miyazaki, Y., et al., (2016). Application of combinational supercritical CO2 techniques to the preparation of inhalable particles. *J. Drug Delv. Sci. Tec., 36*, 1–9. doi: 10.1016/j. jddst.2016.08.010.

Miyazaki, Y., et al., (2017). Improved respirable fraction of budesonide powder for dry powder inhaler formulations produced by advanced supercritical CO_2 processing and use of a novel additive. *Int. J. Pharm., 528*(1&2), 118–126. doi: 10.1016/j. ijpharm.2017.06.002.

Molina, C., et al., (2019). The crucial role of leucine concentration on spray dried mannitol-leucine as a single carrier to enhance the aerosolization performance of Albuterol sulfate. *J. Drug Delv. Sci. Tec., 49*, 97–106. doi: 10.1016/j.jddst.2018.11.007.

Momin, M. A. M., et al., (2018). High dose dry powder inhalers to overcome the challenges of tuberculosis treatment. *Int. J. Pharm., 550*, 398–417. doi: 10.1016/j. ijpharm.2018.08.061.

Momin, M. A. M., Tucker, I. G., et al., (2018). Manipulation of spray-drying conditions to develop dry powder particles with surfaces enriched in hydrophobic material to achieve high aerosolization of a hygroscopic drug. *Int. J. Pharm., 543*(1&2), 318–327. doi: 10.1016/j.ijpharm.2018.04.003.

Myrdal, P. B., et al., (2014). Advances in metered dose inhaler technology: Formulation development. *AAPS Pharm. Sci. Tech., 15*(2), 434–455. doi: 10.1208/s12249–013–0063-x.

Newman, S. P., (2005). Principles of metered-dose inhaler design. *Respir. Care., 50*(9), 1177–1190.

O'Donnell, K. P., & Williams III, R. O., (2013). Pulmonary dispersion formulations: The impact of dispersed powder properties on pressurized metered dose inhaler stability. *Drug Dev. Ind. Pharm., 39*(3), 413–424. doi: 10.3109/03639045.2012.664145.

Ober, C. A., et al., (2013). Preparation of rifampicin/lactose microparticle composites by a supercritical antisolvent-drug excipient mixing technique for inhalation delivery. *Powder Technol., 236*, 132–138. doi: 10.1016/j.powtec.2012.04.057.

Parisini, I., et al., (2015). Mathematical approach for understanding deagglomeration behavior of drug powder in formulations with coarse carrier. *Asian J. of Pharm. Sci., 10*, 501–512. doi: 10.1016/j.ajps.2015.08.007.

Paul, M., Young, M., et al., (2008). Advances in pulmonary therapy. In: Williams, III, R. O., et al., (eds.), *Advanced Drug Formulation Design to Optimize Therapeutic Outcomes* (pp. 1–52). Informa Healthcare, NY.

Preedy, E. C., & Prokopovich, P., (2013). History of inhaler devices. In: *Inhaler Devices: Fundamentals, Design and Drug Delivery* (pp. 13–28). Elsevier Inc. Woodhead Publishing Limited, Cambridge.

Price, D., et al., (2013). Real-life comparison of beclometasone dipropionate as an extra fine or larger-particle formulation for asthma. *Respir Med., 107*, 987–1000. doi: 10.1016/j. rmed.2013.03.009.

Pritchard, J. N., (2001). The influence of lung deposition on clinical response. *J. Aerosol. Med., 14*(1), S19–S26. doi: 10.1089/08942680150506303.

Qu, L., et al., (2015). Particle engineering via mechanical dry coating in the design of pharmaceutical solid dosage forms. *Curr. Pharm. Des., 21*(40), 5802–5814. doi: 10.217 4/1381612821666151008151001.

Rangaraj, N., et al., (2019). Insight into pulmonary drug delivery: Mechanism of drug deposition to device characterization and regulatory requirements. *Pulm. Pharmacol. Ther., 54*, 1–21. doi: 10.1016/j.pupt.2018.11.004.

Rasenack, N., et al., (2003). Micronization of anti-inflammatory drugs for pulmonary delivery by a controlled crystallization process. *J. Pharm. Sci., 92*, 35–44. doi: 10.1002/ jps.10274.

Riley, T., et al., (2012). Challenges with developing *in vitro* dissolution tests for orally inhaled products (OIPs). *AAPS Pharm. Sci. Tech., 13*(3), 978–989. doi: 10.1208/ s12249-012-9822-3.

Robinson, C. A., & Tsourounis, C., (2013). Inhaled corticosteroid metered-dose inhalers: How do variations in technique for solutions versus suspensions affect drug distribution? *Ann. Pharmacother., 47*, 416–420. doi: 10.1345/aph.1R480.

Rogueda, P., (2005). Novel hydrofluoroalkane suspension formulations for respiratory drug delivery. *Expert Opin. Drug Deliv., 2*(4), 625–638. doi: 10.1517/17425247.2.4.625.

Rudén, J., et al., (2019). Linking carrier morphology to the powder mechanics of adhesive mixtures for dry powder inhalers via a blend-state model. *Int. J. Pharm., 561*, 148–160. doi: 10.1016/j.ijpharm.2019.02.038.

Saim, S., & Horhota, S. T., (2002). Process for overcoming drug retention in hard gelatin inhalation capsules. *Drug Dev. Ind. Pharm., 28*(6), 641–654. doi: 10.1081/ DDC-120003855.

Sallam, A., (2019). Quality by design considerations for product development of dry-powder inhalers. In: Beg, S., & Hasnain, M. S., (eds.), *Pharmaceutical Quality by Design* (pp. 173–192). Academic Press, Elsevier Inc, AC.

Sanders, M., (2007). Inhalation therapy: An historical review. *Prim. Care Respir. J., 16*(2), 71–81. doi: 10.3132/pcrj.2007.00017.

Santosh, R., Thorat, L., & Sarika, M., (2015). Meshram: Review on quality by designing for metered dose inhaler product development. *Sch. Acad. J. Pharm., 4*(6), 324–330.

Sheth, P., Grimes, M. R., et al., (2017). Impact of droplet evaporation rate on resulting *in vitro* performance parameters of pressurized metered dose inhalers. *Int. J. Pharm., 528*, 360–371. doi: 10.1016/j.ijpharm.2017.06.014.

Sheth, P., Sandell, D., et al., (2017). Influence of formulation factors on the aerosol performance of suspension and solution metered dose inhalers: A systematic approach. *The AAPS Journal, 19*(5), 1396–1410. doi: 10.1208/s12248-017-0095-3.

Shoyele, S. A., & Cawthorne, S., (2006). Particle engineering techniques for inhaled biopharmaceuticals. *Adv. Drug Deliv. Rev.*, *58*(9), 1009–1029. doi: 10.1016/j.addr.2006.07.010.

Shur, J., et al., (2016). From single excipients to dual excipient platforms in dry powder inhaler products. *Int. J. Pharm.*, *514*, 374–383. doi: 10.1016/j.ijpharm.2016.05.057.

Sibum, I., et al., (2018). Challenges for pulmonary delivery of high powder doses. *Int. J. Pharm.*, *548*, 325–336. doi: 10.1016/j.ijpharm.2018.07.008.

Singh, B., & Beg, S., (2015). Attaining product development excellence and federal compliance employing Quality by Design (QbD) paradigms. *The Pharma Review.* 13(9), 35–44.

Singh, B., & Beg, S., (2014). Product development excellence and federal compliance via QbD. *Chronicle PharmaBiz.* 15(10), 30–35.

Singh, D. J., et al., (2015). Preparation and evaluation of surface modified lactose particles for improved performance of fluticasone propionate dry powder inhaler. *J. Aerosol. Med. Pulm. Drug Deliv.*, *28*(4), 254–267. doi: 10.1089/jamp.2014.

Smith, I. J., et al., (2003). The inhalers of the future? A review of dry powder devices on the market today. *Pulm. Pharmacol. Ther.*, *16*, 79–95. doi: 10.1016/S1094–5539(02)00147–5.

Solvay Special Chemicals. Solkane Solvay Special Chemicals® 227 pharma and Solkane® 134a pharma. https://www.solvay.com/en/brands/solkane (Accessed on 19 November 2019).

Stein, S. W., & Gabrio, B. J., (2000). Understanding throat deposition during cascade impactor testing. *Respir. Drug Deliv.*, *2*, 287–290.

Stein, S. W., & Myrdal, P. B., (2006). The relative influence of atomization and evaporation on metered dose inhaler drug delivery efficiency. *Aerosol. Sci. Technol.*, *40*, 335–347. doi: 10.1080/02786820600612268.

Stein, S. W., et al., (2015). Modeling and understanding combination pMDI formulations with both dissolved and suspended drugs. *Mol. Pharmaceutics.*, *12*(9), 3455–3467. doi: 10.1021/acs.molpharmaceut.5b00467.

Sun, Y., (2016). Carrier free inhaled dry powder of budesonide tailored by supercritical fluid particle design. *Powder Technol.*, *304*, 248–260. doi: 10.1016/j.powtec.2016.07.036.

Tarara, T. E., et al., (2004). Characterization of suspension-based metered dose inhaler formulations composed of spray-dried budesonide microcrystals dispersed in HFA-134a. *Pharm. Res.*, *21*(9), 1607–1614. doi: 10.1023/B:PHAM.0000041455.13980.f1.

Taylora, G., et al., (2018). Gamma scintigraphic pulmonary deposition study of glycopyrronium formoterol metered dose inhaler formulated using co-suspension delivery technology. *Eur. J. Pharm. Sci.*, *111*, 450–457. doi: 10.1016/j.ejps.2017.10.026.

Thalberg, K., et al., (2012). Modeling dispersion of dry powders for inhalation. The concepts of total fines, cohesive energy and interaction parameters. *Int. J. Pharm.*, *427*, 224–233. doi: 10.1016/j.ijpharm.2012.02.009.

Traini, D., et al., (2006). Investigation into the influence of polymeric stabilizing excipients on inter-particulate forces in pressurized metered dose inhalers. *Int. J. Pharm.*, *320*, 58–63. doi: 10.1016/j.ijpharm.2006.04.016.

Tsapis, N., et al., (2002). Trojan particles: Large porous carriers of nanoparticles for drug delivery. *PNAS.*, *99*(19), 12001–12005. doi: 10.1073/pnas.182233999.

Vehring, R., (2008). Pharmaceutical particle engineering via spray drying. *Pharm. Res.*, *25*(5), 999–1022. doi: 10.1007/s11095–007–9475–1.

Wang, W., et al., (2015). Effects of surface composition on the aerosolization and dissolution of inhaled antibiotic combination powders consisting of colistin and rifampicin. *The AAPS J., 18*(2), 372–384. doi: 10.1208/s12248–015–9848-z.

Wang, Y. B., et al., (2014). The impact of pulmonary diseases on the fate of inhaled medicines—A Review. *Int. J. Pharm., 461*, 12–128. doi: 10.1016/j.ijpharm.2013.11.042.

Weers, J. G., et al., (2010). Pulmonary formulations: What remains to be done? *J. Aerosol. Med. Pulm. Drug Deliv., 23*(2), S5–S23. doi: 10.1089/jamp.2010.0838.

Weers, J., & Tarara, T., (2014). The PulmoSphere™ platform for pulmonary drug delivery. *Ther. Deliv., 5*(3), 277–295. doi: 10.4155/tde.14.3.

Williams III, R. O., et al., (1999). Application of co-grinding to formulate a model pMDI suspension. *Eur. J. Pharm. Biopharm., 48*, 131–140. doi: 10.1016/S0939–6411(99)00027–2,

Wu, H. T., et al., (2018). Characterization and aerosolization performance of mannitol particles produced using supercritical assisted atomization. *Chem. Eng. Res. Des., 137*, 308–318. doi: 10.1016/j.cherd.2018.07.024.

Yang, F., et al., (2015). The effects of surface morphology on the aerosol performance of spray-dried particles within HFA 134a based metered dose formulations. *Asian J. Pharm. Sci., 10*, 513–519. doi: 10.1016/j.ajps.2015.07.006.

Yang, M. Y., et al., (2014). Pulmonary drug delivery by powder aerosols. *J. Control Release, 193*, 228–240. doi: 10.1016/j.jconrel.2014.04.055.

Young, P. M., et al., (2007). Recent advances in understanding the influence of composite-formulation properties on the performance of dry powder inhalers. *Physica B., 394*, 315–319. doi: 10.1016/j.physb.2006.12.058.

Yurdasiper, A., et al., (2018). Nanopharmaceuticals: Application in inhaler systems. In: *Emerging Nanotechnologies in Immunology: The Design, Applications and Toxicology of Nanopharmaceuticals and Nanovaccines* (pp. 165–201). Elsevier Inc.

Zhou, Q. T., et al., (2015). Inhaled formulations and pulmonary drug delivery systems for respiratory infections. *Adv. Drug Deliv. Rev., 85*, 83–99. doi: 10.1016/j.addr.2014.10.022.

Zhou, Q. T., et al., (2016). How much surface coating of hydrophobic azithromycin is sufficient to prevent moisture-induced decrease in aerosolization of hygroscopic amorphous colistin powder? *The AAPS J., 18*(5), 1213–1224. doi: 10.1208/s12248–016–9934-x.

Zhu, K., et al., (2008). Analysis of the influence of relative humidity on the moisture sorption of particles and the aerosolization process in a dry powder inhaler. *J. Aerosol Sci., 39*(6), 510–524. doi: 10.1016/j.jaerosci.2008.02.003.

CHAPTER 9

Recent Advances in the Development of Novel Ocular Drug Delivery Systems

MOHAMMED JAFAR,[1*] SYED SARIM IMAM,[2] and
SYED AZIZULLAH GHORI[3]

[1]Department of Pharmaceutics, College of Clinical Pharmacy,
Imam Abdulrahman Bin Faisal University, P.O. Box 1982,
Dammam-31441, Saudi Arabia, Mobile: +966502467326

[2]Department of Pharmaceutics, College of Pharmacy,
King Saud University, Riyadh-11451, Saudi Arabia

[3]Department of Pharmacy Practice, College of Clinical Pharmacy,
Imam Abdulrahman Bin Faisal University, P.O. Box 1982,
Dammam-31441, Saudi Arabia

*Corresponding author. E-mail: mjomar@iau.edu.sa

ABSTRACT

Quality by Design (QbD) is an approach encouraged by regulatory bodies and applied by pharmaceutical industries to improve the quality of the final product. The objective of this chapter is to describe via a QbD approach to increase the available knowledge of ocular formulation. Many ocular drug delivery systems have been intensively explored by using the QbD approach by many researchers. The anatomical barriers and physiological conditions of the eye are also important parameters that control the designing of novel drug delivery systems. There are various QbD-based nanosized ocular drug delivery carriers like micelle, liposome, lipid nanoparticle, polymeric nanoparticles approach that have been developed for this purpose. These novel systems offer manifold advantages over conventional systems as they increase the efficiency of drug delivery by improving the release profile and also reduce drug toxicity.

9.1 INTRODUCTION

The eye is considered as an essential part of the body that comprises of two major anatomical part: the anterior as-well-as the posterior region. The posterior region mainly composed of choroid, vitreous chamber, macula, retina and importantly the posterior area of the sclera is located interior to the lens (Janagam et al., 2017). The majority of eye-related illnesses seem to be arised from the posterior part of the eye, thereby increasing the number and intensity in a consistent manner (Thrimawithana et al., 2011). If left untreated, these problems may cause permanent eye damage resulting in loss of complete vision. According to the recent data reports, it was revealed that around 39 million people were affected because of age-associated macular degeneration (AMD), Retinopathy due to diabetes, and disease of glaucoma of the posterior region of the eye resulting in complete visual loss (International Federation, 2013; McGrath et al., 2017).

Presently, the use of invasive procedures and topical administration of drugs in the form of an ocular gel, ointment, etc. to the posterior and anterior regions of the eye is the only available option for managing these disorders. Yet, posterior side topical drug delivery abides a point of confrontation because of diverse static and dynamic barriers, like nasolacrimal drainage, tear clearance, the cornea, conjunctiva, and scleral barriers. The current advancement in the field of nanotechnology and nano-drug studies laid down a great provision and access by overwhelming the restrictions of the conventional treatments, due to their protecting capability for encapsulated medications that ease their transport to a particular site of tissue (Weng et al., 2017; Kaur and Kakkar 2014). Additionally, nanoparticles aids as a favorable vehicle for topical drug delivery due to prolonged drug duration, higher ocular drug absorption, and posterior area drug delivery via controlled rate (Delplace et al., 2015). Varied nano-vehicles such as, lipid nanoparticles, liposomes, emulsions, spanlastics, micelles, polymeric nanoparticles, layered double hydroxides (LDH), dendrimers, cyclodextrins, and pro-active medication with built-in quality has been employed in order to achieve drug delivery to the desired ocular site (Madni et al., 2017).

At the commencement of the radical millennium, Food and Drug Regulatory Authority (FDA) proposed trending quality by design (QbD) plan, which involves lesser experimental trial-runs and may only include three or four independent variables (factors) recognizing that the "quality cannot be tested into products but it should be built in by design" (Pramod et al., 2016; Beg et al., 2017a,b and 2019, Singh et al., 2014 and 2015). The careful 'screening' of significant variables and subsequent response surface analysis using experimental designs is attained through systematic experimental optimization of delivery systems. For optimization of delivery systems, a variety of experimental designs has been adopted and the steps involved in optimization are depicted in Figure 9.1. Among all of these experimental designs, factorial and central composite designs are extensively employed for the optimization of different ocular formulations (Reha et al., 2016; Singh et al., 2013). For the purpose of systematic optimization of the formulations varied experimental design approach like the factorial design (FD), central composite design (CCD), and fractional factorial design (FFD) have been often utilized. This chapter is focused with regards to QbD-based ocular drug delivery systems, which are highly utilized in managing the posterior eye disorders as shown in Table 9.1.

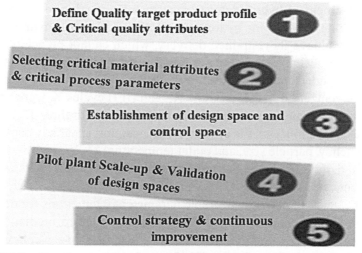

FIGURE 9.1   Steps involved in using quality by design approach for developing ocular drug delivery systems.

9.2   QBD-BASED OCULAR DELIVERY SYSTEMS

9.2.1   LIPID NANO-MEDICINES

Solid lipid nanoparticles (SLN), as well as nanostructured lipid carriers (NLC), are considered to be regularly investigated lipid nanoparticles that are used for ocular drug delivery. These nano-drugs usually contain a solid lipid core, which has the potential in accumulating medications with hydrophilic and lipophilic nature into lipid fabric (Figure 9.2). SLN is accurately embraced with more than a single solid lipid, which shows a melting point of 40°C and even higher. Subsequently, at the beginning of the 1990s, the benefits of control release property of SLNs have been emerged (Souto and Doktorovova 2009), including cellular toxicity, augmented compatibility, and high *in vivo* tolerance (Doktorovova et al., 2014; Doktorovova et al., 2016). Compared to SLN, NLCs, which contain suitable blends of both liquid and solid lipids seem to possess the benefits of high drug doses carrying potential, improved storage steadiness and efficient drug discharging characteristics (Das et al., 2012; Liu et al., 2017). The QbD approach has been precisely opted in developing the nanoparticles by performing crucial analysis of the material attributes affecting the product performance. Khurana et al., (2018) executed the Quality by Design (QbD) principles on process parameter optimization for the development of hybrid delivery system (combination of (SLNs) and in-situ gelling system) for hydrophilic drug moxifloxacin hydrochloride (MOX) to achieve its restrained delivery, which cannot be achieved via single type of technology. In the design of experiments (DoE), the process parameters (independent variables), i.e., chiller temperature X_1, high pressure homogenization (HPH) pressure X_2, and HPH cycles X_3 were ameliorated using face-directed central composite design with three-factors and two levels by simplifying the effect on three responses, namely encapsulation efficiency, particle size, and outlet temperature Y_1, Y_2, and Y_3, respectively. To demonstrate a second-order polynomial equation for full-model both dependent and independent variables were thoroughly assayed. To affirm the deletion of in considerable parameters/interactions for deriving a reduced-model polynomial equation has been opted to predict Y_1, Y_2, and Y_3 for optimized moxifloxacin in situ gelled nanosuspension, F value has been employed. The effects of X_1, X_2, and X_3 are exhibited through the suitability plots on Y_1, Y_2 and Y_3, respectively. The design space is created to acquire the optimized process parameters viz. chiller temperature (–5°C), HPH pressure 800–900 bar and 8 cycles that ended in a nanosuspension with ≈500 nm size, encapsulation efficiency >65% and final formulation temperature <23°C that were required to sustain the formulation in a liquid condition. The regulatory bodies currently recognized and encouraged the method following Quality by Design (QbD) in order to enhance the quality of the finished product. This plan has been substantiated to be a useful device in the development of robust nanosuspension for extremely hydrophilic agents with refined efficacy. In order to control the release of SLNs from the application site and extend their action in a sustained manner, the hybrid gel systems are highly recommended. Additionally, in another recent study that was conducted by Wang et al. (2018) on ocular solid lipid nanoparticles involves optimized chitosan-coated solid lipid nanoparticles (chitosan-SLNs) encapsulated with methazolamide by systematic screening of formulation elements. Both orthogonal and Box-Behnken design with entrapment proficiency, particle size, and zeta potential as the indexes have been utilized for screening the optimized formula of preparation. The optimized composition (methazolamide-chitosan-SLNs) entanglement efficiency was identified as $(58.5 \pm 4.5)\%$, particle size (247.7 ± 17.3) nm and zeta potential (33.5 ± 3.9) mV. The result clearly confirms that the combination of orthogonal as well as Box-Behnken design seems to be efficacious and reliable in the optimization of nano-carriers, and chitosan-SLNs, a dormant vehicle for ophthalmic administration.

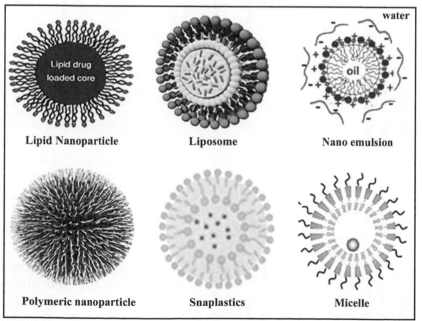

FIGURE 9.2 Various ocular nanoformulations used to target the posterior segment of the eye.

TABLE 9.1 QbD Applied Ocular Drug Delivery System with Used Independent and Dependent Variables

S.No.	QbD Design	Drug	Formulation	Independent variables	Dependent variables	Reference
1	Factorial optimization	Dorzolamide	Self-assembly nanostructures	Effects of pH (X_1); drug to polymer ratio (P/D: X_2)	Drug content (Y_1), particle size (Y_2), polydispersity index (Y_4), zeta potential (Y_3), partition coefficient (Y_5), release half-life (Y_6), release extent (Y_7).	Afify et al., 2018
2	5^2 full factorial design	Dorzolamide-HCl via	Proniosomes	Cholesterol and surfactant	Entrapment efficiency, particle size, drug released after 8h.	Fouda et al., 2018
3	Box–Behnken model	Tenoxicam	Nanovesicles	Glyceryl tripalmitate (A), pluronic F127 (B), gellan gum (C)	Particle size, zeta potential, encapsulation efficiency, gelation temperature.	Elsayed et al., 2017
4	Central composite design	Curcumin	Nanostructured lipid carrier	X_1; the total mass of medium-chain triglyceride (MCT) and glyceryl monostearate (GMS); X_2; GMS/MCT mass ratio; and X_3; the amount of Solutol HS15	Y_1: particle size; Y_2: polydispersity index; Y_3: zeta potential; Y_4: entrapment efficiency.	Liu et al., 2016
5	Two-level full factorial design	Prednisolone	Nanoparticle-laden contact lens	Concentration of PLGA (0.1%–0.4% w/v); Concentration of PVA (4%–7.5% w/v); Concentration of prednisolone (0.5–2.0 mg/mL); Homogenization time (10 and 20 min.)	Size and PDI	El Shaer et al., 2016
6	3^2 full factorial design	Norfloxacin	Nanoparticulate in-situ gel	Chitosan and TPP concentration(s)	Particle size, % entrapment efficiency, % cumulative drug release.	Upadhayay et al., 2016
7	Box–Behnken statistical design	Levofloxacin	Solid lipid nanoparticles	Stearic acid (X_1), Tween 80 (X_2), Sodium deoxycholate (X_3)	Particle size (Y_1), entrapment efficiency (Y_2)	Baig et al., 2016

TABLE 9.1 (*Continued*)

S.No.	QbD Design	Drug	Formulation	Independent variables	Dependent variables	Reference
8	Box–Behnken statistical design	Bevacizumab	PLGA nanoparticles	Chitosan concentration, PLGA content, polyvinyl alcohol (PVA) concentration, sonication time.	Particle size, polydispersity index (PDI), entrapment efficiency (EE), in vitro release.	Pandit et al., 2016
9	Central composite design	Curcumin	Thermoresponsive in situ gel	Pluronic F127 (X_1), pluronic F68 (X_2).	Sol-gel transition temperatures before (R_1) and after dilution (R_2)	Lou et al., 2014
10	Box–Behnken model	Methazolamide	Solid-lipid nanoparticles	Amount of GMS, amount of phospholipid, the concentration of surfactant.	Entrapment efficiency, dosage loading, particle size.	Wang et al., 2014
11	Box–Behnken statistical design	Moxifloxacin	Nanoparticles	CS concentration (X_1), DS concentration (X_2), amount of Mox (X_3).	Particle size (Y_1), encapsulation efficiency (Y_2), zeta potential (Y_3).	Kakoos, 2014
12	Box–Behnken statistical design	Gatifloxacin	Solid-lipid nanoparticles	Lipid(mix) concentration (X_1), poloxamers-188 (X_2), sodium-taurocholate (X_3).	Drug release (Y_1), encapsulation efficiency (Y_2), particle size (Y_3).	Kalam et al., 2013
13	Box–Behnken statistical design	Chloramphenicol	Solid-lipid nanoparticles	Solid lipid (X_1), surfactant (X_2), drug/lipid ratio (X_3).	Entrapment efficiency (EE), drug loading (DL), turbidity.	Hao et al., 2011
14	Box–Behnken statistical design	Gatifloxacin	Chitosan-sodium alginate nanoparticles	Amount of the bioadhesive polymers: CS, ALG and the amount of drug in the formulation.	Particle size, zeta potential, encapsulation efficiency burst release.	Motwani et al., 2008

Baig et al. (2016) also conducted another study that reported promising results with regards to augmentation of levofloxacin loaded stearic acid solid lipid nanoparticles, by implementing Box–Behnken experimental design. Stearic acid as lipid (X_1), Tween 80 as a surfactant (X_2) and sodium deoxycholate as a co-surfactant (X_3), is recognized as independent variables while particle size (Y_1) and entrapment efficiency (Y_2) as dependent variables. Design-Expert software (Design-Expert 8.0.5.2, State-Ease Inc., Minneapolis, USA) is utilized for constructing 17 trial experiments. Responses have been noticed in almost 17 formulations, which were prepared concurrently fixed to first order, second order and quadratic models through Box-Behnken design. The synergistic effects of all the three independent variables with that of the two dependent variables (responses), was found evident and it was also noticed that the linear model to be the well-suited model for the two dependent variables. Improved levofloxacin formulations offer about 237.82 nm of particle size with 78.71% of entrapment efficiency. To investigate the preparation process for SLN, Box–Behnken design has been implemented that revealed as an essential appliance, permitting and demonstrating the association between the elements and quality attributes is reflected through this study. For promoting ocular drug delivery, Fangueiro et al. (2014) opted 3^3 full factorial design in the development and optimization of cationic lipid nanoparticles (LN). A 3^3 full factorial design approach comprising of three variables were fixed at 3-positions, that applied to optimize the experimental effectiveness performed within minimal experimental trials. To achieve this, three different variables and outcomes with regards to physicochemical characteristics of the LN generated were scrutinized. Approximately, 11 experiments were planned for the purpose of design. The solid lipid S100, lecithin (Lipoid®S75) and the hydrophilic surfactant P188 concentrations have been recognized via independent variables. Whereas, the established dependent variables identified were mean particle size (Z-Ave), polydispersity index (PI) and zeta potential (ZP). In case of individual factor, the lower, medium and higher values specific to the lower, medium and upper levels were figured out as (-1), a (0) and a $(+1)$ signs. With the aid of STATISTICA 7.0 (Staf soft, Inc.) software the data were analyzed and reported. The factorial design showed a promising result, recognizing the specific parameters effecting the dispersions of LN, depending on the multi-emulsion technique. A cationic nanostructured hetero lipid matrices has been developed by Youshia et al. (2012) applied in promoting methazolamide ocular delivery which was built via a 3^2 full factorial design in order to determine impact of two independent variables, the ratio of cetostearyl alcohol (CSA): Compritol along with the Tween 80 concentration, at three variant positions. The dependent variables identified were entrapment efficiency percentages (EE%), mean particle size (PS), polydispersity index (PDI), and zeta potential (ZP). The results reveal that higher EE% and PS are achieved with an increase in the CSA-Compritol ratio, whereas higher Tween 80 concentration, results in reduced PS with an in-significant EE% effect. Values for ZP regarding each formula were found to be affirmative and better than 30 mV as well. 4% CSA, 2% Compritol, 0.15% stearyl amine, and 2% Tween 80, EE% of 25.62%, PS of 207.1 nm, PDI of 0.243, and ZP of 41.50 mV, formulas are known to be the preferred option for optimization. Novel research has been conducted by Kalam et al. (2013) aiming to enhance the bioavailability of gatifloxacin inside the eye through solid-lipid nanoparticles (SLN). Oil and water (o/w), micro-emulsion technique with stearylamine was adopted for generating cationic SLNs. The produced formulations were improved via three-factor, Box–Behnken statistical design of Grade three. The lipid mix concentration (X_1), poloxamers-188 (X_2), and sodium-taurocholate (X_3) were identified as independent variables, while drug release (Y_1), encapsulation efficiency (EE) (Y_2), and particle size (Y_3) with applied restraints for augmenting the drug release and EE and reducing the particulate size as dependent variables. The optimization process was authenticated, response surface plots were appropriately figured, statistical legitimacy of the polynomials was fixed, optimized formulations were chosen depending on the prob-ability and grid search. Quadratic model was known to be the best suitable design for the three dependent variables which was reflected through the responses of different models. With the aid of polynomial equations, the quantitative effect of the stated factors at different positions on the greatest entrapment and release and reduced particulate dimensions has been determined. The linearity noticed between both original and expected values of the response variables determines the predictive capability of the design. Therefore, the elevated grade of prediction seems to be pretty effectual in improving the delivery systems of drugs, exhibiting non-linear responses. This is achieved by employing response surface methodology. González-Mira et al. (2011) adopted a central composite factorial design to optimize flurbiprofen loaded NLC for promoting ocular drug delivery. Two-level factorial design points, axial or star points, and center points are the known components of central composite design. Thus, three independent variables [liquid lipid concentration in the total lipid phase (X_1), surfactant concentration (X_2), and drug concentration (X_3)] were chosen and examined at five variant positions coded as $-\alpha$, -1, 0, 1, and $+\alpha$. The alpha value is determined as (1.682) in order to execute the rotatability of Design. Physicochemical properties of the formed FB–NLC, i.e., particle size (measured either by photon correlation spectroscopy or laser diffraction), polydispersity index (PI) and encapsulation efficiency (EE) were included as dependent variables or responses. The experimental responses which were determined reflect the outcome of the distinct effect and the three independent variable connections. For designing the responses, a full second-order polynomial equation is employed. Statgraphics Plus 5.1 (Sigma Plus) software is applied for data analysis. Analysis of variance (ANOVA) test was performed for the individual parameter, determining the importance of effects and interactions between them. A P-value lower than 0.05 was considered to be statistically significant. The obtained results of the design indicate and reveal a significant effect of Oil/L (wt%) on the mean particle size calculated via PCS (p-value <0.05). This established negative effect, shows an inverse proportionality and association with the particulate dimensions. Due to greater Oil/L (wt%), a new trend towards lesser particle size was identified. The extrapolated polynomial equations and Pareto charts seem to be satisfactory in anticipating the values of the dependent variable for deriving optimum NLC with required particulate dimensions, polydispersity index, and encapsulation efficiency aiding ocular instillation.

9.2.2   LIPOSOMES

Liposomes are colloidal vesicular transporters, which are produced by the hydration of phospholipids. The nanosized liposomes are made up of phospholipids composed of the polar head as well as nonpolar fatty acid chains (Figure 9.2), which aids them accommodated in individual minor structural phospholipid units both the hydrophilic and hydrophobic drug molecules accessing their delivery to the targeted sites (Peptu et al., 2015). Phosphatidylcholine (PC), phosphatidylserine (PS), soya phosphatidylcholine, and phosphatidylethanolamine, containing indistinguishable nature with the lipid present on the surface of the cell membrane, generally opted for liposomal preparations that lead to enhance pre-corneal absorption (Agarwal et al., 2016). The newer generation surface-modified liposomes possessing both mucoadhesive and improved penetration properties, not only capable of entrapping the drug molecules but can also aims to specific sites through cornea binding (Fangueiro et al., 2016). Various effects of the used penetration enhancers have been examined which are opted for preparing hybridized vesicles (PEHVs) with enhanced porosity comprises of soya bean phosphatidylcholine and a blend of surfactants. Using the Design-Expert 7.0 software (Stat-Ease Inc., Minneapolis, MN) Naguib et al. (2017) have conducted a new study by establishing a D-optimal design mixture design. The independent variables such as the discrete quantity for each labrafac lipophile WL, Transcutol, Tween 80, and Labrasol have been identified. Whereas the dependent variables (responses) include particle size, entrapment efficiency percentage and the percentage of drug released after 24 h. The design points include vertices, centers of edges, axial check blends, interior blends and overall centroid, through which the total number of 16 points consisting of three recreated points were generated. The particle size (P.S.), entrapment efficiency (EE%) and the percentage of drug discharge preceding 24 h (Q 24 h%), identified as dependent variables values that were allowed to apply on the design and subsequent equations establishing a relationship between dependant and the independent variables. The quadratic model with an anticipated non-significant lack of fix is found to be the suitable model obtained for overall responses. Therefore, to attain a favorable delivery system for an anti-glaucoma drug, the PEHVs were adapted and proven to possess all the necessary characteristics such as appropriate particle size, elevated entrapment efficiency, sustentation of drug discharge, exceptional stability, sterilization tolerability, high drug bioavailability and lack of irritancy nature.

Mehanna et al. (2009) opted for a 2^5 full factorial design for achieving ocular drug delivery depending on five independent variables involved in developing and optimizing the reverse phase of evaporation ciprofloxacin (CPF) HCl liposomes. The five factors determined comprise of Molar concentration of cholesterol, initial concentration of CPF, pH of the aqueous phase, sonication time, and lastly the type of surface charge. A design matrix composed of 32 experimental trials built through a Design Expert® (Version 7.3.1, State-Ease Inc., Minneapolis, MN, USA), for which the interactive statistical first-order computer-generated equation was described. The ANOVA software was utilized to set-up the statistical affirmation of the linear equations generated via Design Expert®. ANOVA. The principles of F ratios, and correlation coefficients are used for the model validation. In all cases, $p < 0.05$ was accepted to resemble the importance. Apart from statistical confirmation, the model dependability can also be conflicted by correlating with anticipated response values with that of the observed (actual). In order to affirm the tie-up between the expected values and the actual data, the ratio between actual and expected values as well as bias was investigated.

9.2.3   EMULSIONS

Micro or nano-emulsions are some of the most rising liquid globules applied onto the ocular anterior surface with some exclusive nature (enhanced bioavailability, ocular tissue compatibility, high drug loading) (Kumar and Sinha, 2014). Emulsions can be defined as biphasic liquid drug delivery systems where two immiscible liquids are made to become miscible by adding an emulgent (surfactant or co-surfactant) (Figure 9.2). The emulsion droplets behave like a drug pool for liberating hydrophilic as well as hydrophobic agents in the corneal layer. Droplets of emulsions are formed by blending the oil phase with the aqueous phase and surface-active agents, which possess lower energy absorption (Vandammee, 2002). Microemulsions ranging between sizes of 5 nm to 200 nm shows immense drug absorption and also improves the pre-corneal penetration.

Patel et al. (2016) formulated Loteprednoletabonate (LE) loaded nano-emulsions according to the experimental design using a two-factor, three-level (3^2) factorial design by choosing independent variables as the percentage of oil Capryol 90 (X_1), and Smix (X_2), while mean globule size (measured in nm) (Y_1) and polydispersity index (Y_2) (responses) as the dependent variables. To recognize the importance of various independent variables on the experimental responses, response surface analyses were studied and determined. Design-Expert software (version 8.0.5, Stat-Ease, Inc., Minneapolis, MN) was employed to achieve and assess the 3^2 facto-rial design matrixes. The second-order quadratic or polynomial equation is produced based on the responses. To determine the certainty of the para-digm, Design-Expert software ANOVA, lack-of-fit and multiple correlation coefficient (R^2) tests were performed and in addition to this, optimization was accompanied via a desirability function. Derringer and Suich (Vojnoic et al., 1993) used the regular linear scale desirability function to upgrade all the responses concurrently. With the aid of desirability function the leading optimistic and collaborating spot in the design location which promotes in achieving expected target outcomes in case of dependent variables.

9.2.4   POLYMERIC NANOPARTICLES

Polymers show different characteristics in their composition. For attaining favorable ocular drug delivery to the targeted area, the best suitable option is the polymeric nanoparticles of colloidal nanosized systems (1 nm < d < 1000 nm) (Ghangoria et al., 2016). Based on the structural differences, the polymeric nanoparticles are classified as: nanospheres and nanocapsules (Figure 9.2). Nanospheres generally consist of a polymeric matrix with three drug-loading patterns: (1) to encapsulate drugs into the spheres; (2) to absorb drugs onto the surface; (3) to disperse drugs within the polymeric network. In contrast to nanospheres, nanocapsule score-shell possess the ability to dissolve drugs in the core or to absorb drugs on the shell when present in the drug-loading form (Meyer et al., 2012; Tekade et al., 2014). Khan et al. (2018) developed Chitosan coated PLGA nanoparticles that resemble to enhance the ocular hypotensive effect of forskolin. Four factors, four responses Box-Behnken Statistical Design Expert® (Software Version 10) with 29 experimental trials were considered for achieving CS-PLGA NP's augmentation. The independent variables identified are PVA concentration (%w/v), PLGA amount (mg), CS concentration (%), and sonication time (min) whereas the particulate size, PDI, drug loading (DL), and entrapment efficiency (EE) has been coded as dependent variables.

Indomethacin chitosan nanoparticles (NPs) were developed by Abul Kalam et al. (2016) involving ionotropic gelation and enhanced chitosan and tripolyphosphate (TPP) concentrations as well as stirring time by using 3-factor, 3-level Box–Behnken experimental design. Maximal chitosan (A) concentration and TPP (B) were noted as 0.6 mg/ml and 0.4 mg/ml with 120 mins of stirring time (C), followed by applied restraints of reducing the particle size (R_1), increasing the encapsulation efficiency (R_2), and drug liberation (R_3). Based on the 3D response surface plots, factors A, B, and C were established that provide a collusive effect on R_1, and additionally factor A produces a negative influence on R_2 and R_3. Interaction of AB found to be negative on R_1 and R_2 but positive in the case of R_3. A synergistic effect has been noticed through factor AC on R_1 and R_3, although with a similar combination negative effect on R_2 has been exhibited. In the case of all responses, the interaction BC seems to be positive. After 6 months of sustentation, with zeta potentials (+ 25 to + 32 mV), the NPs with a size range of 321–675 nm has been formed. Encapsulation, drug release, and content were found in the range of 56–79%, 48–73%, and 98–99%, respectively.

A polymer-surfactant nanoparticle of doxycycline hydrochloride has been constructed by Pokharkar et al., (2015) for achieving ocular drug delivery. By using 2^3 factorial design, different clusters were generated for the purpose of investigating the variable responses based on the nanoparticulate performance and characteristics. The gellan gum, Aerosol OT, and doxycycline hydrochloride concentrations were selected as preparation variables. All other processing variables and formulations were kept to be constant throughout the research time. The percentage encapsulation efficiency, particle size, and zeta potential are designated as response variables. With the aid of Design-Expert Software (Version 8.0.5, Stat-Ease, Inc., Minneapolis, USA), experimental design and statistical data analysis have been established. Achouri et al. (2015) employed emulsification and a homogenization process for promoting self-assembled liquid crystalline nanoparticles as a drug delivery system for keratoconus treatment, in which a formulation containing riboflavin a water-soluble drug, with two surfactants (poloxamer 407 and mono acyl glycerol – monoolein) and water was optimized and processed. A fractional factorial design was implemented for evaluating the major responses as well as interaction effects involving five parameters on two responses, such as particle size and encapsulation efficiency. The temperature of both phases, emulsification time, homogenization process with heating, the number of passes and pressure are considered as the five core elements. The inclusion of heating during the homogenization process and the pressure that results in nanoparticle generation with 145 nm of average size and 46% average encapsulation efficiency and known as the most suitable effective parameters. In line with the above study, Achouri et al. (2015) enhanced further self-assembled liquid crystalline nano-drugs for attaining effective ocular drug delivery. For the purpose of ternary mixtures, a newer study was conducted by selecting a simplex lattice experimental design of restrained areas. In case of optimizing the dependent variables systematically including encapsulation efficiency and the particle size, the quantity of three items: poloxamer 407 (Z_1), water (Z_2)

and MO (Z_3) has been chosen as input variables. Almost every formulation and processing variable were fixed to be constant during the complete study duration. Two optimized formulations produced were F1 and F2. In the ternary phase diagram, their position seems to be very closure containing poloxamer 407; 44.18%, and 42.03% of monoolein; 46.29% and 48.44% of water for F1 and F2. The preparations leaded with an effective accommodation between inputs and outputs explored.

9.2.5   SNAPLASTICS

Spanlastics are considered as newer elastic micro-vesicular carriers comprises of spans and non-ionic surfactants that possess considerable elasticity nature in structure and quantity. Hydrophilic, hydrophobic, and amphiphilic drugs can be loaded into its multi-lamellar micro-vesicles with the aid of snaplastics (Figure 9.2). Non-ionic surfactants like tweens play an eminent role in reducing interfacial tension, enhancing fluid nature and deformability, which results in improved diffusion of spanlastics (Deol et al., 2015). Broadly, the application of surfactants is encouraged for expanding the pores of the bio-membrane encouraging the temporary entry of huge spanlastics (Kakkar and Kaur 2011). To facilitate the posterior eye segment drug delivery, spanlastics is highly recommended and considered favorable and efficient ophthalmic nanodevice. For easing topical ocular drug-delivery used in the management of posterior eye diseases, Farghaly et al., (2017) adapted and optimized fenoprofen calcium (FPCa) spanlastics. In order to determine the impact of preparation variables, on the vesicle features using Design-Expert® software, Full factorial design has been employed in forming FPCa-loaded spanlastics. In this design, three factors were assessed, each at two levels, and experimental trial runs are performed on eight feasible combinations. The level of Span 60 (F1), the type of EA (F2) and the type of cosolvent in the hydration media (F3) were chosen as independent variables, while the %EE (R1), particle size (PS) (R2), deformability index (DI) (R3) and % FPCa released after 24 h (Q24h) (R4) are denominated as dependent variables.

9.2.6   MICELLES

Nano-micelles consisting of polymeric and surfactant nano-micelles are known to be as rising novel carrier systems for posterior eye drug delivery.

Apart from their smaller size, improved drug solubility and stability (Alvarez et al., 2016), enhanced corneal permeation (Prosperi-Porta et al., 2016), lower adverse effects and high biocompatibility (Vadlapudi et al., 2014) aids them to become potential candidates for poorly aqueous soluble drug delivery. Fewer amphiphilic molecules, when added to special solvents, adapt to self-assemble and results in core-shell monomers called nano-micelles (Cholkar et al., 2012) (Figure 9.2). Duan et al. (2015) utilized central composite design-response surface methodology (CCD-RSM) to enhance the formation mechanics used in in-situ gel systems based on P123/ TPGS mixed micelles (MM) and gellan gum for ophthalmic delivery of curcumin (CUR), because of the fact that it requires minimal experimental runs and will efficiently create a second-phase reaction paradigm involving two to six components. For the purpose of nominating the main influential elements for CCD-RSM, a sequential single-element experimental run are required for the research using drug loading (DL%) and entrapment efficiency (EE%) as indexes. In recapitulation, CUR-MMs, produced via thin-film dispersed method, were found as spherical, micro-sized and proportionately aerosolized with increased DL and EE percentage. The decreased values of CMC represent the enhancement of self-assembled micellar ability contrast with that of the individual micelles.

9.3 CONCLUSION AND FUTURE PROSPECTS

Eye possesses tenacious, evasive basic structures and physical barriers that result in reduced bioavailability of drug molecules. Effective and favorable drug delivery system through the topical route targeting posterior region of the eye, must constitute the following characteristics: (i) sustaining and extending the detention time on the corneal layer, (ii) augmenting the drug invasion in ocular tissues, and (iii) effectively targeting the medications to desired and expected location. A number of novel drug delivery system and approaches are designed depending on state of the art nanotechnology using quality by design approach like Box-Behnken, Factorial, and central composite designs, in the sense to improve the clinical implication and performance of the drug in the deep-rooted ocular tissues by imparting quality in these novel formulations as needed by the FDA and other regulatory bodies. Thus, for now, it seems to be essential for Good Manufacturing Practice (GMP) to plan a guide for the above novel ocular systems, which will surely speed up the commercialization of the novel drug formulation in the near future. QbD-based multifunctional nano-sized topical drug delivery structure targeting the posterior eye region seems promising for fast marketing and may accomplish the growing demand that emanates from the distention of the geriatric population and the overindulging of digital devices.

KEYWORDS

- emulsion
- lipid nano-medicines
- liposomes
- micelle
- ocular delivery systems
- polymeric nanoparticle
- snaplastics

REFERENCES

Abul, K. M., Khan, A. A., Khan, S., Almalik, A., & Alshamsan, A., (2016). Optimizing indomethacin-loaded chitosan nanoparticle size, encapsulation, and release using Box-Behnken experimental design. *Int. J. Biol. Macromol., 87*, 329–340.

Achouri, D., Hornebecq, V., Piccerelle, P., Andrieu, V., & Sergent, M., (2015). Self-assembled liquid crystalline nanoparticles as an ophthalmic drug delivery system. Part I: Influence of process parameters on their preparation studied by experimental design. *Drug Dev. Ind. Pharm., 41*(1), 109–115.

Achouri, D., Sergent, M., Tonetto, A., Piccerelle, P., Andrieu, V., & Hornebecq, V., (2015). Self-assembled liquid crystalline nanoparticles as an ophthalmic drug delivery system. Part II: Optimization of formulation variables using experimental design. *Drug Development and Industrial Pharmacy, 41*, 3, 493–501.

Afify, E. A. M., Elsayed, I., Gad, M. K., Mohamed, M. I., & Afify, M. A. R., (2018). Enhancement of pharmacokinetic and pharmacological behavior of ocular dorzolamide after factorial optimization of self-assembled nanostructures. *PLoS One., 13*(2), e0191415.

Agarwal, R., Iezhitsa, I., Agarwal, P., et al., (2016). Liposomes in topical ophthalmic drug delivery: An update. *Drug Deliv., 23*(4), 1075–1091.

Alvarez-Rivera, F., Fernández-Villanueva, D., Concheiro, A., et al., (2016). α -Lipoic acid in Soluplus® polymeric nanomicelles for ocular treatment of diabetes-associated corneal diseases. *J. Pharm. Sci., 105*(9), 2855–2863.

Baig, M. S., Ahad, A., Aslam, M., Imam, S. S., Aqil, M., & Ali, A., (2016). Application of Box-Behnken design for preparation of levofloxacin-loaded stearic acid solid lipid nanoparticles for ocular delivery: Optimization, *in vitro* release, ocular tolerance, and antibacterial activity. *Int. J. Biol. Macromol., 85*, 258–270.

Beg, S., Rahman, M., Kohli, K., (2019). Quality-by-design approach as a systematic tool for the development of nanopharmaceutical products. *Drug Discovery Today.* 24(3), 717–725.

Beg, S., Akhter, S., Rahman, M., Rahman, Z., (2017a). Perspectives of Quality by Design approach in nanomedicines development. *Current Nanomedicine*, 7, 1–7.

Beg, S., Rahman, M., Panda, S.S., (2017b). Pharmaceutical QbD: Omnipresence in the product development lifecycle. *European Pharmaceutical Review.* 22(1), 2–8.

Cholkar, K., Patel, A., Vadlapudi, A. D., et al., (2012). Novel nanomicellar formulation approaches for anterior and posterior segment ocular drug delivery. *Recent Pat. Nanomed., 2*(2), 82–95.

Das, S., Ng, W. K., & Tan, R. B., (2012). Are nanostructured lipid carriers (NLCs) better than solid lipid nanoparticles (SLN): Development, characterizations and comparative evaluations of clotrimazole-loaded SLN and NLCs? *Eur. J. Pharm. Sci., 47*(1), 139–151.

Delplace, V., Payne, S., & Shoichet, M., (2015). Delivery strategies for the treatment of age-related ocular diseases: From a biological understanding to biomaterial solutions. *J. Control Release, 219*, 652–668.

Deol, P., Kaur, I. P., Sharma, G., et al., (2015). Potential of nanomaterials as movers and packers for drug molecules. *Solid State Phenom., 222*, 159–178.

Doktorovová, S., Kovačević, A. B., Garcia, M. L., et al., (2016). Preclinical safety of solid lipid nanoparticles and nanostructured lipid carriers: Current evidence from *in vitro* and *in vivo* evaluation. *Eur. J. Pharm. Biopharm., 108*(C), 235–252.

Doktorovova, S., Souto, E. B., & Silva, A. M., (2014). Nanotoxicology applied to solid lipid nanoparticles and nanostructured lipid carriers—A systematic review of *in vitro* data. *Eur. J. Pharm. Biopharm., 87*(1), 1–18.

Duan, Y., Cai, X., Du, H., & Zhai, G., (2015). Novel in situ gel systems based on P123/ TPGS mixed micelles and gellan gum for ophthalmic delivery of curcumin. *Colloids and Surfaces B: Biointerfaces., 128*, 322–330.

Elsayed, I., & Sayed, S., (2017). Tailored nanostructured platforms for boosting transcorneal permeation: Box-Behnken statistical optimization, comprehensive *in vitro*, *ex vivo* and *in vivo* characterization. *Int. J. Nanomedicine, 12*, 7947–7962.

ElShaer, A., Mustafa, S., Kasar, M., Thapa, S., Ghatora, B., & Alany, R. G., (2016). Nanoparticle-laden contact lens for controlled ocular delivery of prednisolone: Formulation optimization using statistical experimental design. *Pharmaceutics, 8*(2), 14.

Fangueiro, J. F., Andreani, T., Egea, M. A., Garcia, M. L., Souto, S. B., Silva, A. M., & Souto, E. B., (2014). Design of cationic lipid nanoparticles for ocular delivery: Development, characterization and cytotoxicity. *Int. J. Pharm., 461*(1&2), 64–73.

Fangueiro, J. F., Veiga, F., Silva, A. M., et al., (2016). Ocular drug delivery - new strategies for targeting anterior and posterior segments of the eye. *Curr. Pharm. Des., 22*(9), 1135–1146.

Farghaly, D. A., Aboelwafa, A. A., Hamza, M. Y., et al., (2017). Topical delivery of fenoprofen calcium via elastic nano-vesicular spanlastics: Optimization using experimental design and *in vivo* evaluation. *AAPS Pharm. Sci. Tech., 18*, 2898.

Fouda, N. H., Abdelrehim, R. T., Hegazy, D. A., & Habib, B. A., (2018). Sustained ocular delivery of Dorzolamide-HCl via proniosomal gel formulation: *In-vitro* characterization, statistical optimization, and *in-vivo* pharmacodynamic evaluation in rabbits. *Drug Deliv., 25*(1), 1340–1349.

Ghanghoria, R., Tekade, R. K., Mishra, A. K., et al., (2016). Luteinizing hormone-releasing hormone peptide tethered nanoparticulate system for enhanced antitumoral efficacy of paclitaxel. *Nanomedicine, 11*(7), 797–816.

Gonzalez-Mira, E., Egea, M. A., Souto, E. B., Calpena, A. C., & García, M. L., (2011). Optimizing flurbiprofen-loaded NLC by central composite factorial design for ocular delivery. *Nanotechnology, 28, 22*(4), 045101.

Hao, J., Fang, X., Zhou, Y., Wang, J., Guo, F., Li, F., & Peng, X., (2011). Development and optimization of solid lipid nanoparticle formulation for ophthalmic delivery of chloramphenicol using a Box-Behnken design. *Int. J. Nanomedicine, 6*, 683–692.

International Federation on Ageing, (2013). *The High Cost of Low Vision: The Evidence on Ageing and the Loss of Sight*. LT Publication.

Janagam, D. R., Wu, L., & Lowe, T. L., (2017). Nanoparticles for drug delivery to the anterior segment of the eye. *Adv. Drug Deliv. Rev., 122*, 31–64.

Kakkar, S., & Kaur, I. P., (2011). Spanlastics—A novel nanovesicular carrier system for ocular delivery. *Int. J. Pharm., 413*(1), 202–210.

Kalam, M. A., Sultana, Y., Ali, A., Aqil, M., Mishra, A. K., Aljuffali, I. A., & Alshamsan, A., (2013). Part I: Development and optimization of solid-lipid nanoparticles using Box-Behnken statistical design for ocular delivery of gatifloxacin. *J. Biomed. Mater. Res. A., 101*(6), 1813–1827.

Kaskoos, R. A., (2014). Investigation of moxifloxacin loaded chitosan-dextran nanoparticles for topical installation into eye: *In-vitro* and *ex-vivo* evaluation. *Int. J. Pharm. Investig., 4*(4), 164–173.

Kaur, I. P., & Kakkar, S., (2014). Nanotherapy for posterior eye diseases. *J. Control Release, 193*, 100–112.

Khan, N., Ameeduzzafar, K. K., Bhatnagar, A., Ahmad, F. J., & Ali, A., (2018). Chitosan coated PLGA nanoparticles amplify the ocular hypotensive effect of forskolin: Statistical design, characterization and *in vivo* studies. *Int. J. Biol. Macromol., S, 116*, 648–663.

Khurana, L. K., Singh, R., Singh, H., & Sharma, M., (2018). Systematic development and optimization of an in-situ gelling system for moxifloxacin ocular nanosuspension using high-pressure homogenization with an improved encapsulation efficiency. *Current Pharmaceutical Design, 24*, 1434.

Kumar, R., & Sinha, V. R., (2014). Preparation and optimization of voriconazole microemulsion for ocular delivery. *Colloids Surf B Biointerfaces, 117*(C), 82–88.

Liu, D., Li, J., Cheng, B., et al., (2017). *Ex vivo* and *in vivo* evaluation of the effect of coating a coumarin-6-labeled nanostructured lipid carrier with chitosan-n-acetylcysteine on rabbit ocular distribution. *Mol Pharm., 14*(8), 2639–2648.

Liu, D., Li, J., Pan, H., He, F., Liu, Z., Wu, Q., Bai, C., Yu, S., & Yang, X., (2016). Potential advantages of a novel chitosan-N-acetylcysteine surface modified nanostructured lipid carrier on the performance of ophthalmic delivery of curcumin. *Sci Rep., 6*, 28796.

Lou, J., Hu, W., Tian, R., Zhang, H., Jia, Y., Zhang, J., & Zhang, L., (2014). Optimization and evaluation of a thermoresponsive ophthalmic in situ gel containing curcumin-loaded albumin nanoparticles. *Int. J. Nanomedicine, 9*, 2517–2525.

Madni, A., Rahem, M. A., Tahir, N., et al., (2017). Non-invasive strategies for targeting the posterior segment of eye. *Int. J. Pharm., 530*(1&2), 326–345.

McGrath, C., Rudman, D. L., Trentham, B., et al., (2017). Reshaping understandings of disability associated with age-related vision loss (ARVL): Incorporating critical disability perspectives into research and practice. *Disabil. Rehabil., 39*(19), 1990–1998.

Mehanna, M. M., Elmaradny, H. A., & Samaha, M. W., (2009). Ciprofloxacin liposomes as vesicular reservoirs for ocular delivery: Formulation, optimization, and *in vitro* characterization. *Drug Development and Industrial Pharmacy, 35*, 583–593.

Meyer, H., Stöver, T., Fouchet, F., et al., (2012). Lipidic nanocapsule drug delivery: Neuronal protection for cochlear implant optimization. *Int. J. Nanomedicine, 7*, 2449–2464.

Motwani, S. K., Chopra, S., Talegaonkar, S., Kohli, K., Ahmad, F. J., & Khar, R. K., (2008). Chitosan-sodium alginate nanoparticles as submicroscopic reservoirs for ocular delivery: Formulation, optimization and *in vitro* characterization. *Eur. J. Pharm. Biopharm., 68*(3), 513–525.

Naguib, S. S., Hathout, R. M., & Mansour, S., (2017). Optimizing novel penetration enhancing hybridized vesicles for augmenting the *in-vivo* effect of an anti-glaucoma drug. *Drug Deliv., 24*(1), 99–108.

Pandit, J., Sultana, Y., & Aqil, M., (2017). Chitosan-coated PLGA nanoparticles of bevacizumab as novel drug delivery to target retina: Optimization, characterization, and *in vitro* toxicity evaluation. *Artif. Cells Nanomed. Biotechnol., 45*(7), 1397–1407.

Patel, N., Nakrani, H., Raval, M., & Sheth, N., (2016). Development of loteprednol etabonate-loaded cationic nanoemulsified in-situ ophthalmic gel for sustained delivery and enhanced ocular bioavailability. *Drug Deliv., 23*(9), 3712–3723.

Peptu, C. A., Popa, M., Savin, C., et al., (2015). Modern drug delivery systems for targeting the posterior segment of the eye. *Curr. Pharm. Des., 21*(42), 6055–6069.

Pokharkar, V., Patil, V., & Mandpe, L., (2015). Engineering of polymer–surfactant nanoparticles of doxycycline hydrochloride for ocular drug delivery. *Drug Deliv., 22*(7), 955–968.

Pramod, K., Tahir, M. A., Charoo, N. A., Ansari, S. H., & Ali, J., (2016). Pharmaceutical product development: A quality by design approach. *Int. J. Pharm. Investig., 6*(3), 129–138.

Preeti, U. P., Kumar, M., & Pathak, K., (2016). Norfloxacin loaded pH triggered nanoparticulate *in-situ* gel for extraocular bacterial infections: Optimization, ocular irritancy and corneal toxicity. *Iran J. Pharm. Res., 15*(1), 3–22.

Prosperi-Porta, G., Kedzior, S., Muirhead, B., et al., (2016). Phenylboronic-acid-based polymeric micelles for mucoadhesive anterior segment ocular drug delivery. *Biomacromolecules, 17*(4), 1449–1457.

Reha, S., & Chodankar, A. D., (2016). Optimization techniques: A futuristic approach for formulating and processing of pharmaceuticals. *Indian J. Pharm. Biol. Res., 4*(2), 32–40.

Singh, B., & Beg, S., (2015). Attaining product development excellence and federal compliance employing Quality by Design (QbD) paradigms. *The Pharma Review.* 13(9), 35–44.

Singh, B., & Beg, S., (2014). Product development excellence and federal compliance via QbD. *Chronicle PharmaBiz.* 15(10), 30–35.

Singh, B., Raza, K., Beg, S., (2013). Developing "Optimized" drug products employing "Designed" experiments. *Chemical Industry Digest.* 23, 70–76.

Souto, E. B., & Doktorovová, S., (2009). Chapter six - solid lipid nanoparticle formulations: Pharmacokinetic and biopharmaceutical aspects in drug delivery. In: Düzgünes, N., (ed.), *Methods in Enzymology* (pp. 105–129). Amsterdam (AMS): Academic Press.

Tekade, R. K., Youngren-Ortiz, S. R., Yang, H., et al., (2014). Designing hybrid onconase nanocarriers for mesothelioma therapy: A Taguchi orthogonal array and multivariate component-driven analysis. *Mol. Pharm., 11*(10), 3671–3683.

Thrimawithana, T. R., Young, S., Bunt, C. R., et al., (2011). Drug delivery to the posterior segment of the eye. *Drug Discov Today., 16*(5&6), 270–277.

Vadlapudi, A. D., Cholkar, K., Vadlapatla, R. K., et al., (2014). Aqueous nanomicellar formulation for topical delivery of biotinylated lipid prodrug of acyclovir: Formulation development and ocular biocompatibility. *J. Ocul. Pharmacol. Ther., 30*(1), 49–58.

Vandamme, T. F., (2002). Microemulsions as ocular drug delivery systems: Recent developments and future challenges. *Prog. Retin. Eye Res., 21*(1), 15–34.

Vojnovic, D., Moneghini, M., Rubessa, F., & Zanchetta, A., (1993). Simultaneous optimization of several response variables in a granulation process. *Drug Dev. Ind. Pharm., 19*, 1479–1496.

Wang, F., Chen, L., Jiang, S., He, J., Zhang, X., Peng, J., Xu, Q., & Li, R., (2014). Optimization of methazolamide-loaded solid lipid nanoparticles for ophthalmic delivery using Box-Behnken design. *J. Liposome Res., 24*(3), 171–181.

Wang, F., Zhang, M., Zhang, D., Huang, Y., Chen, L., Jiang, S., Shi, K., & Li, R., (2018). Preparation, optimization, and characterization of chitosan-coated solid lipid nanoparticles for ocular drug delivery. *J. Biomed Res., 31*, 1–13.

Weng, Y., Liu, J., Jin, S., et al., (2017). Nanotechnology-based strategies for treatment of ocular disease. *Acta Pharmaceutica Sinica B., 7*(3), 281–291.

Youshia, J., Kamel, A. O., El Shamy, A., & Mansour, S., (2012). Design of cationic nanostructured heterolipid matrices for ocular delivery of methazolamide. *Int. J. Nanomedicine, 7*, 2483–2496.

CHAPTER 10

Recent Advances in the Development of Nanopharmaceutical Products

RAHUL SHUKLA, AJIT SINGH, NIDHI SINGH, and DHEERAJ KUMAR

Department of Pharmaceutics, National Institute of Pharmaceutical Education and Research, Raebareli, Lucknow, Uttar Pradesh–226002, India

*Corresponding author. E-mail: rahulshuklapharm@gmail.com

10.1 INTRODUCTION

The name "nano" originated from the Greek word "nanos" and Latin word "nanos" that deals with enormously tiny particles. Nanotechnology is a branch of science and technology that basically manages the nature of matter on the atomic and molecular scale. Nanotechnology is a collective term applied for the proper definition of the products, methods, and characteristics at the nano/micro-scale level. Nanosciences are mainly dependent on particle behavior; smaller the particle size greater number of the particle is on the surface hence increases the surface area for absorption, dissolution profile and in vivo drug release profile (Babu et al., 2014). Various parameters affect the formulation of nanoparticulate systems such as "concentration of surfactant, polymer-drug ratio, sonication time, stirring rate, phase volume ratio, etc." (Kesharwani and Iyer, 2015). Nowadays, nanoparticles are implicated due to several advantages such as minimal side effects, targeted delivery, adaptable degradation kinetic, increase patient amenability by reducing dosing frequency and have the ability to freight multiple drugs in the same formulation. Nanoformulations boost the field of protein and peptide drug delivery by providing an efficient targeted specific system and also reduce the degradation of protein and peptide drugs (Ferrari, 2005). There are different kinds of nanoformulations used in the drug delivery system which include solid lipid nanoparticles, polymeric nanoparticles, liposomes, niosomes, carbon nanotubes, polymeric micelles, nanogels, microspheres, polymer lipid hybrid nanoparticles, cross-linked chitosan nanoparticles, and raft polymeric carriers (Nature Publishing Group, 1965). Fabrication of nanoparticles is mainly performed by top-down approaches, bottom-up approaches, chemical precipitation, solvent injection, precipitation from the solvent-in-water emulsion, co-solvent evaporation, melt homogenization, emulsification process, and sol-gel techniques. The nanopharmaceuticals is characterized for surface morphology [scanning electron microscopy (SEM), transmission electron microscopy (TEM), atomic force micros-copy (AFM)), particle size (master sizer, zeta sizer, x-ray diffraction), zeta potential, and polydispersity index (PDI)] (Acosta, 2009).

10.2   IMPLICATIONS OF NANOPARTICLES IN DRUG DELIVERY

Nanotechnology is a scientific field that collectively relates engineering and pharmaceutical manufacturing principles at the molecular level (Biswas, Islam, and Choudhury, 2014). The effectiveness of most of the drugs is dependent upon the particle size, as lesser the particle size provides a higher surface area that finally results in an increase in solubility and bioavailability. Moreover, its tiny size particles also have the tendency to cross the blood-brain barrier (BBB) and capability to get absorbed via the constricted junction of endothelial cells of the skin (Emerich and Thanos, 2006; Kohane, 2007). Nanotechnology is an emerging field of medical science and nowadays obtaining more consideration because of its libera-tion of medicaments at target location by the use of biodegradable and non-biodegradable polymers, thus, reduces other body tissue toxicity. It also provides appropriate formulation options for the delivery of those drugs that face hurdles during formulation via conventional drug delivery methods due to the poor solubility, poor bioavailability, more toxicity and stability issues related to the drug (Singh, Jr., 2009; Onoue, Yamada, and Chan, 2014). Nanoformulations boost the field of protein and peptide drugs by providing an efficient targeted drug delivery system. It also prevents the degradation of protein and peptides drugs due to the protective shield of the nano-delivery system (Alexis et al., 2008). Most of the nanoformu-lation systems are hydrophobic in nature; this is considered as the hurdle in the nanodelivery system as hydrophobicity facilitates the easy clearance of such a formulation system from blood circulation via the lymphatic system. To address such hurdle surface modification of the system is performed by using hydrophilic excipients such as polymers, surfactants, and copolymers, which include polyethylene glycol, poloxamers, poloxamines, polysorbate 80 and polyethylene oxides. Surface modification with these excipients also reduces the RES (reticuloendothelial system) uptake of drugs by preventing opsonin-NP binding (opsonization) and thus, enhances their blood circulation time and provides prolong the duration of action (Vo, Kasper, and Mikos, 2012). Targeted drug delivery via nanoformulation is achieved by using various ligands, antibodies, and polymers. In sort to develop an optimized nanoformulation the inclusion of suitable targeting ligands, surface modification and reactivity is essential. These approaches prevent the aggregation of drugs, provide stability to the formulation and also may affect the pharmacological behavior of drugs (Rizvi and Saleh, 2017). Nanoparticles avert the active constituents (API) from degradation, facilitate its entry inside the biological membrane, enhance solubility, bioavailability, reduce side effects of drugs to other organs of the body and have potential to load multiple drugs in the same formulation (Lu et al., 2016) (Figure 10.1).

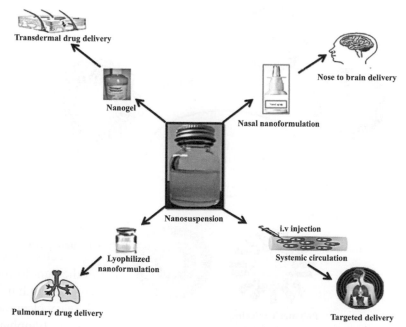

FIGURE 10.1   Role of nanoformulation in targeted drug delivery.

10.3   TYPES OF NANOPHARMACEUTICALS

The recent advancement in the field of drug discovery leads to the expansion of a large number of new, extremely potent drug candidates. Regardless of their potency, they fail to reach the market because of its reduced efficacy, inadequate bioavailability and hurdles related to techniques of successful drug delivery systems. These hurdles lead to the development of a novel drug delivery system that solves the problem related to solubility, bioavailability, stability and effective methods to deliver the drugs (Rigogliuso et al., 2012). The main intent of a novel drug delivery system is to enhance the pharmacokinetic and pharmacodynamic properties of drugs to facilitate their delivery to the predetermined targeted site, at right time and in the accurate quantity (Xiong et al., 2011). The various different types of nanopharmaceuticals used for effective drug delivery system are solid lipid nanoparticles, nanostructured lipid carriers, liposomes, niosomes, carbon nanotubes, polymeric micelles, nanogels, microsphere, polymer lipid hybrid nanoparticles, cross-linked chitosan nanoparticles, raft polymeric carriers, polymeric nanoparticles, and nanocrystals (Yu et al., 2016) (Figure 10.2).

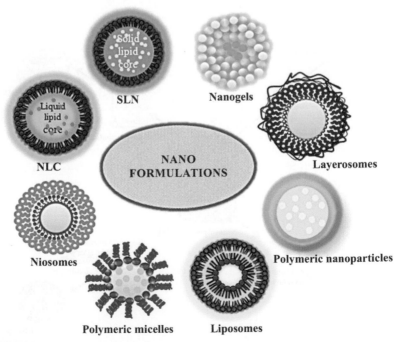

FIGURE 10.2   Types of nanoformulation.

10.3.1 LIPOSOMES

The word liposome derived from the Greek word "liposoma" meaning fat bodies; it mimics the biological membrane of the body. Liposomes are tiny spherical bilayered lipid vesicles allowing the incorporation of both hydrophilic as well as lipophilic drugs. Along with these benefits, liposomes also provide biocompatibility and biodegradability with membrane, which makes it a more acceptable delivery system (Yu et al., 2012). Liposomes mainly consist of naturally obtained phospholipids such as egg phosphatidylethanolamine and an untainted surfactant such as DOPE (dioleoylphosphatidylethanolamine).

Numerous benefits of liposomal formulation are:

*   Facilitates passive targeted delivery to cancer cells.
*   Encapsulation helps in enhancing the stability of drugs.
*   Reduce other body tissue toxicity.
*   Biocompatible and biodegradable in nature.
*   Enhance pharmacokinetic properties such as decreases elimination rate of drugs and enhance their blood circulation time.
*   Provide active targeting by coupling with various target particular ligands.
*   Despite the use of liposome in drug and gene delivery, it is also applied as mediator for the efficient delivery of pesticides for plants, dyes in textiles, cosmeceuticals and for the delivery of nutritional supplements.

Liposomes play a pivotal role in nanocosmetology by various means such as enhancement of penetration and diffusion of active ingredients through skin, targeted delivery of active pharmaceutical ingredients, prolong the drug release time, diminish unnecessary toxicity and provide stability (Dua et al., 2012). The selection of methods for liposome preparation is based on several parameters such as physicochemical properties of drugs as well as other components used in liposome formulation, nature of the solvent used to dissolve lipid and nature of drugs and their toxicity profile. Various methods used for the preparation of liposomes are lipid film hydration, reverse phase evaporation, solvent dispersion method, freeze-thaw cycling of MLV (multilamellar vesicles), extrusion technique and detergent removal method. Usually, three types of liposomes are used in drug delivery, i.e., multilamellar vesicles (MLV), large unilamellar vesicles (LUV), and small unilamellar vesicles (SUV), which mostly falls below the size of 200 nm (Singh, Vengurlekar, and Rathod, 2014). Despite of several advantages, liposomes possess certain drawbacks like low encapsulation efficiency, pitiable stability and drug leakage due to its fragile nature. Stability and leakage problems of liposomes are resolved by using lipids with long-chain hydrocarbon with a low degree of unsaturation and branching that forms a tightly packed Lipid bilayer structure. The stability of liposomes in the hemopoietic system (blood circulation) is improved by the application of cholesterol in permutation with higher melting phospholipids. The characterization of liposomes is done by nuclear magnetic resonance (NMR), cryo-electron microscopy and small-angle X-ray scattering to check lamellarity of liposomes and size of the liposomal formulation are determined by master sizer, zeta sizer (Dua et al., 2012). AmBisomes (Amphotericin B), DaunoXome (Daunorubicin citrate), DepoCyt (Cytarabine), and DepoDur (Morphine sulfate) are some of the liposomal products available in the market (Figure 10.3).

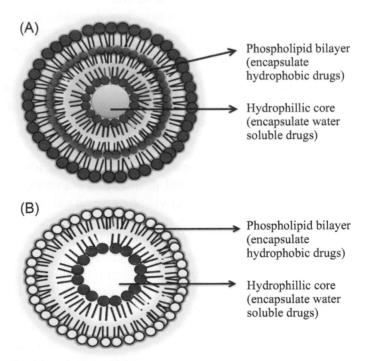

(A)

Phospholipid bilayer (encapsulate hydrophobic drugs)

Hydrophillic core (encapsulate water soluble drugs)

(B)

Phospholipid bilayer (encapsulate hydrophobic drugs)

Hydrophillic core (encapsulate water soluble drugs)

FIGURE 10.3   Liposome (A), multilamellar vesicles, and (B) large unilamellar vesicles.

10.3.2 SOLID LIPID NANOPARTICLES (SLN)

SLN (Figure 10.4) is basically a colloidal lipid carrier with solid lipid core that serves important advantages over other nanoformulations due to their applicability through various routes of administrations (parenteral as well as non-parenteral delivery). Lipophilic drugs with poor water solubility are mainly incorporated in SLN formulations in order to overcome the solubility related problem (Aaltonen et al., 2012). The lipids used in the formulation of SLN must be of generally recognized as safe (GRAS) category and they should not undergo the melting process at normal body temperature. It is composed of solid lipid core enclosing the drug in matrix and this lipidic core is covered by a layer of the stabilizing agent (Rigogliuso et al., 2012). The size of solid lipid nanoparticles is generally less than 100 nm. The matrix material incorporated in their formulation of SLN is usually composed of fatty alcohol, glycerides, and fatty acids. However, the most commonly applied surfactants are poloxamer 188, sodium oleate, polysorbate 80, sorbitantrioleate, and lecithin (Bunjes and Unruh, 2007). SLN formulations are decorated with many advantages such as the aqueous-based methods of preparation which devoid the use of organic solvent, good biocompatibility profile, biodegradability, high stability as compared to other nanocarrier systems and easy and cost-effective methods of preparation than polymeric and other surfactant based formulation. Regardless of many advantages, SLN has some limitation such as low drug loading efficiency, gelation tendency, and chances of polymeric transitions (Jumaa and Muller, 2000). Most commonly employed methods for preparing SLN are melt homogenization technique and precipitation from solvent in water emulsion. Aquasol A (Vitamin A) is an example of SLN, which is available in the market.

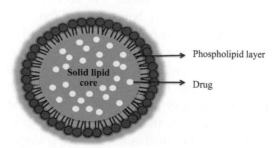

FIGURE 10.4   Solid lipid nanoparticles.

10.3.3 NANOSTRUCTURED LIPID CARRIER (NLC)

NLC is a second-generation colloidal lipid carrier system that differs from SLN in composition and physical state of lipid (liquid lipid as well as a mixture of solid and liquid lipids). NLC serves several advantages over SLN such as provide high encapsulation efficiency of lipophilic drugs in comparison to hydrophilic drugs and avoids drug leakage from formulation (Selvamuthukumar and Velmurugan, 2012). NLC formulations are mainly used for the delivery of topical and dermatological applications and mostly dispensed in the form of lotion, cream, and gels. Ketoderm cream (2% Ketoconazole) is the marketed NLC product (Figure 10.5).

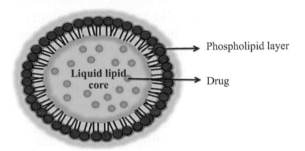

FIGURE 10.5   Nanostructured lipid carrier.

10.3.4 NIOSOMES

The physiology of niosomal formulation is alike liposomes in structure with a spherical bilayered vesicular system. Niosomes differ from liposomes in composition where instead of phospholipids it comprises of nonionic surfactant (Figure 10.6). Niosomes demonstrate superior stability in comparison to liposomes with simple and cost-effective preparation methods (Nagalakshmi et al., 2016). Niosomes exhibit amphiphilic properties similar to liposomes they are having both polar head and a non-polar tail group of the nonionic surfactant molecule. Niosomes can easily pass through the skin surface and increases the penetration of drugs via skin. Polar groups used in niosomal formulations consist of ethylene oxides, sugars, amino acid, polyhydroxy groups, glycerol, etc. and the nonionic surfactant incorporated are Span and Brij. Cholesterol is incorporated to reduces agglomeration tendency in niosomes which is supposed to provide stability and also prevents phase conversion of niosomal formulation from coagulate to fluid state and protect drug outflow. Niosomes are formulated by hydration method followed by size reduction using sonication and high-pressure homogenization. Free drug which is not encapsulated within niosomes is separated by employing centrifugation and dialysis methods. The final size of niosomal formulation is dependent on the nature of surfactant, type of nonionic surfactant and lipids (Lo et al., 2010). Lancome, a cosmetic company introduces variety of anti-aging cosmetic products in market which are based on niosomal formulations.

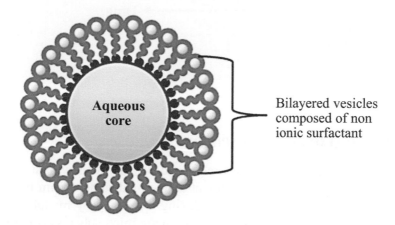

FIGURE 10.6   Niosomes.

10.3.5   *POLYMERIC NANOPARTICLES*

Polymeric nanoparticles refer to the formulation of nanoparticles by incorporating drug into polymer using direct polymerization technique (Figure 10.7). Both natural polymers such as gelatin, chitosan and albumin and synthetic polymer such as poly (lactic acid) (PLA), poly (glycolic acid) (PGA), poly lactic-glycolic acid (PLGA), and poly (Ɛ-caprolactone) (PCL) are used extensively because of their biocompatible and biodegradable nature. PEGylation of nanoparticles improve their surface property by imparting hydrophilicity to surface. These PEGylated nanoparticles does not undergo RES uptake by macrophages and phagocytes thus its blood circulation time improved and it retain in blood circulation for longer period of time and therefore prolongs the duration of action of drug. In some instances, the active drug is directly placed over the surface of nanoformulations to enhance the bioavailability of medicament (Sonia and Sharma, 2012). Eligard (Leuprolide), Genexol (Paclitaxel), Opaxio (Paclitaxelpoliglumex) are some of the clinically approved polymeric nanoparticles.

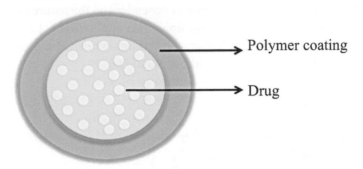

FIGURE 10.7   Polymeric nanoparticle.

10.3.6   POLYMERIC MICROSPHERE

Polymeric microspheres are sphere-shaped tiny particles with size range in varies from 1 to 6 μm that protect active medicament from harsh GI environment, helps in reducing the dosing frequency by modulating the pharmacokinetic properties of drug. Polymeric microspheres also provide several advantages such as decrease other body organ toxicity by facilitating delivery to targeted site and thus boost the system of drug delivery (Kamps et al., 2010). Biodegradable polymers such as PLGA, PLA, and PCL are the backbone in formulation of polymeric microspheres. PLGA undergoes ester hydrolysis in body and produce non-harmful metabolite that gets easily excreted from body. Thus, polymeric microspheres made from biologically acceptable polymers attract many research groups in order to explore its applications in drug delivery. Nutropin Depot (somatropin) and Lupron Depot (leuprolide acetate) are the two marketed injectable products consisting of microsphere as a delivery system.

10.3.7   CARBON NANOTUBES

Carbon nanotubes are cylindrical large molecular structure with diameter ranges from 0.4–40 nm while the length can vary from few nanometers to several centimeters (i.e., from 0.14 nm to 55.5 cm) (Figure 10.8). It plays vital role in drug delivery system by providing numerous advantages such as ability to penetrate in cell membrane, efficient delivery of medicaments, vaccines and some bigger molecules by improving their uptake through biological membrane (Luo et al., 2017). Carbon nanotubes exhibit high drug loading tendency of small as well as larger molecules like peptides and some amino acids. The mechanism of permeation of drug-loaded carbon nanotubes basically involves two modes, i.e., either through passive diffusion across the phospholipids bilayer membrane or via cellular endocytosis. The carbon nanotubes are classified into single-walled carbon nanotubes (SWCNTs) and multi-walled carbon nanotubes (MWCNTs). SWCNT contains hexagonal lattice structural backbone and MWCNT composed of circular arrangements of graphene sheets. The common things between both single wall and multi-wall carbon nanotubes lie at their closing stages as both of them contains molecule similar with fullerene (Gorain et al., 2018).

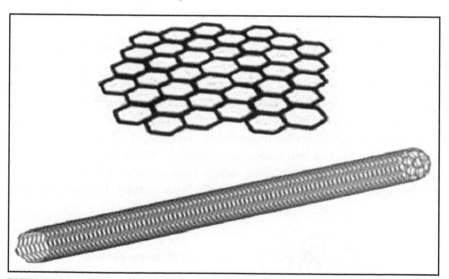

FIGURE 10.8   Carbon nanotubes.

10.3.8   MODIFIED NANOCARRIER SYSTEMS

10.3.8.1   TRANSFERSOMES

Transfersomes are the modified form of liposome with more elasticity. Transfersomes show beneficial activity over liposomes in transdermal preparation, as liposomes cannot penetrate the deep skin layers and thus unable to dispense the medicament in severs skin infection. However, transfersomes have the ability to get to the bottom layer of skin and infuse the whole vesicle into systemic circulation via skin, therefore, increased efficacy observed in this case. Transfersomes formulation consists of phospholipids like phosphatidylcholine and surfactant like deoxycholate, Span80, Tween 80, and sodium cholate. The surfactant performs the function of provision of flexibility to the vesicles, which finally responsible for increased permeation through skin layers (Rigogliuso et al., 2012).

10.3.8.2 LAYEROSOMES

Layersomes are the modification of liposomal system where liposomes are coated with one or more layers of biofeasible polyelectrolytes by the process of layer-by-layer coating technique (Figure 10.9). The concept of layerosomes came to existence in order to improve the stability of liposomes in harsh GI environment and also pertaining to the storage stability enhancement to improve the self-life of liposomal system. The layer-by-layer coating is done by polypeptides and natural polysaccharides because they mimic biological environment and thus enhance stability. The coating polyelectrolyte agents includes poly (L-lysine) (pLL)/chitosan and poly (glutamic acid) (pGA) polypeptides/Na hyaluronate. The size of layerosomes can be determined by photon correlation spectroscopy (PCS) by using zetasizer instrument. The charge obtained while measurement of zeta potential depends upon the charge of polyelectrolyte layer coating. Layerosomes are

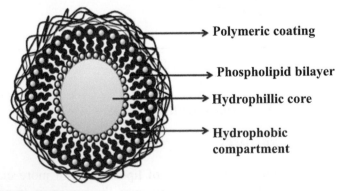

FIGURE 10.9 Layersomes.

reported to affect the drug release rate where drug release for longer duration of time was observed in most of the cases (Liu et al., 2018).

10.3.8.3 BILOSOMES

Bilosomes are similar to liposomes which are described as bilayered nonionic surfactant vesicles containing bile salts. The nature of bile salts are weakly acidic and the apparent pKa value changes with change in environment. Bile salt is amphiphilic molecule having steroids nucleus containing polar side chains with hydroxyl group at the end and non-polar side chains with methyl group at the end. Bilosomes are suitable for the delivery of protein and peptides drug and also have potential for the delivery of vaccines. Bilosomes show excellent stability in comparison to liposomes and niosomes in gastrointestinal fluid. Like liposomes they do not undergoes oxidative degradation and there is no requirement of any special storage condition (Babu et al., 2014; Kesharwani et al., 2018).

10.3.9 POLYMERIC MICELLES

Polymeric micelles are a type of nanocarriers system widely used in pharmaceutical drug delivery for effective delivery of both hydrophilic and lipophilic drugs which attributes to their amphiphilic nature (Ahmad et al., 2014). Micelles play an important role in drug delivery due to their distinctive structure-property, its non-aqueous core-shell facilitates loading of hydrophobic drugs, protein, and DNA and water-soluble part provide a protective layer that protects nonaqueous layer from internal incursion. It also aids several advantages such as the highest drug loading and multiple drug loading at a time (Kim et al., 2018). Despite of several advantages, polymeric micelles have some pitfalls related to its stability in systemic circulation after parenteral administration. Polymeric micelles are available in the market with brand names of Genexol PM (Paclitaxel), Estrasorb (Estradiol cream for topical), etc.

10.3.10 RECENTLY DEVELOPED NANOFORMULATIONS

Recently many nanocarriers were developed in the area of nanotechnology and boost drug delivery systems and these nanocarriers are nanocrystals, nanogels, nanobeads, nanomesh, nanofibers, etc.

10.3.10.1   NANOCRYSTALS

Nanocrystals are the nano range colloidal drug delivery system with less or minimum requirements of excipients or in other words we can say that it is a carrier-free system that requires only stabilizer to stabilize the system (Gao et al., 2008). Nanocrystals are a new and fascinating approach to enhance the solubility of BCS class II and class IV drugs. Instead of enhancing solubility, nanocrystals also facilitate several benefits such as dissolution velocity improvement, enhancement of bioavailability, targeted drug delivery, increase payload of drug, increase surface adhesiveness, decrease dose and reduce nonspecific toxicity and thus helps in enhancing the pharmacokinetic and pharmacodynamic property of drugs (Ankita and Anil, 2010). Nanocrystals were formulated by using various methods such as bottom-up process, top-down process, high-pressure homogenization, precipitation, milling and combination method like precipitation-lyophilization-homogenization (PLH) technology, and nano-edge technology. Nanocrystals can be dispensed in the form of nanosuspension and administered in the body via various routes like as parenteral, oral, ocular, nasal and dermal delivery. There are certain marketed nanocrystalline products occupying the market, which includes Megace ES (Megestrol acetate), Rapamune (Rapamycin), and Tricor (Fenofibrate).

10.3.10.2   NANOBEADS, NANOGELS, AND NANOFIBERS

Nanogels and nanobeads are the smart polymeric nanocarriers having the tendency to recognize infected tissue or cells and prompt optimistic response of cells (Figure 10.10). Nanobeads are also called as quantum beads or nanodots. These are the nano-range polymeric beads serving the advantages for the concurrent measurement of thousands of biological interactions at a time and also have a potential role in drug discovery and clinical diagnostic (Kammona and Kiparissides, 2012). Nanogels are the three-dimensional nano-range hydrogels formulated by the cross-linking assembly of polymers and it serves benefits in the area of controlled drug delivery system. Nanofibers are the polymeric fibers having a diameter in nano-range or less than 1 μm and useful for the targeted delivery of anticancer and antiviral drugs (Kabanov and Vinogradov, 2009). Some marketed products of these nanoformulations include Zyclin (Clindamycin nanogels), Adalene (Adapalene nano gel), chito flex (chitosan nanofibers dressing), permacol (collagen nanofibers for skin regeneration), etc (Table 10.1).

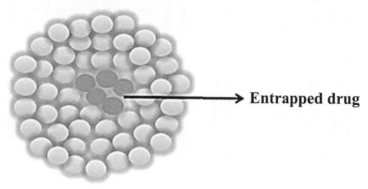

Entrapped drug

FIGURE 10.10   Nanogels.

10.3.11   SOLUMATRIX FINE PARTICLE TECHNOLOGY FOR SIZE REDUCTION

Solumatrix technology is developed in 2004 for the purpose to reduce the drug particles to 200–800 nm size range (Figure 10.11). Dry milling process reduces the drugs particles into superfine powder. It exhibits drug particle in sub-micron range in diameter, and converts the particle 20 times smaller than API (active pharmaceutical ingredients) (Wang et al., 2013).

This method improved the efficacy of pharmaceuticals by increasing the drug solubility and dissolution rate for better absorption from the gastrointestinal tract due to the higher surface area to mass ratio of particles. This fine particle tech consists of rationales involving (1) Higher absorption rate and reduction in dose; (2) Improved therapeutic efficacy of pharmaceutical and drug products; and (3) Lower chances of adverse effects due to a lower dose of drug. Solumatrix fine particle technology has been used to deduct the dose without compromising delaying the rate of absorption and provide similar time to peak plasma concentration and also provide lower lesser systemic absorption, which allows for distribution in injured tissues in a timely manner (Phaechamud

TABLE 10.1 Examples of Marketed Nanoformulations Used in Drug Delivery System

Nanoformulation	Properties	Marketed formulation	References
Liposomes	Bilayered lipid vesicles, encapsulate both hydrophilic and lipophilic drug, biocompatible, enhance blood circulation time of drugs.	AmBisomes (Amphotericin B) DaunoXome (Daunorubicin citrate), DepoCyt (Cytarabine), DepoDur (Morphine sulfate), Doxil (Doxorubicin hydrochloride)	Hiemenz and Walsh, 1996 ; Weissig, Pettinger, and Murdock, 2014
Niosomes	Spherical bilayered vesicles comprise of nonionic surfactant, Exhibit a better stability profile than liposomes.	Lancome (anti-aging cream)	Muzzalupo, 2015
Nanocrystal	Colloidal drug delivery system, minimum or less excipients required, enhance solubility of poorly soluble drugs, increase payload, reduction in dose and toxicity.	Megace ES (Megestrol acetate), Rapamune (Rapamycin), Tricor (Fenofibrate)	Junghanns, 2008
SLN	Aqueous based formulation system (pass up the use of organic solvent), good biocompatibility profile, enhance the stability of formulation than other nanocarriers system; method of formulation is easy and less expensive than polymeric and other surfactant based formulation.	Aquasol A (Vitamin A)	Weissig, Pettinger, and Murdock, 2014
NLC	Second generation colloidal lipid carrier system, liquid lipid is used, provide high encapsulation efficiency, avoid drug leakage from formulation.	Ketoderm cream 2% (Ketoconazole)	Weissig, Pettinger, and Murdock, 2014
Polymeric nanoparticles	Biodegradable and biocompatible in nature, enhance blood circulation time and provide prolong duration of action.	Eligard, Genexol, Opaxoio,	McCarthy, 2005
Polymeric micelles	Highest drug loading capacity and have the capability to load more than one drug at a time.	Genexol PM, Estrasorb	Muzzalupo, 2015

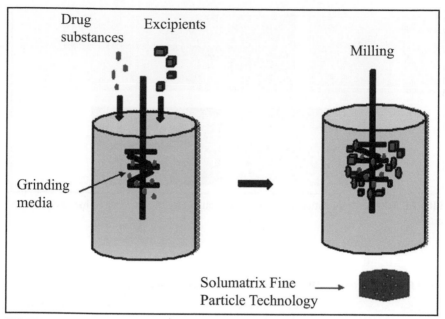

FIGURE 10.11   Method of formulation of product by solumatrix fine particle technology.

and Tuntarawongsa, 2016). This technology is used to formulate new branded medicines with well-established molecules of drug having known product experience and commercial value. The product derived from this technology exhibit clinical benefits for the consumer or patients and accurately defined the regulatory affairs and success in market. Large number of FDA (food and drug administration) approved and late-stage dosage forms in the process of development utilize solumatrix technology (Figure 10.12; Table 10.2).

Utilization of solumatrix technology mostly efficacious in reducing pain and inflammation, it is widely used in the management of complications of arthritis, acute and chronic pain of many etiologies (Sharma et al., 2011).

Three FDA approved NSAIDs (Non-steroidal anti-inflammatory drugs) (Solumatrix diclofenac, Solumatrix indomethacin, and Solumatrix meloxicam) to help the advances the science of responsible pain management (Phaechamud and Tuntarawongsa, 2016) (Table 10.3).

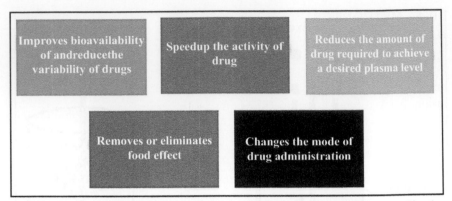

FIGURE 10.12   Implication of solumatrix technology on the drugs pharmacokinetics profile.

TABLE 10.2   Products Derived From Solumatrix Technology

Disease	Drug products	Drug development phases
Anticancer molecules	ICE-1207 LUNG	Preclinical trial
	ICE-1208 LUKEMIA	
Respiratory disease	ICE-1202	Preclinical trials
	ICE-1203	
	ICE-1204	
Pain and inflammation	ZORVOLEX	Phase-1
	TIVORBEX	Phase-1
	VIVLODEX	Phase-1
	ICE-1201	Preclinical trial
	SOLUMATRIX NARPOXEN	Phase-1

TABLE 10.3   Dose of FDA Approved NSAIDS Formulated by Solumatrix Technology

Drugs	Conventional dose in tablets	Dose in Solumatrix formulation
Diclofenac	75 mg	35 mg (ZORVOLEX)
Indomethacin	75 mg	20 mg (TIVROBEX)
Meloxicam	7.5 mg	5 mg (VIVLODEX)

10.4   METHODS OF PREPARATION OF NANOPHARMACEUTICALS

Nanoformulation is an important carrier for novel drug delivery system and prepared via several methods such as melt homogenization, precipitation from solvent in water emulsion, solvent evaporation, co-solvent evaporation, emulsification process, etc.

10.4.1   *MELT HOMOGENIZATION*

Melt homogenization is a simple and easy method of preparation of nanoparticles by use of high-pressure homogenization followed by size reduction using ultrasonication (Hussaini, Solorio, and Young, 2016). This method is generally used in formulation of solid lipid nanoparticle and nanostructure lipid carriers (Figure 10.13).

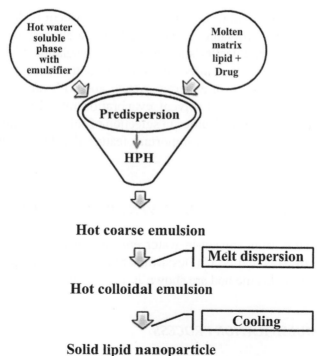

FIGURE 10.13   Preparation of nanoparticle by hot melt homogenization technique.

10.4.2   SOLVENT EVAPORATION METHOD

In solvent evaporation technique, the drug along and polymer are dissolved in organic solvent having minimum boiling point then further this solution containing polymer and drug is subjected to evaporation to remove the organic solvent to form the thin film, this is followed by dehydration of formed film to form the nanoparticles. The formation of nanoparticles by this method dependent on various factors such as concentration of drug and polymer, nature of solvent and evaporation rate (Desjardins et al., 2015). The main limitations of this process are that there is limited option available for solvent selection and redispersibility of formulation with the aqueous medium has to be considered during formulation. This technique is mainly used in the formulation of polymeric micelle.

10.4.3   CO-SOLVENT EVAPORATION

In co-solvent evaporation technique the aqueous system is directly pour into the non-aqueous (organic) solvent that ultimately results in formation of self-assembled micelles and promote encapsulation of drugs. The formation of nanoparticle is affected by many factors such as nature of solvent, the concentration of aqueous system and API, ratio of aqueous and non-aqueous solvent and solvent evaporation rate. The main drawback of this technique is difficulties in selection of solvent. Along with this drawback this technique has an important feature that high drug loading efficiency can be achieved.

10.4.4   PRECIPITATION FROM SOLVENT-IN-WATER EMULSION

The precipitation from solvent-in-water emulsion method is preferred in formulation of SLN and NLC (Desjardins et al., 2015). The process and steps involved in this method are shown in Figure 10.14.

10.4.5   EMULSIFICATION PROCESS

This method is generally used in formulation of nanoparticle either by single emulsion process or by double emulsion process.

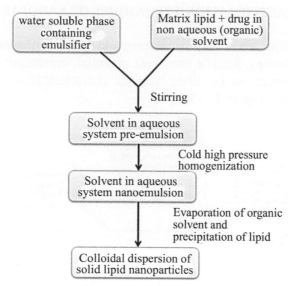

FIGURE 10.14   Precipitation from solvent-in-water emulsion.

10.4.5.1   SINGLE EMULSION

In single emulsion technique firstly polymer and drug are solublize in non-aqueous solvent. This solution is further emulsified with water-miscible solvents containing a surfactant. This method can be used to encapsulate the lipophilic drug moieties. Emulsification process is done by using high-pressure homogenization and sonication and the oil-in-water emulsion (O/W) is formed subsequently as soon as the organic solvent is evaporated from the system (Olugemo et al., 2015).

10.4.5.2   DOUBLE EMULSION

The double emulsion technique is generally applicable for the incorporation of hydrophilic drugs and water-in-oil-in-water (W/O/W) emulsion is formed. Hydrophilic drug is solubilized in an aqueous solvent followed by incorporation aqueous drug solution in polymer solution that leads to the formation of primary emulsion (Olugemo et al., 2015). This prepared primary emulsion is then added into the water-miscible system containing a surfactant to form a secondary emulsion and eventually subsequent evaporation of organic solvent leads to the formation of the desired emulsion.

10.5 CHARACTERIZATION TECHNIQUES OF NANOPARTICLES

Nanoformulations are usually characterized to seek information regarding surface morphology, particle size, zeta potential, crystallinity, and drug excipients interactions by using various characterization methods as described below (Figure 10.15).

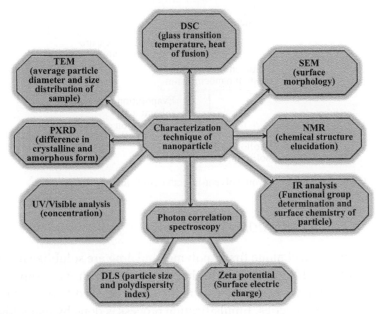

FIGURE 10.15 Characterization technique of nanoparticles.

10.5.1 PHOTON CORRELATION SPECTROSCOPY (PCS)

a) **Particle Size Determination and Particle Distribution Index**

Dynamic light scattering (DLS) analyses the constant changing pattern of laser light due to the diffraction which is attributes to the Brownian motion of nanoparticle. The particle size and the poly-dispersity index (PDI) of are determined using DLS on the basis of fluctuations in intensity of laser light (Zeng et al., 2010). In the case of lyophilized samples, it is first diluted to an appropriate concentration with triple distilled deionized water. The samples are analyzed at 25°C temperature with an angle of detection of 173 degrees. The particle size and PDI were determined by the instrument zeta sizer (Malvern Instruments, Malvern, UK), which works with the principle of DLS.

b) **Zeta Potential**

Zeta potential measures electrical charges lying on the surface of nanoparticle. Zeta potential is representative of stability of dispersion systems (Goldburg, 1999). It measures the potential difference between the bulk of fluid in which particles are dispersed and surface of nanoparticle containing opposite charge. Zeta potential with value more than ±40 indicates high stability of the dispersion system (Hänggi et al., 2016).

10.5.2   UV-VISIBLE ANALYSIS

The UV-Visible spectrophotometer is an important technology and mostly used for optimization of gold and silver nanocomposites. It is having capability to measure shape, concentration, size, refractive index and agglomeration state (Desai et al., 2012). This technique is also used to quantify and measure the active pharmaceutical ingredient entrapped in the nanoparticle (Goldburg, 1999). Bimetallic nanoparticle is characterized by comparing the spectrum with physical mixtures of monometallic nanoparticles (Contreras-Caceres et al., 2013).

10.5.3   FOURIER TRANSFORM INFRARED SPECTROSCOPY (FTIR)

FTIR technique is important for investigation of the surface chemistry of nanoparticles and functional group determination of those materials involved nanoparticle preparation (Movasaghi et al., 2008). The FTIR spectrum reveals information about nature of bond, existence of specific functional groups and interaction between nonfunctional groups in 400–4000 cm^{-1} wavelength region. IR spectroscopy is useful to characterize the multifunctional Fe hybrid, Ag and Au nanoparticles (Sheny, et al., 2011).

10.5.4   NUCLEAR MAGNETIC RESONANCE (NMR)

NMR is very essential analytical technique which is having application for elemental structure determination of nano-scale substances (Rangareddy, Mohanaraju, and Subbaramireddy, 2013). It is useful for the characterization of ferric and ferromagnetic materials due to the large magnetic saturation of such materials and applied for monitoring adsorbed gases diffusion from metallic nanoparticles. It is very decisive tool for reaction steps monitoring during polymer synthesis which is an integral materials for nanoparticle fabrication (Guo, Zhou and Lv, 2013).

10.5.5   TRANSMISSION ELECTRON MICROSCOPY (TEM)

TEM is a high power image magnification tool. Images are magnified by using beam of electrons that are transmitted through the sample. Rather than using light, electrons are used for illuminating the particles which result in high resolution of images (Folarin, Sadiku, and Maity, 2011). Transmission electron microscopy helps in the determination of the particle size of metallic nanoparticle (Gutowski, 1954). For the determination of the size of solid lipid nanoparticles, at the first aqueous diluted suspension will be prepared followed by TEM analysis. TEM imaging also applied for the measurement of average particle diameter and size distribution of formulated samples (Johnson, 1999).

10.5.6   SCANNING ELECTRON MICROSCOPY (SEM)

SEM involves focusing of high-energy beam electrons on the sample which provokes a variety of signals at the outer layer of a solid sample, these scattered signals are collected by the detector for the imaging purpose. SEM discloses the information about the sample such as chemical composition, surface morphology and crystalline nature of the sample (Williams and Carter, 1996). SEM is used to investigate the outer surface of nanoparticles. The area which can be observed under SEM is around 5 μm to 1 cm in width. The sample preparation for SEM analysis, gold-plated conductors are used to sputter-coat at 11 mA for 50 s to deposit a thin layer on top of the sample (McDowell et al., 2012).

10.5.7   X-RAY SPECTROSCOPIC ANALYSIS

10.5.7.1   POWDERED X-RAY DIFFRACTION (PXRD)

PXRD is an unique analytical method, which is used chiefly in research and development for the determination of crystallinity traits of a compound or nanomaterial and capable to supply exact information on single-cell magnitude (Wang, 2000). The *analyzed* material is finely crushed and the size is reduced, followed by the determination of average bulk composition (Sokolova et al., 2011). The intensity of peak within the lattice is determined as a function of atom dispersion in the subjected sample (Liu, 2005). In XRD analysis, generated properties of x-ray diffraction patterns provide an exclusive "fingerprint" of the crystals within the presented sample. Consequently, interpretation of peak intensities is compared to reference materials pattern accompanied by measurements, this fingerprint allows researchers to identify the crystallinity (Bunjes and Unruh, 2007).

10.5.7.2   SMALL-ANGLE X-RAY SCATTERING (SAXS)

The small angle x-ray scattering studies mainly used for phase identification in the internal structure of nanoparticles and reveals information about nanoparticle size distribution and nanoparticles pore size. It works on the principle of elastic scattering behavior of x-rays when travel through materials at 0° to 10° angle. SAXS has enormous advantages over other crystallographic techniques (Akbari, Tavandashti, and Zandrahimi, 2011).

10.5.8   DIFFERENTIAL SCANNING CALORIMETRY (DSC)

Differential scanning calorimetry is a thermal technique applied for multiple purposes in various research and scientific organization to carry out quality in research work. It provides structural relevant information on the dispersed particles in a given sample. DSC offers several scientific measurements including glass transition temperature, reaction temperature, heat of the fusion, melting temperature, etc. (Ingham, 2015). This technique is more popular in pharmaceuticals industries especially in research and development where large number of sample has to be investigated like analysis of number of chemicals, drugs analysis, polymers attributes, rubbers, metals, crystals in liquid samples followed by oxidative stability studies. It exhibits many crucial properties such as nature and crystallinity of the samples when compared to other existence calorimetric techniques (Bunjes and Unruh, 2007). DSC is able to screen and quantify the little changes in the thermal events in the sample. The measurement of energy absorbed or liberated by the particular sample during heating and cooling operation is based on DSC. In DSC, the sample of reference material and representative material are exposed at the same level of temperatures and the differences between the heat flow rate of the formulated sample and reference materials are measured and the result is interpreted.

10.5.9 THERMOGRAVIMETRIC ANALYSIS (TGA)

Thermogravimetric analysis is a technique applied to measure the thermal stability of samples (i.e., nanoparticles). The small modifications in physical and chemical properties of nanomaterials can be assessed either as a function of temperature where temperature varied with the constant heating rate or as a function of time where time is varied with constant temperature (Lin et al., 2014). The graph of TGA is a plot of mass change vs temperature or time which is categorized into seven types of curves based on stages of mass loss (Ingham, 2015) (Table 10.4).

TABLE 10.4 Techniques for Characterization of Nanoparticles

Technique	Parameters	References
XRD	Nature of crystal their composition and structure, size	Wang, 2000
FTIR	Nature of hydrogen bonding, ligands binding, and surface composition	Sheny et al., 2011
NMR	Atomic composition of formulation, ligands density, and arrangement, effects of ligands on nanoparticles shapes, elemental and chemical composition, growth kinetics	Rangareddy, Mohanaraju, and Subbaramireddy, 2013
TGA	Stabilizer composition	Lin et al., 2014
DLS	Hydrodynamic size of particles and information about agglomerates	Hänggi et al., 2016
XPS	Composition of elements, electronic structure, and oxidative states.	Miele et al., 2009
TEM	Detect formulation monodispersity, shape, aggregation states, internal structural information, dispersion of NPs in matrices, growth kinetics	Folarin, Sadiku, and Maity, 2011; Gutowski, 1954
AFM	Detect structure and shape in 3D mode	Hänggi et al., 2016
SEM	Information about morphology, detection of nanoparticles, size distribution	Johnson, 1999
PCS	Surface charge, agglomeration states, polydispersity index, size	Zeng et al., 2010
DSC	Detect density, size	Ingham, 2015
BET	Specific surface area	Zeng et al., 2010

10.6   STABILITY EVALUATION OF NANOFORMULATIONS

The nanoparticulate system is chiefly classified into the following main categories such as microparticles, nanoparticles, micelles, and other nanoparticulate systems are micro/nanogels, hydrogels, and polymer-drug conjugates. The stability is depending on the type of drug delivery system used (Figure 10.16). The drug delivery system is selected by considering the pharmacokinetics and pharmacodynamics of drug which includes chemistry, solubility, potency, site of action, and clearance rate of the drug. Along with these properties drug loading capacity, release kinetics, and the route of administration also decide the choice of drug delivery system. In regards to the nanoparticulate system, the stability is greatly influenced by particle size, particle size distribution, and surface charge. Storage stability for freeze-dried nanoformulations has to be tested in accordance with the ICH stability guidelines (Q1A (R2). This guideline describes the storage conditions for accelerated stability as a storage temperature of 4°C and 25°C for six months. After the completion of the storage period, the formulations are evaluated for particle size, PDI, zeta potential and % encapsulation efficiency after reconstitution in order to assess the effect of storage condition on these critical evaluation parameters.

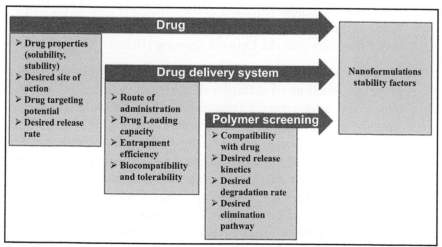

FIGURE 10.16   Process of selection of formulation in the drug delivery system.

10.6.1   STABILITY ISSUES WITH NANOFORMULATION

Stability of nanoparticles is a major concern though these systems are said to be stabilized by the use of surfactants and polymers. As these nano-delivery systems are usually prepared by high-energy methods of preparation, the energy is consumed to break the particles into nano-size range. These nano-size particles are highly energetic in terms of kinetics energy, thus they tend to stabilize by forming the agglomerates, which pertains to the stability issue in nanoformulations. These types of formulation systems are thermodynamically unstable due to high surface area and surface energy of small particles. Most commonly observed instability problems are nucleation and crystal growth that ultimately leads to agglomeration. Other stability issues are sedimentation, polymorphic transformations of crystals and chemical incompatibility.

- **Ostwald ripening:** The phenomenon in which larger particles grow at the expense of the smaller particles is called Ostwald ripening. There are two preconditions for Ostwald ripening phenomena to occur: (i) When the system is polydisperse; and (ii) when the dispersed phases have finite solubility in the dispersion medium. Both these conditions are frequently encountered in nanosuspension formulations. In addition, most of the stabilizers used in the preparation of nanosuspensions also increase the solubility of drug and hence they may provoke Ostwald ripening (Urandur et al., 2018).

Ostwald ripening kinetics in disperse systems is governed by basic processes, such as (i) diffusion of the solute molecules; and (ii) attachment or detachment (crystal growth and dissolution) to and from the particle surface. If crystal growth/dissolution at the particle surface is rapid then diffusion becomes the rate-determining step (diffusion-controlled growth). Whereas, if diffusion of the solute molecules is faster than their incorporation or removal to or from the solid particles then coarsening of the system is governed by the mechanisms of crystal growth (including surface energy and presence of defects interface controlled growth) (Corcione and Frigione, 2012).

Depending upon the nature of the interface and crystal growth mechanism three different types of interface coarsening can be identified: (i) continuous growth, (ii) surface nucleation, and (iii) twisted growth (Schirmer, Kim, and Klemm, 2001).

The kinetics of diffusion-controlled growth and interface controlled growth are given by the following equation:

$$d^n - d_0^n = k \times t$$

where, d = average diameter at time t; d_0 = average initial diameter; k = ripening rate; n = 3 (for Lifshitz, Slyozov and Wagner (LSW) diffusion controlled processes); and n = 2 (for twisted growth). However, the ripening rate is given by the equation:

$$k = \frac{64DC\infty Vm\gamma}{9RT}$$

where, D = translational diffusion coefficient of the dissolved solute molecules; C_∞ = bulk solubility of the dispersed phase; γ = interfacial tension; V_m = molar volume of the dispersed phase; R = gas constant; and T = temperature.

• **Sedimentation:** As nanosuspensions are colloidal dispersion they are more prone to sedimentation as compared to true solutions, which are homogenous. Sedimentation is unavoidable when dispersed particle gravity is higher than the buoyancy force provided by the suspension. Sedimentation is irreversible; hence, the stabilizers should be chosen keeping sedimentation tendency in view.

Flocculation is also a kind of sedimentation, which is a result of dominant attractive forces among the particles. Possible mechanisms of flocculation include surface charge neutralization, polymer bridging, polymer-particle surface complex or a combination of these factors (Kabalnov, 2001).

• **Crystalline Transformation:** Preparation processes such as high-pressure homogenization and milling as well as solidification processes such as freeze-drying and surface drying may cause an alteration in the crystalline properties or crystal habit of the drug (Baldan, 2002). The crystalline drug may also transform into amorphous form during these processes or vice versa may also happen. Amorphous form of drug is thermodynamically unstable compared to crystalline form and thus show higher dissolution. Amorphous form also tends to convert to crystalline form at a faster rate as compared to crystalline thus crystalline form is always preferred over amorphous form (Mixtures, 1992). Amorphous form of drug may undergo transformation to crystalline state during storage and affect the therapeutic effect of drug (Mixtures, 1992).

10.7 CONCLUSION

Advancement in the field of drug delivery by nanotechnology is very lucrative area of sciences and technology. Understanding the properties of nanomaterial in field of medicine will take discipline of therapy quantum leap forward. Nanoparticle have potential to reduce toxicity, increase efficacy, controlled the release rate of drugs. Nanoformulations provides targeted approach for disease treatment, enhances the solubility of hydrophobic drug, increase the payload of drug to the targeted site in body and increase the retention time of drug in the body. Liposome, polymeric nanoparticles, nanocrystals, solid lipid nanoparticles and nanoemulsions are some of nanoformulations entered to the market and playing very significant role in management of various types of diseases like cancer, Alzheimer's and other chronic diseases. Recently reported experiments mentioned the potential fullerenated nanoparticles, layerosomes, nano-lipid carrier, nanofibers, and bilosomes are used as drug delivery system for the delivery of protein and peptide to the specific site of the body. These nano-delivery systems can easily cross the physiological barrier due to their nano-size range and their surface modification activity with cellular membrane. Therefore nanoparticles also involve potential of cell surface targeting and biochemical mechanisms of cell signaling. During nanoparticle formulation, selection of excipients, compatible drug and efficient preparation methods are very important for the achieving the desired physical parameters of nanoparticle such as drug loading, entrapment efficiency and particle size distribution index. Low energy consuming methods like nanoprecipitation method and solvent evaporation methods are cheap and economical for nano-formulation preparation as compared to high-energy method.

Characterizations of nanoparticles during product development is crucial aspect for understanding surface chemistry, morphology, size, charges, molecular structure, compatibility of excipients with drug and its stability in *in-vitro* and *in-vivo* environments of nanoformulation. Cutting edge techniques that involve PCS, SEM, TEM, NMR, FTIR, XRDs, and DSC are available which are employed for the analysis of nano-engineered particles. Stability issues are associated with nanoformulation that may cause alteration in potency of drug and reduce the effectiveness or therapeutic efficacy of whole delivery system. During formulation process, different physicochemical properties of drug, screening of polymer and drug-polymer interaction are critical quality control factor to decide the stability of nanoparticle during shelf life. Stability cases like Ostwald ripening, crystalline transformation and sedimentation of nanoparticle are the key indicators of unstable formulation. Thus, thorough evaluation of stability shall be carried out by performing the stability test as per ICH guideline before releasing it for the commercialization purpose. In future, nanoproducts will become important part in therapeutics and medicine as drug delivery system as well as for diagnostic purposes as there is exponential rise in market value of nanoformulation and also it increases the attention of pharma industry due to their attractive commercial and therapeutic benefits over other traditional delivery systems.

KEYWORDS

- atomic force microscopy
- nanoparticles in drug delivery
- nanopharmaceuticals drug delivery system
- nanopharmaceuticals products
- polydispersity index
- scanning electron microscopy
- transmission electron microscopy
- zeta potential

REFERENCES

Aaltonen, J., Allesø, M., Mirza, S., Koradia, V., Gordon, K. C., Rantanen, J., Ab, C., Abramovič, H., Klofutar, C., Administración, D. E., et al., (2012). Dissolution rate of poorly soluble drugs potencial influence on dissolution rate using calcium sulfate as carrier in drug formulations. *Tesis. Int. J. Pharm., 13*(2), 1–10.

Acosta, E., (2009). Bioavailability of nanoparticles in nutrient and nutraceutical delivery. *Curr. Opin. Colloid Interface Sci., 14*(1), 3–15.

Ahmad, Z., Shah, A., Siddiq, M., & Kraatz, H. B., (2014). Polymeric micelles as drug delivery vehicles. *RSC Adv., 4*(33), 17028–17038.

Akbari, B., Tavandashti, M. P., & Zandrahimi, M., (2011). *Particle Size Characterization of Nanoparticles—A., 8*(2), 48–56.

Alexis, F., Pridgen, E., Molnar, L. K., & Farokhzad, O. C., (2008). *Reviews Factors Affecting the Clearance and Biodistribution of Polymeric Nanoparticles, 5*(4), 505–515.

Ankita, R., & Anil, B. B. K., (2010). Polymers in drug delivery: A review. *Int. J. Pharma. Res. Dev. – Online, 2*(8), 9–20.

Babu, A., Templeton, A. K., Munshi, A., & Ramesh, R., (2014). Nanodrug delivery systems: A promising technology for detection. *Diagnosis and Treatment of Cancer, No. 7.*

Baldan, A., (2002). Progress in Ostwald ripening theories and their applications to nickel-base superalloys. Part I: Ostwald ripening theories. *J. Mater. Sci., 37*(11), 2171–2202.

Biswas, A. K., Islam, R., & Choudhury, Z. S. (2014). *Nanotechnology Based Approaches in Cancer Therapeutics, 043001.*

Bunjes, H., & Unruh, T., (2007). Characterization of lipid nanoparticles by differential scanning calorimetry, x-ray and neutron scattering. *Adv. Drug Deliv. Rev., 59*(6), 379–402.

Contreras-Caceres, R., Dawson, C., Formanek, P., Fischer, D., Simon, F., Janke, A., Uhlmann, P., & Stamm, M., (2013). Polymers as templates for Au and Au@ Ag bimetallic nanorods: UV-vis and surface enhanced Raman spectroscopy. *Chemistry of Materials, 25*(2), 158–169.

Corcione, C. E., & Frigione, M., (2012). Characterization of nanocomposites by thermal analysis. *Materials (Basel)., 5*(12), 2960–2980.

Desai, R., Mankad, V., Gupta, S. K., & Jha, P. K., (2012). Size distribution of silver nanoparticles: UV-visible spectroscopic assessment. *Nanoscience and Nanotechnology Letters, 4*(1), 30–34.

Desjardins, P. J., Olugemo, K., Solorio, D., & Young, C. L., (2015). Pharmacokinetic properties and tolerability of low-dose solu matrix diclofenac. *Clin. Ther., 37*(2), 448–461.

Dua, J. S., Rana, A. C., & Bhandari, A. K., (2012). Liposome: methods of preparation and applications. *Int. J. Pharm. Stud. Res., 3*(2), 14–20.

Emerich, D. F., & Thanos, C. G., (2006). *The Pinpoint Promise of Nanoparticle-Based Drug Delivery and Molecular Diagnosis, 23,* 171–184.

Ferrari, M., (2005). Cancer nanotechnology: opportunities and challenges, *Nature Reviews Cancer, 5*(3), 161–171.

Folarin, O. M., Sadiku, E. R., & Maity, A., (2011). Polymer-noble metal nanocomposites: Review. *Int. J. Phys. Sci., 6*(21), 4869–4882.

Goldburg, W. I., (1999). Dynamic light scattering. *Am. J. Phys., 67*(12), 1152–1160.

Gorain, B., Choudhury, H., Pandey, M., Kesharwani, P., Abeer, M. M., Tekade, R. K., & Hussain, Z., (2018). Carbon nanotube scaffolds as emerging nanoplatform for myocardial tissue regeneration: A review of recent developments and therapeutic implications. *Biomed. Pharmacother., 104*, 496–508.

Guo, C., Zhou, L., & Lv, J., (2013). Effects of expandable graphite and modified ammonium polyphosphate on the flame-retardant and mechanical properties of wood flour-polypropylene composites. *Polym. Polym. Compos., 21*(7), 449–456.

Gutowski, (1954). *Nuclear Magnetic Resonancel., No. 9.*

Hänggi, D., Etminan, N., Steiger, H. J., Johnson, M., Peet, M. M., Tice, T., Burton, K., Hudson, B., Turner, M., Stella, A., et al., (2016). *A Site-Specific, Sustained-Release Drug Delivery System for Aneurysmal Subarachnoid Hemorrhage.*

Hiemenz, J. W., & Walsh, T. J. (1996). *Lipid Formulations of Amphotericin B : Recent Progress and Future Directions.*

Hussaini, A., Solorio, D., & Young, C., (2016). Pharmacokinetic properties of low-dose solumatrix meloxicam in healthy adults. *Clin. Rheumatol., 35*(4), 1099–1104.

Ingham, B., (2015). X-ray scattering characterization of nanoparticles. *Crystallogr. Rev., 21*(4), 229–303.

Johnson, Jr., C. S., (1999). Diffusion ordered nuclear magnetic resonance spectroscopy: Principles and applications. *Prog. Nucl. Magn. Reson. Spectrosc., 34*, 203–256.

Jumaa, M., & Muller, B. W., (2000). *Lipid Emulsions as a Novel System to Reduce the Hemolytic Activity of Lytic Agents: Mechanism of the Protective Effect, 9*, 285–290.

Junghanns, J. A. H., (2008). *Nanocrystal Technology, Drug Delivery and Clinical Applications, 3*(3), 295–309.

Kabalnov, A., (2001). Ostwald ripening and related phenomena. *J. Dispers. Sci. Technol., 22*(1), 1–12.

Kabanov, A. V., & Vinogradov, S. V., (2009). Nanogels as pharmaceutical carriers: Finite networks of infinite capabilities. *Angew. Chemie Int. Ed., 48*(30), 5418–5429.

Kammona, O., & Kiparissides, C., (2012). Recent advances in nanocarrier-based mucosal delivery of biomolecules. *Journal of Controlled Release*, 781–794.

Kamps, A. C., Sanchez-Gaytan, B. L., Hickey, R. J., Clarke, N., Fryd, M. & Park, S. J., (2010). Nanoparticle-directed self-assembly of amphiphilic block copolymers. *Langmuir, 26*(17), 14345–14350.

Kesharwani, P., & Iyer, A. K., (2015). Recent advances in dendrimer-based nanovectors for tumor-targeted drug and gene delivery. *Drug Discov. Today, 20*(5), 536–547.

Kesharwani, P., Gorain, B., Low, S. Y., Tan, S. A., Ling, E. C. S., Lim, Y. K., Chin, C. M., Lee, P. Y., Lee, C. M., Ooi, C. H., et al., (2018). Nanotechnology-based approaches for anti-diabetic drugs delivery. *Diabetes Res. Clin. Pract., 136*, 52–77.

Kim, G., Piao, C., Oh, J., & Lee, M., (2018). Self-assembled polymeric micelles for combined delivery of anti-inflammatory gene and drug to the lungs by inhalation. *Nanoscale, 10*(18), 8503–8514.

Kohane, D. S., (2007). *Microparticles and Nanoparticles for Drug Delivery, 96*(2), 203–209.

Lin, P. C., Lin, S., Wang, P. C., & Sridhar, A. R., (2014). Techniques for physicochemical characterization of nanomaterials. *Biotechnol. Adv., 32*(4), 711–726.

Liu, J., (2005). Scanning transmission electron microscopy and its application to the study of nanoparticles and nanoparticle systems. *J. Electron Microsc. (Tokyo), 54*(3), 251–278.

Liu, K., Li, H., Williams, G. R., Wu, J., & Zhu, L. M., (2018). PH-responsive liposomes self-assembled from electrosprayed microparticles, and their drug release properties. *Colloids Surfaces A Physicochem. Eng. Asp., 537*, 20–27.

Lo, C. T., Jahn, A., Locascio, L. E., & Vreeland, W. N., (2010). Controlled self-assembly of monodisperse niosomes by microfluidic hydrodynamic focusing. *Langmuir, 26*(11), 8559–8566.

Lu, H., Wang, J., Wang, T., Zhong, J., Bao, Y., & Hao, H., (2016). *Recent Progress on Nanostructures for Drug Delivery Applications*, 2016.

Luo, S., Luo, Y., Wu, H., Li, M., Yan, L., Jiang, K., Liu, L., Li, Q., Fan, S., & Wang, J., (2017). Self-assembly of 3D carbon nanotube sponges: A simple and controllable way to build macroscopic and ultralight porous architectures. *Adv. Mater., 29*(1), 1603549.

McCarthy, J. R., Perez, J. M., Brückner, C., & Weissleder, R., (2005). Polymeric nanoparticle preparation that eradicates tumors. *Nano Letters, 5*(12), 2552–2556.

McDowell, M. T., Ryu, I., Lee, S. W., Wang, C., Nix, W. D., & Cui, Y., (2012). Studying the kinetics of crystalline silicon nanoparticle lithiation with in situ transmission electron microscopy. *Adv. Mater., 24*(45), 6034–6041.

Miele, E., Spinelli, G. P., Miele, E., Tomao, F., & Tomao, S., (2009). *Albumin-Bound Formulation of Paclitaxel (Abraxane ® ABI-007) in the Treatment of Breast Cancer*, 99–106.

Movasaghi, Z., Rehman, S., & urRehman, D. I., (2008). Fourier transform infrared (FTIR spectroscopy of biological tissues. *Applied Spectroscopy Reviews, 43*(2), 134–179.

Muzzalupo, R., (2015). *Niosomal Drug Delivery for Transdermal Targeting : Recent Advances*, 23–33.

Nagalakshmi, S., Krishnaraj, K., Jothy, M. A., Chaudhari, P. S., Pushpalatha, H., & Shanmuganthan, S., (2016). Fabrication and characterization of herbal drug-loaded nonionic surfactant based niosomal topical gel. *J. Pharm. Sci. Res., 8*(11), 1271–1278.

Olugemo, K., Solorio, D., Sheridan, C., & Young, C. L., (2015). Pharmacokinetics and safety of low-dose submicron Indomethacin 20 and 40 Mg compared with Indomethacin 50 Mg. *Postgrad. Med., 127*(2), 223–231.

Onoue, S., Yamada, S., & Chan, H., (2014). *Nanodrugs : Pharmacokinetics and Safety*, 1025–1037.

Phaechamud, T., & Tuntarawongsa, S., (2016). Transformation of eutectic emulsion to nanosuspension fabricating with solvent evaporation and ultrasonication technique. *Int. J. Nanomedicine, 11*, 2855–2865.

Rangareddy, P., Mohanaraju, K., & Subbaramireddy, N., (2013). A review on polymer nanocomposites: Monometallic and bimetallic nanoparticles for biomedical, optical and engineering applications. *Che. Sci. Rev. Lett., 1*(4), 228–235.

Rigogliuso, S., Sabatino, M. A., Adamo, G., Grimaldi, N., Dispenza, C., & Ghersi, G., (2012). Nanocarriers for drug delivery application. *Chem. Eng. Trans., 27*, 247–252.

Rizvi, S. A. A., & Saleh, A. M., (2017). Applications of nanoparticle systems in drug delivery technology. *Saudi Pharm. J., 26*(1), 64–70.

Schirmer, J., Kim, J. S., & Klemm, E., (2001). Catalytic degradation of polyethylene using thermal gravimetric analysis and a cycled-spheres-reactor. *J. Anal. Appl. Pyrolysis, 60*(2), 205–217.

Gao, L., Zhang, D., & Chen, M., (2008). Drug nanocrystals for the formulation of poorly soluble drugs and its application as a potential drug delivery system. *Journal of Nanoparticle Research, 10*(5), 845–862.

Selvamuthukumar, S., & Velmurugan, R., (2012). *Nanostructured Lipid Carriers : A Potential Drug Carrier for Cancer Chemotherapy*, 1–8.

Sharma, P., Zujovic, Z. D., Bowmaker, G. A., Denny, W. A., & Garg, S., (2011). Evaluation of a crystalline nanosuspension: Polymorphism, process induced transformation and *in vivo* studies. *Int. J. Pharm., 408*(1&2), 138–151.

Sheny, D. S., Mathew, J., & Philip, D. (2011). Phytosynthesis of Au, Ag and Au–Ag bimetallic nanoparticles using aqueous extract and dried leaf of Anacardiumoccidentale. *Spectrochimica Acta Part A: Molecular and Biomolecular Spectroscopy. 79*(1), 254–262.

Singh, A., Vengurlekar, P., & Rathod, S., (2014). *Design, Development and Characterization of Liposomal Neem Gel., 5*(04), 140–148.

Singh, R., & Jr, J. W. L., (2009). Nanoparticle-based targeted drug delivery. *Exp. Mol. Pathol., 86*(3), 215–223.

Sokolova, V., Ludwig, A. K., Hornung, S., Rotan, O., Horn, P. A., Epple, M., & Giebel, B., (2011). Characterisation of exosomes derived from human cells by nanoparticle tracking analysis and scanning electron microscopy. *Colloids Surfaces B Biointerfaces, 87*(1), 146–150.

Sonia, T. A., & Sharma, C. P., (2012). An overview of natural polymers for oral insulin delivery. *Drug Discov. Today, 17*(13&14), 784–792.

Urandur, S., Banala, V. T., Shukla, R. P., Mittapelly, N., Pandey, G., Kalleti, N., Mitra, K., Rath, S. K., Trivedi, R., Ramarao, P., et al., (2018). Anisamide-anchored lyotropic nano-liquid crystalline particles with AIE effect: A smart optical beacon for tumor imaging and therapy. *ACS Appl. Mater. Interfaces, 10*(15), 12960–12974.

Vo, T. N., Kasper, F. K., & Mikos, A. G., (2012). Strategies for controlled delivery of growth factors and cells for bone regeneration. *Adv. Drug Deliv. Rev.*

Voorhees, P. W., (1992). Ostwald ripening of two-phase mixtures. *Annual Review of Materials Science, 22*(1), 197–215.

Wang, Y., Zheng, Y., Zhang, L., Wang, Q., & Zhang, D., (2013). Stability of nanosuspensions in drug delivery. *J. Control. Release, 172*(3), 1126–1141.

Wang, Z. L., (2000). Transmission electron microscopy of shape-controlled nanocrystals and their assemblies. *J. Phys. Chem. B, 104*(6), 1153–1175.

Weissig, V., Pettinger, T. K., & Murdock, N., (2014). Nanopharmaceuticals (Part 1): Products on the market. *International Journal of Nanomedicine, 4357*–4373.

Williams, D. B., & Carter, C. B., (1996). The transmission electron microscope. *Transm. Electron Microsc., 3*–17.

Xiong, X., Falamarzian, A., Garg, S. M., & Lavasanifar, A., (2011). Engineering of amphiphilic block copolymers for polymeric micellar drug and gene delivery. *J. Control. Release, 155*(2), 248–261.

Yu, D. G., Yang, J. H., Wang, X., & Tian, F., (2012). Liposomes self-assembled from electrosprayed composite microparticles. *Nanotechnology, 23*(10), 105606.

Yu, X., Trase, I., Ren, M., Duval, K., Guo, X., & Chen, Z., (2016). Design of nanoparticle-based carriers for targeted drug delivery. *J. Nanomater., 1*–15.

Zeng, Z. W., Zhou, G. L., Wang, J. J., Li, F. Z., & Wang, A. M., (2010). *Recent Advances in PEG – PLA Block Copolymer Nanoparticles, 1057*–1065.

CHAPTER 11

Recent Advances in the Development of Nanoparticles for Oral Delivery

MD. RIZWANULLAH,[1] MOHD. MOSHAHID ALAM RIZVI,[2] and SAIMA AMIN[1*]

[1]Formulation Research Lab, Department of Pharmaceutics, School of Pharmaceutical Education and Research, Jamia Hamdard, New Delhi, India

[2]Genome Biology Lab, Department of Biosciences, Faculty of Natural Sciences, Jamia Millia Islamia, New Delhi, India

*Corresponding author. E-mail: samin@jamiahamdard.ac.in

11.1 INTRODUCTION

Among all drug delivery routes, the oral route is regarded as one of the most preferred, most comfortable, cost-effective and patient-compliant routes of drug administration. The selection of a drug delivery route is primarily focused on patient acceptability, physicochemical properties of the drug, and target area (Ahmad et al., 2013; Moss et al., 2018). Despite the potential advantages, some disadvantages are also associated with oral drug delivery. Most of the drugs are lipophilic and showed poor aqueous solubility. In addition, most of the drugs are either substrate for P-glycoprotein (P-gp) or metabolizing enzyme, cytochrome P450 or both that result in a decrease in oral bioavailability and therapeutic efficacy due to their expulsion or pre-systemic metabolism. Furthermore, the hostile environment of the gastrointestinal (GI) tract also limits the successful drug delivery via the oral route (Cheng et al., 2008; Ahmad et al., 2015). The oral bioavailability of the drug is also influenced by some other factors like chemical degradation of the drug in GI fluid, gastric emptying rate, and intestinal motility. There are a large number of physicochemical factors encountered in the GIT that limit the successful oral drug delivery (Daugherty and Mrsny, 1999).

After oral administration, the drug must survive the essential demanding parameters for oral bioactive delivery. It can be achieved by developing some novel drug delivery strategies such as (i) coating with permeation enhancers; (ii) co-administration of P-gp inhibitors to inhibit drug efflux; (iii) addition of some enzyme inhibitors to suppress the activity of proteolytic enzymes, (iv) avoiding pre-systemic metabolism; and (v) fabrication of highly efficient nanoparticles as a drug delivery system to overcome the intestinal permeation barriers and to increase the oral bioavailability of drugs (Agrawal et al., 2014; Peng et al., 2018).

Oral delivery of nanoparticles offers some potential benefits. Nanoparticles permits (i) encapsulation of both lipophilic and hydrophilic drugs; (ii) encapsulation of more than one drugs; (iii) drug targeting to the specific part of GIT; (iv) endocytosis of drug through different passive and active mechanisms across the GIT; and (v) intracellular delivery of macromolecules (Lin et al., 2017; Gedawy et al., 2018). In addition, nanoparticles can enhance intestinal permeability, oral bioavailability, therapeutic efficacy, and therapeutic index of encapsulated drugs. Furthermore, the robust structure of the nanoparticles can modulate the drug release profile thereby improve residence time in the GIT. The surface of nanoparticles can be decorated with hydrophilic molecules, e.g., polyethylene glycol, ligands, e.g., lectin and glycoproteins to enhance interactions with the GI mucosa. It helps the nanoparticles to deliver the drug at the specific cells, tissues or areas of the GIT (Agrawal et al., 2014). The ligands utilized to decorate the nanoparticles for oral drug delivery include lectins (Mishra et al., 2011); folic acid (Jain et al., 2012); and bile acids (Ahmad et al., 2017).

11.2   GASTROINTESTINAL BARRIERS IN ORAL DELIVERY OF NANOPARTICLES

For the successful development of nanoparticle as a drug delivery system for enhanced oral delivery, it is necessary to understand the proper mechanism of the digestion environment. But, there are still some significant challenges remained in the successful development of oral nanoparticles, such as barriers available in the GIT, which are categorized as chemical, enzymatic, and physical barriers.

11.2.1   CHEMICAL BARRIER

The stability of nanoparticles over a wide range of pH variation in the GIT is most important. Nanoparticles reach the stomach after administration through the mouth. There is a sudden change in pH from 6.8 to 1.2 and such a transition happens again from an extremely acidic environment (pH 1.2) of the stomach to a slightly alkaline environment (pH 6.5 to 8.0) of the small intestine (Al Rubeaan et al., 2016).

The mean residence time of nanoparticles in the stomach and small intestine is about 2.5 and 3-4 h respectively (Davis et al., 1984). Many studies reported that the dissociation of the nanoparticulate structure takes place due to the deprotonation or protonation of nanoparticle components (like polymer or lipids) in different pH environments. The dissociation of nanoparticles results in the burst release effect and degradation of encapsulated drugs (Wang et al., 2017a; Zhou et al., 2016a). Therefore, the developed nanoparticles should have good GI stability across a wide range of pH (pH 1.2 to 8.0) to protect the encapsulated drug throughout the entire GI transition.

11.2.2   ENZYMATIC BARRIER

Enzymatic degradation of the nanoparticle is another crucial challenge for successful oral drug delivery. The susceptibility of nanoparticles to different digestive enzymes present in the GIT poses a significant hurdle to achieve a desired therapeutic efficacy after oral administration. Decomposition of the lipid-based nanoparticles begins in the stomach by lipase and pepsin enzyme, respectively (Olbrich and Müller, 1999; Zhou et al., 2016b). The degradation of nanoparticles continues in the small intestinal lumen by enzymes, including lipase, trypsin, α-chymotrypsin (Liu et al., 2018).

11.2.3   PHYSICAL BARRIER

After the successful transit of nanoparticles from the stomach to the intestinal lumen by overcoming the chemical and enzymatic barriers, they are exposed to the intestinal epithelium layer that covers the surface of the GIT. Intestinal epithelium layer consists of enterocytes, goblet cells, Paneth cells, and micro-fold cells creates another significant barrier before the absorption of the nanoparticles (Pathak and Raghuvanshi, 2015). Goblet cells can produce mucus and form a mucous layer that covers and protects the underlying epithelium (Ensign et al., 2012a). The mucous layer is a negatively charged viscous mixture of mucin, antiseptic enzymes, immunoglobulins, and salts. The mucous layer is capable of trapping the molecules with high molecular weight and low permeability, as well as nanoparticles possessing a strong positive charge (Lai et al., 2009). Many studies revealed that nanoparticles with the neutral and hydrophilic surfaces are the ideal candidate for mucus permeation (Ensign et al., 2012b; Shan et al., 2015). There are two absorption mechanisms by which nanoparticles cross the epitheliums and enter into the systemic circulation after diffusion through the mucus layer (Shahbazi and Santos, 2013).

11.3   MECHANISM OF TRANSPORT OF NANOPARTICLES

11.3.1   PARACELLULAR PATHWAY

Paracellular pathway helps in the transport of nanoparticles via the space between two epithelial cells as illustrated in Figure 11.1 (Snoeck et al., 2005). The two adjacent epithelial cells connected with the tight junctions provide strength to the cell lining (Pappenheimer, 2001). The tight junctions are reversibly opened by two different mechanisms i) down-regulation of tight junction protein, and ii) decreasing the Ca^{2+} concentration (Yeh et al., 2011).

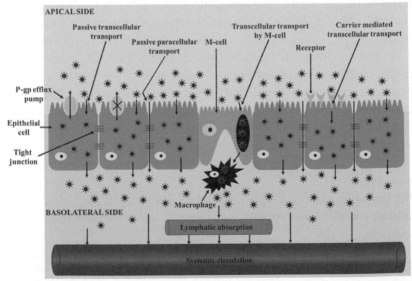

FIGURE 11.1   Schematic diagram illustrating the transport mechanisms of nanoparticles after oral delivery.

11.3.2   TRANSCELLULAR PATHWAY

The transcellular pathway involves the transport of drug molecules across the lipophilic membrane of the epithelial cells via passive diffusion, active transport or endocytosis (Figure 11.1).

In the small intestine, absorption of macromolecules usually occurs via endocytosis pathways, including phagocytosis, pinocytosis and receptor-mediated endocytosis (Mandracchia et al., 2017). Pinocytosis has the same endocytic mechanisms as phagocytosis, but the ingested substances are liquid materials along with the dissolved moieties, rather than solid materials. Macropinocytosis also belongs to pinocytosis, providing an effective way for non-selective endocytosis of extracellular nutrients and liquid macromolecules. This process depends on the activation of clathrin, attributing to the formation of large vesicular structures (0.15–5 μm) (Lukyanenko et al., 2011). The cut-off size of nanoparticles that could be uptaken by epithelial cells has been reported to be 300 nm (He et al., 2012). Apart from particle size, the surface properties also play a vital role in the absorption of nanoparticles through the transcellular pathway. It is known that nanoparticles with a positive charge and hydrophobic surface properties are ideal for the high interaction with the negatively charged epithelial cell membrane, which is in contradiction to mucus permeation theory (Verma and Stellacci, 2010).

11.3.2.1   TRANSCELLULAR TRANSPORT BY ENTEROCYTES

The transport of nanoparticles across enterocytes is an energy-dependent process, mainly occurred by macropinocytosis, clathrin, or caveolae-mediated endocytosis and clathrin and caveolae-independent endocytosis (Neves et al., 2016). Clathrin and caveolae-independent endocytosis are related to the motion of lipid rafts. The possible transcellular internalization by enterocytes seems to occur via the contribution of multiple pathways (Liu et al., 2018). Nowadays, efforts on studying the pathways involved in the internalization of particles have focused on using specific endocytic inhibitors through Caco-2 cell monolayers (Liu et al., 2018).

11.3.2.2   TRANSCELLULAR TRANSPORT BY M CELLS

The gastrointestinal tract is characterized by particular gut-associated lymphoid tissue (GALT) and M cells that reside in the follicle-associated epithelium on the surface of Peyer's patches in the ileum (Kiyono and Fukuyama, 2004). Compared to enterocytes, M cells are characterized by flattened apical surfaces, limited lysosomes and lack of mucus layers. They are specialized in translocation of antigens and intact nano- and microparticles, macromolecules, as well as mucosal vaccination from the lumen to GALT by pinocytosis and phagocytosis (Kadiyala et al., 2010).

11.4 NANOPARTICLES FOR ORAL DELIVERY

Nanoparticles as drug delivery system have gained much impressive attention for oral drug delivery in the last two decades. Nanoparticles are meant to deliver therapeutic drugs at a nanosized range (generally <1000 nm), leading to an increase in the surface area. Nanoparticles are reported to improve cellular uptake, modulate Pg-p efflux of the drug, bypass pre-systemic metabolism thereby increase the oral bioavailability of the drug. Nanoparticles release the drug in a sustained manner that helps in maintaining the therapeutic concentration in the systemic circulation for a long time period. Therefore, the half-life of the drug can be improved and dose frequency can be reduced. In addition, nanoparticles increase GI stability of the encapsulated drug by protecting them from the hostile environment of the GIT. Compared to the other oral bioavailability enhancement techniques, nanoparticles as a drug delivery system can be more efficiently taken up by the lymphatic system and deliver the drug directly to the systemic circulation (Agarwal et al., 2014; Pathak and Raghuvanshi, 2015). Different types of nanoparticles for efficient oral delivery are summarized in Table 11.1.

11.4.1 NANOCRYSTALS

Nanocrystal technology is the most interesting technique to increase aqueous solubility and oral bioavailability of lipophilic drugs. Nanocrystals are carrier-free colloidal nanoplatform and have been widely used for oral bioavailability enhancement of BCS class II drug by increasing their saturation solubility, dissolution rates in the GI fluid and adhesion to intestinal mucosa (Keck and Müller, 2006; Junyaprasert and Morakul, 2015). Nanocrystals composed of pure crystalline drug particles with a minute quantity of stabilizers absorbed onto the surfaces of the drug particles

TABLE 11.1 Recent Studies on Nanoparticles for Improved Oral Delivery

Nanoparticles	Drug	Excipients	Animal/Cell line	Outcomes	Reference
Nanocrystals	Nimodipine	Poloxamer F127, hydroxypropylmethyl cellulose	Beagle dogs	Improved aqueous solubility and dissolution rate, 2.6 fold improved oral bioavailability compared to marketed preparation	Fu et al., 2013
Nanocrystals	Curcumin	Hydroxypropyl cellulose SL, sodium dodecyl sulfate	Male Sprague–Dawley rats	16 fold higher oral bioavailability compared to free drug suspension	Onoue et al., 2010
Liposomes	Capsaicin	Soybean lecithin, sodium cholate, isopropyl myristate	Male Sprague–Dawley	Liposome was non-irritant to gastric mucosa and safe for oral administration, 3.34 fold improved oral bioavailability compared to free drug	Zhu et al., 2015
Liposomes	Lopinavir	Hydrogenated soya phosphatidylcholine, Cholesterol	Female albino Wistar rats	2.24 and 1.16 fold improved oral bioavailability compared to free drug and marketed formulation	Patel et al., 2017
Nanoemulsion	Curcumin	Ethyl oleate, cremorphor EL 35 and polyethylene glycol 400	Male Sprague-Dawely rats, A549 cell line	Significantly higher cytotoxicity against A549 cells compared to free drug, 4 and 7.3 fold improved intestinal permeability and oral bioavailability respectively compared to free drug	Wan et al., 2016
Nanoemulsion	Mebudipine	Ethyl oleate, Tween 80, Span 80, polyethylene glycol 400	Male albino Wistar rats	2.6 fold improved oral bioavailability compared to free drug suspension	Khani et al., 2016
SNEDDS	Ondansetron hydrochloride	Capmul MCM, Labrasol, Tween 20	Unisex albino Wistar rats	3.01 and 5.34 fold improved C_{max} and AUC compared to free drug	Beg et al., 2013
SNEDDS	Darunavir	Capmul MCM C8, Tween 80, Transcutol P	Male albino Wistar rats	Nearly 3 fold improved relative oral bioavailability compared to pure drug	Inugala et al., 2015
SLN	Aripiprazole	Tristearin, soy lecithin, sodium taurocholate	Male albino Wistar rats	1.6 fold improved oral bioavailability and better therapeutic efficacy	Silki and Sinha, 2018

TABLE 11.1 (Continued)

SLN	Docetaxel	Glycerylmonostearate, soybean lecithin, Tween 80, chitosan,	Male Sprague-Dawley rats	SLN was non-irritant to gastric mucosa and safe for oral administration, 2.24 fold improved AUC compared to free drug	Shi et al., 2017
NLC	Carvedilol	Stearic acid, oleic acid, tween 80	Albino Wistar rats	3.95-fold improved oral bioavailability compared to free drug suspension, significant reduction in mean systolic blood pressure compared to free drug	Mishra et al., 2016
NLC	Simvastatin	Stearic acid, oleic acid, lecithin, Pluronic F-68	Male albino Wister rats	4 fold improved oral bioavailability, better antihyperlipidemic efficacy	Fathi et al., 2018
Polymeric NPs	Daunorubicin hydrochloride	Chitosan, PLGA, Polyvinyl alcohol	Albino Wistar rats	3.89 and 10 fold higher permeability across rat ilium and oral bioavailability compared to free drug solution respectively	Ahmad et al., 2019
Polymeric NPs	Epirubicin	PLGA, Polyvinyl alcohol	Male albino Wistar rats	2.76 fold improved uptake in Caco-2 cell monolayer compared to free drug solution, 4.49 and 3.9 fold higher permeability across rat ilium and oral bioavailability compared to free drug solution respectively	Tariq et al., 2015
Polymeric NPs	Trans-resveratrol	Eudragit RL 100, Tetradecyltrimethyl ammonium bromide	Male Wistar rat	7.25-fold improved relative oral bioavailability compared to pure drug	Singh and Pai, 2014
Polymeric NPs	Rosuvastatin	Cyclodextrins, pyromellitic dianhydride	Sprague Dawley rats	2.2 and 5.15 fold improved oral bioavailability compared to drug suspension and marketed formulation	Gabr et al., 2018

(Pawar et al., 2014). Nanocrystal technology provides a high level of drug loading. Therefore, nanocrystals have ability to deliver a high dose of the drug to the systemic circulation thereby improve their bioavailability and therapeutic efficacy (Gao et al., 2012). In a study, Quan et al. (2012) developed nanocrystals of nitrendipine to improve oral bioavailability. Nitrendipine nanocrystals showed improved *in vitro* dissolution rate compared to the pure drug and marketed tablet. Pharmacokinetic study in male Wistar rats revealed 15 and 10 fold higher C_{max} of nanocrystals compared to free drug and marketed tablet respectively. In addition, nanocrystals showed 41 and 10 fold improved $AUC_{0 \rightarrow 24}$ compared to free drug and marketed tablet respectively. Similarly, fenofibrate nanocrystals showed 4.73 fold higher relative bioavailability in New Zealand white rabbit compared to the pure drug (Ige et al., 2013). In another study, lutein nanocrystals demonstrated 29.5 times higher saturated solubility in water and significantly higher dissolution rate compared to free drug (Chang et al., 2018). In addition, the pharmacokinetic study using Sprague-Dawley rats revealed that lutein nanocrystals exhibited 3.24 and 2.28 fold higher C_{max} and $AUC_{0 \rightarrow 24}$ compared to the drug suspension.

11.4.2   LIPOSOMES

Liposomes are biodegradable and biocompatible nanocarriers widely used to improve oral bioavailability of lipophilic as well as hydrophilic drugs since the last two decades. Due to the unique lipid bilayer structure, liposomes can better adhere to the mucosal membrane of the GIT. Liposomes form a mixed-micelle structure with bile salts present in the GI lumen to enhance the solubility of lipophilic drugs. In addition, literature strongly suggests that liposomes are one of the most suitable nanoparticle systems for lymphatic targeting (Roger and Anderson, 1998; Wu et al., 2015; Daeihamed et al., 2017). Stability of liposomes in the GI environment is the primary concern for oral delivery of liposomes. However, many effective approaches have been suggested to improve GI stability of liposomes. These include (i) addition of stabilizing lipids to liposomal structures; (ii) coating with polymers; (iii) development of double liposomes, proliposomes and bilosomes (Manconi et al., 2013; Nguyen et al., 2016; Ahmad et al., 2017). In a study, naringenin encapsulated liposomes were developed to enhance oral bioavailability (Wang et al., 2017b). Pharmacokinetic study in Kunming mice revealed 13.44-fold improved oral bioavailability of liposomes compared to free drug. Similarly, pluronic P85-coated brevicapine loaded liposomes showed 5.6 fold higher oral bioavailability in male Sprague-Dawley rat compared to free drug (Zhou et al., 2014). In addition, liposomal formulation exhibited significantly higher permeability in Caco-2 cell monolayer. In another study, valsartan loaded liposomes demonstrated significantly enhanced GI permeability and oral bioavailability (Nekkanti et al., 2015). *Ex vivo* intestinal perfusion study showed significantly higher permeability across ilium compared to free drug. This result was further confirmed by *in vitro* cellular uptake study in male Sprague-Dawley rat that revealed 2.2 fold higher relative oral bioavailability compared to pure drug.

11.4.3   NANOEMULSION

Nanoemulsions (NE) are heterogeneous mixture consists of oil droplets dispersed in an aqueous medium which results in very small droplets in nanometric size (20-200 nm) with narrow nanodroplet distribution. NE is a transparent or translucent isotropic emulsified mixture, stabilized by surfactants (Gao et al., 2011). NE represents extremely low interfacial tensions and great oil/water interfacial areas. Higher thermodynamic stability, long shelf life and significantly higher solubilization capacity of NE provide advantages over unstable dispersions, such as emulsions and suspensions. Nanoemulsions showed significant enhancement in oral bioavailability and bioactivity of lipophilic compounds (Singh et al., 2017). In a study, Yen et al. (2018) developed andrographolide loaded nanoemulsion to improve intestinal permeability and oral bioavailability. *Ex vivo* intestinal permeability using male Sprague–Dawley rat ilium revealed 8.21 and 1.4 fold higher intestinal permeability of nanoemulsion compared to pure drug suspension and ethanolic solution of drug respectively. After a single dose oral administration, nanoemulsion showed 5.9 fold improved relative oral bioavailability compared to pure drug suspension in male Sprague–Dawley rat. In another study, Olmesartanmedoxomil (OM) loaded nanoemulsion was developed to improve oral bioavailability and antihypertensive efficacy (Gorian et al., 2014). OM-NE exhibited significantly higher permeability in Caco-2 cell monolayer compared to free drug suspension. Furthermore, OM-NE showed 2.8 fold higher relative oral bioavailability in male Albino Wistar rats compared to free drug suspension. In addition, OM-NE exhibited 3-fold reduction in blood pressure in experimentally induced hypertension in rats compared to free drug suspension. Recently, Desai and Thakkar (2019) developed darunavir encapsulated nanoemulsion (D-NE) to enhance oral bioavailability and brain uptake. Pharmacokinetic study in male Albino Wistar rats revealed 2.23 fold improved oral bioavailability of D-NE compared to pure drug suspension. In addition, organ biodistribution study showed 2.65-fold improved brain uptake of D-NE compared to pure drug suspension.

11.4.4 SELF-NANOEMULSIFYING DRUG DELIVERY SYSTEMS (SNEDDS)

Since the last decades, SNEDDS gained much interest from researchers as a drug delivery platform to enhance the oral bioavailability of lipophilic drugs belonging to BCS classes II and IV (Thomas et al., 2012). SNEDDS significantly improve the absorption of a drug molecule through enhancement in gastrointestinal solubilization, therefore, overcoming physical and chemical barriers (Porter et al., 2007, 2008). The key factors that can influence oral bioavailability from SNEDDS include: (i) lipid digestion; (ii) droplet size; (iii) lipophilicity of the drugs; and (iv) the types of lipids used (Nangwade et al., 2011). SNEDDS are isotropic mixtures of liquid lipids, a surfactant, a cosurfactant and the drug, which, in the presence of an aqueous phase, form an o/w nanoemulsion under gentle agitation (Date et al., 2010). SNEDDS provides a large interfacial surface area due to the small size, thus improving the dissolution of the drug in GI fluid. This makes SNEDDS a suitable nano-drug delivery platform for oral delivery of highly lipophilic drugs to enhance oral bioavailability and therapeutic efficacy (Ahmad et al., 2014). In a study, Kalam et al. (2017) prepared thymoquinone (TQ) encapsulated SNEDDS to improve oral bioavailability and hepatoprotective efficacy. TQ-SNEDDS exhibited much greater oral absorption compared to TQ suspension. In addition, *an in vivo* study in male Wistar rats revealed that oral administration of TQ-SNEDDS exhibited 3.87 fold higher relative oral bioavailability and better therapeutic efficacy compared to TQ suspension at the same dose. Similarly, ibrutinib encapsulated SNEDDS showed 2.64-fold higher relative oral bioavailability in female Albino Wistar rats compared to pure drug suspension (Shakeel et al., 2016). In another study, cyclovirobuxine-D encapsulated

SNEDDS showed significantly enhanced permeability across Caco-2 cell monolayer compared to marketed tablet of cyclovirobuxine-D (Ke et al., 2016). Furthermore, pharmacokinetic study in New Zealand rabbits showed 2 fold higher relative oral bioavailability of SNEDDS compared to marketed formulation.

11.4.5   SOLID LIPID NANOPARTICLES (SLN)

SLN made from biodegradable and biocompatible solid lipids exists in the submicron size range and has attracted increasing attention in the last two decades. The colloidal nanoparticles which are made of solid lipids (solid at 37°C or below) are called SLN. The use of solid lipids as a matrix prevents the immediate release of encapsulated drugs (Ahmad et al., 2015). Furthermore, SLN protects encapsulated drugs against chemical degradation, does not exhibit biotoxicity and large scale production of SLN is quite easy (Mehnert and Mäder, 2001; Müller et al., 2002). Potential advantages of SLN include improved solubility and GI stability, improved intestinal permeability, prolonged circulation half-life, improved bioavailability, and reduced dose-related toxicity. The above-mentioned advantages make the SLN as potential drug delivery platform for successful oral delivery of both lipophilic as well as hydrophilic compounds (Lin et al., 2017). In a study, Baek and Cho (2017) developed N-carboxymethyl chitosan (NCC) coated curcumin (Cur) encapsulated SLN (NCC-Cur-SLN) to enhance intestinal permeability and oral bioavailability. NCC-Cur-SLN exhibited enhanced cellular uptake and cytotoxicity in MCF-7 breast cancer cell line. *In vivo* study in male, Sprague Dawley rats revealed 6.3 and 9.5 fold improved lymphatic absorption and relative oral bioavailability of NCC-Cur-SLN compared to free Cur solution. Similarly, N-trimethyl chitosan (TMC) decorated palmitic acid (TMC-g-PA) mucoadhesive copolymer grafted resveratrol encapsulated SLN showed 3.8 fold increased relative oral bioavailability in male Balb/c mice compared to resveratrol suspension (Ramalingam and Ko, 2016). In another study, Dudhipala and Veerabrahma (2016) demonstrated improved oral bioavailability, and antihypertensive efficacy of candesartan cilexetil (CC) encapsulated SLN (CC-SLN) to improve oral bioavailability and antihypertensive efficacy. CC-SLN showed 2.75 fold improved relative oral bioavailability as well as significant decrease in systolic blood pressure in male Albino Wistar rats compared to CC suspension at the same therapeutic dose.

11.4.6   NANOSTRUCTURED LIPID CARRIERS (NLC)

Nanostructured lipid carriers (NLC), also known as the second-generation SLN, are attracting foremost consideration from the researchers as potential colloidal drug nanocarrier for oral delivery. These biodegradable and biocompatible nanocarriers are composed of a mixture of two spatially different lipid molecules; i.e. the liquid lipid (oil) is mixed with solid lipid to overcome the problems encountered with SLN. The differences in the structures of the liquid and solid lipids, lead to formation of an imperfect crystal mixture (i.e. imperfect lipid matrix). The imperfect lipid matrix encapsulates the drugs in molecular form or in amorphous clusters (Rizwanullah et al., 2016; Akhter et al., 2018; Rizwanullah et al., 2018). Unique advantages of NLC include (i) high drug loading capacity for both lipophilic and hydrophilic drug molecules; (ii) inhibit leakage of drug during storage (unlike SLN); (iii) modulation of dissolution rate of drug due to imperfect lipid matrix; and (iv) high GI stability (Beloqui et al., 2016; Jaiswal et al., 2016; Rizwanullah et al., 2016). In a study, Tian et al. (2017) developed N-acetyl-L-cysteine-polyethylene glycol (100)-monostearate (NAPG) decorated curcumin (Cur) encapsulated NLC (Cur-NAPG-NLC) to enhance mucus penetration and mucoadhesion for improved bioavailability after oral administration. *In situ* intestinal perfusion study showed significantly enhanced absorption of Cur-NAPG-NLC compared to untargeted Cur-NLC and Cur solution respectively. In addition, a pharmacokinetic study in male Sprague–Dawley rats revealed 116.89 and 499.45 fold higher AUC of Cur-NAPG-NLC compared to untargeted Cur-NLC and Cur solution respectively. Similarly, Fang et al. (2015) prepared cysteine modified docetaxel (DTX) encapsulated NLC (C-DTX-NLC) to facilitate the intestinal transport of DTX by interaction with mucin of the intestinal mucus layer. The results indicated that C-DTX-NLC exhibited enhanced mucoadhesion properties and showed significantly higher intestinal absorption. A pharmacokinetic study in male Sprague-Dawley rats demonstrated that C-DTX-NLC exhibited 1.64 and 12.4 fold enhanced oral bioavailability compared to unmodified DTX-NLC and DTX solution respectively. In another study, rosuvastatin (ROS) encapsulated NLC (ROS-NLC) was developed to improve oral bioavailability and antihyperlipidemic efficacy in albino Wistar rats (Rizwanullah et al., 2017). Confocal microscopy confirmed the deeper penetration of NLC and showed 5.4-fold improved oral bioavailability compared to ROS suspension at the same therapeutic dose. In addition, ROS-NLC showed higher lipid-lowering efficacy in hyperlipidemic rats compared to ROS suspension.

11.4.7 POLYMERIC NANOPARTICLES

Polymeric nanoparticles, prepared from biodegradable and biocompatible polymers, have a wide range of advantages compared to the other nanoparticles and are widely used as a novel oral drug delivery platform. Polymeric nanoparticles offer much better GI stability due to the capability of protecting the encapsulated drug from digestive enzymes present in the GIT. Additional advantages of polymeric nanoparticles include surface functionality, controlled drug release, mucoadhesion, mucopenetration, higher intestinal permeation, prolonged blood circulation, specific tissue targeting and many other adjustable characteristics (Ensign et al., 2012; Pridgen et al., 2015). Several polymers, such as poly(lactideco-glycolide) (PLGA), polylactide (PLA), polycaprolactone (PCL), polyglycolide, poly(d,l-lactide) and chitosan, have been developed for oral drug delivery (Ensign et al., 2012; Pridgen et al., 2014 &2015). In a study, Joshi et al. (2014) developed Gemcitabine HCl encapsulated PLGA-NPs to enhance oral bioavailability. *In vitro* permeability study using Caco-2 cell monolayer demonstrated 6.37 fold higher permeability of PLGA-NPs compared to pure drug solution. In addition, a pharmacokinetic study in male Albino Wistar rats revealed 21.47-fold higher oral bioavailability of PLGA-NPs compared to free drug solution. In another study, the same researchers demonstrated 3.04, and 13.9 fold improved Caco-2 cell monolayer permeability and oral bioavailability in male Albino Wistar rats of lopinavir encapsulated PLGA-NPs compared to free drug solution respectively (Joshi et al., 2016).

Anwar et al. (2011) developed chitosan-atorvastatin (CH-AT) conjugate nanoparticles to improve aqueous solubility and oral bioavailability. CH-AT conjugate nanoparticles showed nearly 100 fold enhanced solubility compared to free AT. Further, a pharmacokinetic study in Albino Wistar rats revealed 5 fold enhanced oral bioavailability of CH-AT conjugate nanoparticles compared to free AT suspension. In a study, curcumin (Cur) encapsulated cationic copolymer Eudragit E 100 nanoparticles (Cur-EE-NPs) showed excellent anticancer efficacy and improved oral bioavailability (Chaurasia et al., 2016). *In vitro* cytotoxicity using colon-6 cancer cells demonstrated a 19 fold reduction in IC_{50} compared to pure Cur solution. In addition, *in vivo* anticancer efficacy study in murine colon-26 tumor-bearing BALB/c mice revealed a significantly higher reduction in tumor volume and increase survival rate when treated with Cur-EE-NPs. Further, a pharmacokinetic study in albino Wistar rats demonstrated 91 and 95 fold improved C_{max} and $AUC_{0\rightarrow12}$ after oral administration of Cur-EE-NPs. In another study, Bu et al. (2015) developed heptaarginine, a cell-penetrating peptide (CPP), and docetaxel (DTX) cyclodextrin inclusion-loaded PLGA-NPs to improve cytotoxicity and oral bioavail-ability. The developed CPP-DTX-CD-PLGA-NPs exhibited significantly improved cellular uptake and cytotoxicity in MCF-7 cells compared to DTX-CD-PLGA-NPs and pure DTX solution, respectively. Further, pharmacokinetic study demonstrated 5.57 and 9.43 fold improved oral bioavailability of CPP-DTX-CD-PLGA-NPs compared to DTX-CD-PLGA-NPs and pure DTX suspension, respectively.

11.4.8   POLYMER LIPID HYBRID NANOPARTICLES (PLHNPS)

PLHNPs are one of the most advanced nano-drug delivery platform composed of biodegradable and biocompatible polymers and lipids. PLHNPs demonstrate the advantages of both lipid-based nanoparticles as well as polymer-based nanoparticles. The hybrid architecture of PLHNPs provides some potential benefits such as controllable particle size, high drug loading, surface functionality, tunable and controlled drug release profile, improved stability in the different environment of GIT, prolonged blood circulation and oral bioavailability (Rao and Prestidge, 2016; Bose et al., 2017). PLHNPs have significant potential to co-encapsulate different therapeutic and imaging agents. In addition, the lipid used in the development of PLHNPs can also prevent the pre-systemic metabolism of the drug. PLHNPs display a higher capacity for *in vivo* cellular drug delivery than other polymer-based nanoparticles as well as lipid-based nanoparticles. The most commonly used polymers for preparation of PLHNPs include PLGA, chitosan, polycaprolactone (PCL), polylactic acid (PLA) while phospholipids, glyceryl monostearate, and stearic acid are most commonly used lipid (Hadinoto et al., 2013; Hallan et al., 2016). In a study, Liu et al. (2017) prepared wheat germ agglutinin (WGA) grafted polymer-lipid hybrid nanoparticles (WGA-PLHNPs) to improve oral bioavailability and anticancer efficacy. *In vitro*, cellular uptake study showed significantly improved uptake of WGA-PLHNPs in Caco-2 cell monolayer compared to unmodified PLHNPs. Further, pharmacokinetic study in male Sprague-Dawley rats revealed 1.96 fold improved relative oral bioavailability of WGA-PLHNPs compared to unmodified PLHNPs. In addition, after oral administration of WGA-PLHNPs showed higher tumor growth inhibition in HepG-2 tumor-bearing male BALB/c nude mice. In another study, Liang et al. (2018) developed silymarin encapsulated PLHNPs (SIL-PLHNPs) to improve oral bioavailability and hepatoprotective efficacy. SIL-PLHNPs showed 1.92-fold improved uptake reduction in triglyceride level in fatty liver cells compared to free drug suspension. Further, a pharmacokinetic study in male Albino Wistar rats revealed 14.38-fold improved relative oral bioavailability compared to a free drug suspension. Recently, enoxaparin loaded chitosan-based PLHNPs revealed 4.5 fold improved AUC in male Sprague-Dawley rats compared to enoxaparin solution (Dong et al., 2018).

11.5   CONCLUSION

In this chapter, we discussed a recent update on the oral delivery of nanoparticles. We also discussed the principles of oral drug delivery systems, as well as their mechanisms, challenges, and benefits. Therapeutic oral delivery of different nanoparticles, such as nanocrystals, liposomes, nanoemulsion, self-nanoemulsifying drug delivery system, solid lipid nanoparticles, nanostructured lipid carriers, polymeric nanoparticles, and polymer lipid hybrid nanoparticles are also summarized. Poor aqueous solubility and substrate for P-gp or metabolizing enzyme, cytochrome P450 are some of the reasons for low oral bioavailability and therapeutic efficacy of drugs. Nanoparticles can improve the oral bioavailability, gastrointestinal stability, intestinal permeation, and efficacy of lipophilic as well as hydrophilic drugs. Nanoparticle systems enhance the oral bioavailability of drug molecules by a number of possible pathways, including P-gp inhibition, bypassing the first-pass metabolism, and resist the drug metabolism by cytochrome P450 family of enzymes present in the gastrointestinal tract and liver. Despite several benefits, nanoparticle technology has some limitations including scale-up difficulties, toxicity issues, and storage stability.

Further research and efforts to break through the challenges are required to maximize the applications of oral delivery of nanoparticles.

KEYWORDS

- **gastrointestinal (GI) tract**
- **gastrointestinal barriers**
- **oral delivery**
- **transport of nanoparticles**

REFERENCES

Agrawal, U., Sharma, R., Gupta, M., & Vyas, S. P., (2014). Is nanotechnology a boon for oral drug delivery? *Drug Discov. Today, 19*(10), 1530–1546.

Ahmad, J., Amin, S., Rahman, M., Rub, R. A., Singhal, M., Ahmad, M. Z., Rahman, Z., Addo, R. T., Ahmad, F. J., Mushtaq, G., Kamal, M. A., & Akhter, S., (2015). Solid matrix based lipidic nanoparticles in oral cancer chemotherapy: Applications and pharmacokinetics. *Curr. Drug Metab., 16*(8), 633–644.

Ahmad, J., Kohli, K., Mir, S. R., & Amin, S., (2013). Lipid based nanocarriers for oral delivery of cancer chemotherapeutics: An insight in the intestinal lymphatic transport. *Drug Deliv. Lett., 3*(1), 38–46.

Ahmad, J., Mir, S. R., Kohli, K., & Amin, S., (2014). Quality by design approach for self nanoemulsifying system of paclitaxel. *Sci. Adv. Mat., 6*, 1778–1791.

Ahmad, J., Singhal, M., Amin, S., Rizwanullah, M., Akhter, S., Kamal, M. A., Haider, N., Midoux, P., & Pichon, C., (2017). Bile salt stabilized vesicles (Bilosomes): A novel nano-pharmaceutical design for oral delivery of proteins and peptides. *Curr. Pharm. Des., 23*(11), 1575–1588.

Ahmad, N., Ahmad, R., Alam, M. A., Ahmad, F. J., Amir, M., Pottoo, F. H., Sarafroz, M., Jafar, M., & Umar, K., (2019). Daunorubicin oral bioavailability enhancement by surface coated natural biodegradable macromolecule chitosan based polymeric nanoparticles. *Int. J. Biol. Macromol., 128*, 825–838.

Akhter, M. H., Rizwanullah, M., Ahmad, J., Ahsan, M. J., Mujtaba, M. A., & Amin, S., (2018). Nanocarriers in advanced drug targeting: Setting novel paradigm in cancer therapeutics. *Artif. Cells Nanomed. Biotechnol., 46*(5), 873–884.

Al Rubeaan, K., Rafiullah, M., & Jayavanth, S., (2016). Oral insulin delivery systems using chitosan-based formulation: A review. *Expert Opin. Drug Deliv., 13*(2), 223–237.

Anwar, M., Warsi, M. H., Mallick, N., Akhter, S., Gahoi, S., Jain, G. K., Talegaonkar, S., Ahmad, F. J., & Khar, R. K., (2011). Enhanced bioavailability of nano-sized chitosan-atorvastatin conjugate after oral administration to rats. *Eur. J. Pharm. Sci., 44*(3), 241–249.

Baek, J. S., & Cho, C. W., (2017). Surface modification of solid lipid nanoparticles for oral delivery of curcumin: Improvement of bioavailability through enhanced cellular uptake, and lymphatic uptake. *Eur. J. Pharm. Biopharm., 117*, 132–140.

Beg, S., Jena, S. S., Patra, C. N., Rizwan, M., Swain, S., Sruti, J., Rao, M. E., & Singh, B., (2013). Development of solid self-nanoemulsifying granules (SSNEGs) of ondansetron hydrochloride with enhanced bioavailability potential. *Colloids Surf. B Biointerfaces, 101*, 414–423.

Beloqui, A., Solinís, M. Á., Rodríguez-Gascón, A., Almeida, A. J., & Préat, V., (2016). Nanostructured lipid carriers: Promising drug delivery systems for future clinics. *Nanomedicine, 12*(1), 143–161.

Bose, R. J. C., Ravikumar, R., Karuppagounder, V., Bennet, D., Rangasamy, S., & Thandavarayan, R. A., (2017). Lipid-polymer hybrid nanoparticle-mediated therapeutics delivery: Advances and challenges. *Drug Discov. Today, 22*(8), 1258–1265.

Bu, X., Zhu, T., Ma, Y., & Shen, Q., (2015). Co-administration with cell penetrating peptide enhances the oral bioavailability of docetaxel-loaded nanoparticles. *Drug Dev. Ind. Pharm., 41*(5), 764–771.

Chang, D., Ma, Y., Cao, G., Wang, J., Zhang, X., Feng, J., & Wang, W., (2018). Improved oral bioavailability for lutein by nanocrystal technology: Formulation development, *in vitro* and *in vivo* evaluation. *Artif. Cells Nanomed. Biotechnol., 46*(5), 1018–1024.

Chaurasia, S., Chaubey, P., Patel, R. R., Kumar, N., & Mishra, B., (2016). Curcumin-polymeric nanoparticles against colon-26 tumor-bearing mice: Cytotoxicity, pharmacokinetic and anticancer efficacy studies. *Drug Dev. Ind. Pharm., 42*(5), 694–700.

Cheng, Y., Xu, Z., Ma, M., & Xu, T., (2008). Dendrimers as drug carriers: Applications in different routes of drug administration. *J. Pharm. Sci., 97*(1), 123–143.

Daeihamed, M., Dadashzadeh, S., Haeri, A., & Akhlaghi, M. F., (2017). Potential of liposomes for enhancement of oral drug absorption. *Curr. Drug Deliv., 14*(2), 289–303.

Date, A. A., Desai, N., Dixit, R., & Nagarsenker, M., (2010). Self-nanoemulsifying drug delivery systems: Formulation insights, applications and advances. *Nanomedicine (Lond), 5*(10), 1595–1616.

Daugherty, A. L., & Mrsny, R. J., (1999). Transcellular uptake mechanisms of the intestinal epithelial barrier Part one. *Pharm. Sci. Technol. Today, 4*(2), 144–151.

Davis, S., Hardy, J., Taylor, M., Whalley, D., & Wilson, C., (1984). The effect of food on the gastrointestinal transit of pellets and an osmotic device (Osmet). *Int. J. Pharm., 21*(3), 331–340.

Desai, J., & Thakkar, H., (2019). Enhanced oral bioavailability and brain uptake of Darunavir using lipid nanoemulsion formulation. *Colloids Surf. B Biointerfaces, 175*, 143–149.

Dong, W., Wang, X., Liu, C., Zhang, X., Zhang, X., Chen, X., Kou, Y., & Mao, S., (2018). Chitosan based polymer-lipid hybrid nanoparticles for oral delivery of enoxaparin. *Int. J. Pharm., 547*(1&2), 499–505.

Dudhipala, N., & Veerabrahma, K., (2016). Candesartan cilexetil loaded solid lipid nanoparticles for oral delivery: Characterization, pharmacokinetic and pharmacodynamic evaluation. *Drug Deliv., 23*(2), 395–404.

Ensign, L. M., Cone, R., & Hanes, J., (2012a). Oral drug delivery with polymeric nanoparticles: The gastrointestinal mucus barriers. *Adv. Drug Deliv. Rev., 64*(6), 557–570.

Ensign, L. M., Schneider, C., Suk, J. S., Cone, R., & Hanes, J., (2012b). Mucus penetrating nanoparticles: Biophysical tool and method of drug and gene delivery. *Adv. Mater., 24*(28), 3887–3894.

Fang, G., Tang, B., Chao, Y., Xu, H., Gou, J., Zhang, Y., Xu, H., & Tang, X., (2015). Cysteine-functionalized nanostructured lipid carriers for oral delivery of docetaxel: A permeability and pharmacokinetic study. *Mol. Pharm., 12*(7), 2384–2395.

Fathi, H. A., Allam, A., Elsabahy, M., Fetih, G., & El-Badry, M., (2018). Nanostructured lipid carriers for improved oral delivery and prolonged antihyperlipidemic effect of simvastatin. *Colloids Surf. B Biointerfaces, 162*, 236–245.

Fu, Q., Sun, J., Zhang, D., Li, M., Wang, Y., Ling, G., Liu, X., Sun, Y., Sui, X., Luo, C., Sun, L., Han, X., Lian, H., Zhu, M., Wang, S., & He, Z., (2013). Nimodipine nanocrystals for oral bioavailability improvement: Preparation, characterization and pharmacokinetic studies. *Colloids Surf. B Biointerfaces, 109*, 161–166.

Gabr, M. M., Mortada, S. M., & Sallam, M. A., (2018). Carboxylate cross-linked cyclodextrin: A nanoporous scaffold for enhancement of rosuvastatin oral bioavailability. *Eur. J. Pharm. Sci., 111*, 1–12.

Gao, F., Zhang, Z., Bu, H., Huang, Y., Gao, Z., & Shen, J., (2011). Nanoemulsion improves the oral absorption of *Candesartan cilexetil* in rats: performance and mechanism. *J. Control. Release, 149*, 68–74.

Gao, L., Liu, G., Ma, J., Wang, X., Zhou, L., & Li, X., (2012). Drug nanocrystals: *In vivo* performances. *J. Control. Release, 160*(3), 418–430.

Garinot, M., Fiévez, V., Pourcelle, V., Stoffelbach, F., Des Rieux, A., Plapied, L., Theate, I., Freichels, H., Jérôme, C., Marchand-Brynaert, J., Schneider, Y. J., & Préat, V., (2007). PEGylated PLGA-based nanoparticles targeting M cells for oral vaccination. *J. Control. Release, 120*(3), 195–204.

Gedawy, A., Martinez, J., Al-Salami, H., & Dass, C. R., (2018). Oral insulin delivery: Existing barriers and current counter-strategies. *J. Pharm. Pharmacol., 70*(2), 197–213.

Gorain, B., Choudhury, H., Kundu, A., Sarkar, L., Karmakar, S., Jaisankar, P., & Pal, T. K., (2014). Nanoemulsion strategy for olmesartanmedoxomil improves oral absorption and extended antihypertensive activity in hypertensive rats. *Colloids Surf. B Biointerfaces, 115*, 286–294.

Hadinoto, K., Sundaresan, A., & Cheow, W. S., (2013). Lipid-polymer hybrid nanoparticles as a new generation therapeutic delivery platform: A review. *Eur. J. Pharm. Biopharm., 85*, 427–443.

Hallan, S. S., Kaur, P., Kaur, V., Mishra, N., & Vaidya, B., (2016). Lipid polymer hybrid as emerging tool in nanocarriers for oral drug delivery. *Artif. Cells Nanomed. Biotechnol., 44*(1), 334–349.

He, C., Yin, L., Tang, C., & Yin, C., (2012). Size-dependent absorption mechanism of polymeric nanoparticles for oral delivery of protein drugs. *Biomaterials, 33*(33), 8569–8578.

Ige, P. P., Baria, R. K., & Gattani, S. G., (2013). Fabrication of fenofibrate nanocrystals by probe sonication method for enhancement of dissolution rate and oral bioavailability. *Colloids Surf. B Biointerfaces, 108*, 366–373.

Inugala, S., Eedara, B. B., Sunkavalli, S., Dhurke, R., Kandadi, P., Jukanti, R., & Bandari, S., (2015). Solid self-nanoemulsifying drug delivery system (S-SNEDDS) of darunavir for improved dissolution and oral bioavailability: *In vitro* and *in vivo* evaluation. *Eur. J. Pharm. Sci., 74*, 1–10.

Jain, S., Rathi, V. V., Jain, A. K., Das, M., & Godugu, C., (2012). Folate-decorated PLGA nanoparticles as a rationally designed vehicle for the oral delivery of insulin. *Nanomedicine (Lond)., 7*(9), 1311–1337.

Jaiswal, P., Gidwani, B., & Vyas, A., (2016). Nanostructured lipid carriers and their current application in targeted drug delivery. *Artif. Cells Nanomed. Biotechnol., 44*(1), 27–40.

Joshi, G., Kumar, A., & Sawant, K., (2014). Enhanced bioavailability and intestinal uptake of Gemcitabine HCl loaded PLGA nanoparticles after oral delivery. *Eur. J. Pharm. Sci., 60*, 80–89.

Joshi, G., Kumar, A., & Sawant, K., (2016). Bioavailability enhancement, Caco-2 cells uptake and intestinal transport of orally administered lopinavir-loaded PLGA nanoparticles. *Drug Deliv., 23*(9), 3492–3504.

Junyaprasert, V. B., & Morakul, B., (2015). Nanocrystals for enhancement of oral bioavailability of poorly water-soluble drugs. *Asian J. Pharm. Sci., 10*, 13–23.

Kadiyala, I., Loo, Y., Roy, K., Rice, J., & Leong, K. W., (2010). Transport of chitosan-DNA nanoparticles in human intestinal M-cell model versus normal intestinal enterocytes. *Eur. J. Pharm. Sci., 39*(1–3), 103–109.

Kalam, M. A., Raish, M., Ahmed, A., Alkharfy, K. M., Mohsin, K., Alshamsan, A., Al-Jenoobi, F. I., Al-Mohizea, A. M., & Shakeel, F., (2017). Oral bioavailability enhancement and hepatoprotective effects of thymoquinone by self-nanoemulsifying drug delivery system. *Mater. Sci. Eng. C. Mater. Biol. Appl., 76*, 319–329.

Ke, Z., Hou, X., & Jia, X. B., (2016). Design and optimization of self-nanoemulsifying drug delivery systems for improved bioavailability of cyclovirobuxine D. *Drug Des. Devel. Ther., 10*, 2049–2060.

Keck, C. M., & Müller, R. H., (2006). Drug nanocrystals of poorly soluble drugs produced by high pressure homogenization. *Eur. J. Pharm. Biopharm., 62*(1), 3–16.

Khani, S., Keyhanfar, F., & Amani, A., (2016). Design and evaluation of oral nanoemulsion drug delivery system of mebudipine. *Drug Deliv., 23*(6), 2035–2043.

Kiyono, H., & Fukuyama, S., (2004). NALT-versus Peyer's-patch-mediated mucosal immunity. *Nat. Rev. Immunol., 4*(9), 699–710.

Lai, S. K., Wang, Y. Y., & Hanes, J., (2009). Mucus-penetrating nanoparticles for drug and gene delivery to mucosal tissues. *Adv. Drug Deliv. Rev., 61*(2), 158–171.

Liang, J., Liu, Y., Liu, J., Li, Z., Fan, Q., Jiang, Z., Yan, F., Wang, Z., Huang, P., & Feng, N., (2018). Chitosan-functionalized lipid-polymer hybrid nanoparticles for oral delivery of silymarin and enhanced lipid-lowering effect in NAFLD. *J. Nanobiotechnology, 16*(1), 64.

Lin, C. H., Chen, C. H., Lin, Z. C., & Fang, J. Y., (2017). Recent advances in oral delivery of drugs and bioactive natural products using solid lipid nanoparticles as the carriers. *J. Food Drug Anal., 25*(2), 219–234.

Liu, C., Kou, Y., Zhang, X., Cheng, H., Chen, X., & Mao, S., (2018). Strategies and industrial perspectives to improve oral absorption of biological macromolecules. *Expert Opin. Drug Deliv., 15*(3), 223–233.

Liu, Y., Liu, J., Liang, J., Zhang, M., Li, Z., Wang, Z., Dang, B., & Feng, N., (2017). Mucosal transfer of wheat germ agglutinin modified lipid-polymer hybrid nanoparticles for oral delivery of oridonin. *Nanomedicine, 13*(7), 2219–2229.

Lukyanenko, V., Malyukova, I., Hubbard, A., Delannoy, M., Boedeker, E., Zhu, C., Cebotaru, L., & Kovbasnjuk, O., (2011). Enterohemorrhagic *Escherichia coli* infection stimulates Shiga toxin 1macropinocytosis and transcytosis across intestinal epithelial cells. *Am. J. Physiol. Cell Physiol., 301*(5), 1140–1149.

Manconi, M., Nácher, A., Merino, V., Merino-Sanjuan, M., Manca, M. L., Mura, C., Mura, S., Fadda, A. M., & Diez-Sales, O., (2013). Improving oral bioavailability and pharmacokinetics of liposomal metformin by glycerolphosphate-chitosan microcomplexation. *AAPS Pharm. Sci. Tech., 14*(2), 485–896.

Mandracchia, D., Rosato, A., Trapani, A., Chlapanidas, T., Montagner, I. M., Perteghella, S., Di Franco, C., Torre, M. L., Trapani, G., & Tripodo, G., (2017). Design, synthesis and evaluation of biotin decorated inulin-based polymeric micelles as long-circulating nanocarriers for targeted drug delivery. *Nanomedicine, 13*(3), 1245–1254.

Mehnert, W., & Mäder, K., (2001). Solid lipid nanoparticles: Production, characterization and applications. *Adv. Drug Deliv. Rev., 47*(2&3), 165–196.

Mishra, A., Imam, S. S., Aqil, M., Ahad, A., Sultana, Y., Ameeduzzafar, & Ali, A., (2016). Carvedilolnano lipid carriers: Formulation, characterization and *in-vivo* evaluation. *Drug Deliv., 23*(4), 1486–1494.

Mishra, N., Tiwari, S., Vaidya, B., Agrawal, G. P., & Vyas, S. P., (2011). Lectin anchored PLGA nanoparticles for oral mucosal immunization against hepatitis B. *J. Drug Target., 19*(1), 67–78.

Moss, D. M., Curley, P., Kinvig, H., Hoskins, C., & Owen, A., (2018). The biological challenges and pharmacological opportunities of orally administered nanomedicine delivery. *Expert Rev. Gastroenterol. Hepatol., 12*(3), 223–236.

Müller, R. H., Radtke, M., & Wissing, S. A., (2002). Solid lipid nanoparticles (SLN) and nanostructured lipid carriers (NLC) in cosmetic and dermatological preparations. *Adv. Drug Deliv. Rev., 54*, 131–155.

Nangwade, B. K., Patel, D. J., Udhani, R. A., & Manvi, F. V., (2011). Functions of lipids for enhancement of oral bioavailability of poorly water-soluble drugs. *Sci. Pharm., 79*(4), 705–725.

Nekkanti, V., Venkatesan, N., Wang, Z., & Betageri, G. V., (2015). Improved oral bioavailability of valsartan using proliposomes: Design, characterization and *in vivo* pharmacokinetics. *Drug Dev. Ind. Pharm., 41*(12), 2077–2088.

Neves, A. R., Queiroz, J. F., Costa, L. S. A., Figueiredo, F., Fernandes, R., & Reis, S., (2016). Cellular uptake and transcytosis of lipid-based nanoparticles across the intestinal barrier: Relevance for oral drug delivery. *J. Colloid. Interface Sci., 463*, 258–265.

Nguyen, T. X., Huang, L., Gauthier, M., Yang, G., & Wang, Q., (2016). Recent advances in liposome surface modification for oral drug delivery. *Nanomedicine (Lond), 11*(9), 1169–1185.

Olbrich, C., & Müller, R. H., (1999). Enzymatic degradation of SLN-effect of surfactant and surfactant mixtures. *Int. J. Pharm., 180*(1), 31–39.

Onoue, S., Takahashi, H., Kawabata, Y., Seto, Y., Hatanaka, J., Timmermann, B., & Yamada, S., (2010). Formulation design and photochemical studies on nanocrystal solid dispersion of curcumin with improved oral bioavailability. *J. Pharm. Sci., 99*(4), 1871–1881.

Pappenheimer, J. R., (2001). Intestinal absorption of hexoses and amino acids: From apical cytosol to villus capillaries. *J. Membr. Biol., 184*(3), 233–239.

Patel, G. M., Shelat, P. K., & Lalwani, A. N., (2017). QbD based development of proliposome of lopinavir for improved oral bioavailability. *Eur. J. Pharm. Sci., 108*, 50–61.

Pathak, K., & Raghuvanshi, S., (2015). Oral bioavailability: Issues and solutions via nanoformulations. *Clin. Pharmacokinet., 54*(4), 325–357.

Pawar, V. K., Singh, Y., Meher, J. G., Gupta, S., & Chourasia, M. K., (2014). Engineered nanocrystal technology: *In-vivo* fate, targeting and applications in drug delivery. *J. Control. Release, 183*, 51–66.

Peng, R. M., Lin, G. R., Ting, Y., & Hu, J. Y., (2018). Oral delivery system enhanced the bioavailability of stilbenes: Resveratrol and pterostilbene. *Biofactors, 44*(1), 5–15.

Porter, C. J. H., Pouton, C. W., Cuine, J. F., & Charman, W. N., (2008). Enhancing intestinal drug solubilization using lipid-based delivery systems. *Adv. Drug Deliv. Rev., 60*(6), 673–691.

Porter, C. J. H., Trevaskis, N. L., & Charman, W. N., (2007). Lipids and lipid-based formulations: Optimizing the oral delivery of lipophilic drugs. *Nat. Rev. Drug Discov., 6*, 231–248.

Pridgen, E. M., Alexis, F., & Farokhzad, O. C., (2014). Polymeric nanoparticle technologies for oral drug delivery. *Clin. Gastroenterol. Hepatol., 12*(10), 1605–1610.

Pridgen, E. M., Alexis, F., & Farokhzad, O. C., (2015). Polymeric nanoparticle drug delivery technologies for oral delivery applications. *Expert Opin. Drug Deliv., 12*(9), 1459–1473.

Quan, P., Xia, D., Piao, H., Piao, H., Shi, K., Jia, Y., & Cui, F., (2011). Nitrendipine nanocrystals: Its preparation, characterization, and *in vitro-in vivo* evaluation. *AAPS Pharm. Sci. Tech., 12*(4), 1136–1143.

Ramalingam, P., & Ko, Y. T., (2016). Improved oral delivery of resveratrol from N-trimethyl chitosan-g-palmitic acid surface-modified solid lipid nanoparticles. *Colloids Surf. B Biointerfaces, 139*, 52–61.

Rao, S., & Prestidge, C. A., (2016). Polymer-lipid hybrid systems: Merging the benefits of polymeric and lipid-based nanocarriers to improve oral drug delivery. *Expert Opin. Drug Deliv., 13*(5), 691–707.

Rizwanullah, M., Ahmad, J., & Amin, S., (2016). Nanostructured lipid carriers: A novel platform for chemotherapeutics. *Curr. Drug Deliv., 13*(1), 4–26.

Rizwanullah, M., Amin, S., & Ahmad, J., (2017). Improved pharmacokinetics and antihyperlipidemic efficacy of rosuvastatin-loaded nanostructured lipid carriers. *J. Drug Target., 25*(1), 58–74.

Rizwanullah, M., Amin, S., Mir, S. R., Fakhri, K. U., & Rizvi, M. M. A., (2018). Phytochemical based nanomedicines against cancer: Current status and future prospects. *J. Drug Target, 26*(9), 731–752.

Rogers, J. A., & Anderson, K. E., (1998). The potential of liposomes in oral drug delivery. *Crit. Rev. Ther. Drug Carrier Syst., 15*(5), 421–480.

Shahbazi, M. A., & Santos, H. A., (2013). Improving oral absorption via drug-loaded nanocarriers: Absorption mechanisms, intestinal models and rational fabrication. *Curr. Drug Metab., 14*(1), 28–56.

Shakeel, F., Iqbal, M., & Ezzeldin, E., (2016). Bioavailability enhancement and pharmacokinetic profile of an anticancer drug ibrutinib by self-nanoemulsifying drug delivery system. *J. Pharm. Pharmacol., 68*(6), 772–780.

Shan, W., Zhu, X., Liu, M., Li, L., Zhong, J., Sun, W., Zhang, Z., & Huang, Y., (2015). Overcoming the diffusion barrier of mucus and absorption barrier of epithelium by self-assembled nanoparticles for oral delivery of insulin. *ACS Nano, 9*(3), 2345–2356.

Shi, L. L., Lu, J., Cao, Y., Liu, J. Y., Zhang, X. X., Zhang, H., Cui, J. H., & Cao, Q. R., (2017). Gastrointestinal stability, physicochemical characterization and oral bioavailability of chitosan or its derivative-modified solid lipid nanoparticles loading docetaxel. *Drug Dev. Ind. Pharm., 43*(5), 839–846.

Silki, & Sinha, V. R., (2018). Enhancement of *in vivo* efficacy and oral bioavailability of aripiprazole with solid lipid nanoparticles. *AAPS Pharm. Sci. Tech., 19*(3), 1264–1273.

Singh, G., & Pai, R. S., (2014). *In-vitro/in-vivo* characterization of trans-resveratrol-loaded nanoparticulate drug delivery system for oral administration. *J. Pharm. Pharmacol., 66*(8), 1062–1076.

Singh, Y., Meher, J. G., Raval, K., Khan, F. A., Chaurasia, M., Jain, N. K., & Chourasia, M. K., (2017). Nanoemulsion: Concepts, development and applications in drug delivery. *J. Control. Release, 252*, 28–49.

Snoeck, V., Goddeeris, B., & Cox, E., (2005). The role of enterocytes in the intestinal barrier function and antigen uptake. *Microbes Infect, 7*(7&8), 997–1004.

Tariq, M., Alam, M. A., Singh, A. T., Iqbal, Z., Panda, A. K., & Talegaonkar, S., (2015). Biodegradable polymeric nanoparticles for oral delivery of epirubicin: *In vitro, ex vivo*, and *in vivo* investigations. *Colloids Surf. B Biointerfaces, 128*, 448–456.

Thomas, N., Holm, R., Mullertz, A., & Rades, T., (2012). *In vitro* and *in vivo* performance of novel supersaturated self nanoemulsifying drug delivery systems (super-SNEDDS). *J. Control. Release, 160*(1), 25–32.

Tian, C., Asghar, S., Wu, Y., Amerigos, D. K., Chen, Z., Zhang, M., Yin, L., Huang, L., Ping, Q., & Xiao, Y., (2017). N-acetyl-L-cysteine functionalized nanostructured lipid carrier for improving oral bioavailability of curcumin: Preparation, *in vitro* and *in vivo* evaluations. *Drug Deliv., 24*(1), 1605–1616.

Verma, A., & Stellacci, F., (2010). Effect of surface properties on nanoparticle-cell interactions. *Small, 6*(1), 12–21.

Wan, K., Sun, L., Hu, X., Yan, Z., Zhang, Y., Zhang, X., & Zhang, J., (2016). Novel nanoemulsion based lipid nanosystems for favorable *in vitro* and *in vivo* characteristics of curcumin. *Int. J. Pharm., 504*(1&2), 80–88.

Wang, T., Xue, J., Hu, Q., Zhou, M., & Luo, Y., (2017a). Preparation of lipid nanoparticles with high loading capacity and exceptional gastrointestinal stability for potential oral delivery applications. *J. Colloid. Interface Sci., 507*, 119–130.

Wang, Y., Wang, S., Firempong, C. K., Zhang, H., Wang, M., Zhang, Y., Zhu, Y., Yu, J., & Xu, X., (2017b). Enhanced solubility and bioavailability of naringenin via liposomal nanoformulation: Preparation and *in vitro* and *in vivo* evaluations. *AAPS Pharm. Sci. Tech., 18*(3), 586–594.

Wu, W., Lu, Y., & Qi, J., (2015). Oral delivery of liposomes. *Ther. Deliv., 6*(11), 1239–1241.

Yeh, T. H., Hsu, L. W., Tseng, M. T., Lee, P. L., Sonjae, K., Ho, Y. C., & Sung, H. W., (2011). Mechanism and consequence of chitosan-mediated reversible epithelial tight junction opening. *Biomaterials, 32*(26), 6164–6173.

Yen, C. C., Chen, Y. C., Wu, M. T., Wang, C. C., & Wu, Y. T., (2018). Nanoemulsion as a strategy for improving the oral bioavailability and anti-inflammatory activity of andrographolide. *Int. J. Nanomedicine., 13*, 669–680.

Zhou, M., Hu, Q., Wang, T., Xue, J., & Luo, Y., (2016b). Effects of different polysaccharides on the formation of egg yolk LDL complex nanogels for nutrient delivery. *Carbohydr. Polym., 153,* 336–344.

Zhou, M., Wang, T., Hu, Q., & Luo, Y., (2016a). Low density lipoprotein/pectin complex nanogels as potential oral delivery vehicles for curcumin. *Food Hydrocoll., 57,* 20–29.

Zhou, Y., Ning, Q., Yu, D. N., Li, W. G., & Deng, J., (2014). Improved oral bioavailability of breviscapine via a Pluronic P85-modified liposomal delivery system. *J. Pharm. Pharmacol., 66*(7), 903–911.

Zhu, Y., Wang, M., Zhang, J., Peng, W., Firempong, C. K., Deng, W., Wang, Q., Wang, S., Shi, F., Yu, J., Xu, X., & Zhang, W., (2015). Improved oral bioavailability of capsaicin via liposomal nanoformulation: Preparation, *in vitro* drug release and pharmacokinetics in rats. *Arch. Pharm. Res., 38*(4), 512–521.

Index

Printed and bound by CPI Group (UK) Ltd, Croydon, CR0 4YY

23/10/2024

01777703-0005